Cardio-Respiratory Signal Processing and Classification

Non-invasive measurements of cardio-respiratory signals has improved diagnosis and prognosis in human health. This edited book invites original theoretical, practical, and review chapters aimed at proposing advancements in cardio-respiratory signal processing methods for healthcare applications. Exemplary themes of interest covered in this title include cardio-respiratory signal processing challenges using complex physiological data, novel HRV analysis, and data extracted from modern wearables and biosensors.

Features:

- Provides a detailed explanation and signal processing analysis of cardio-respiratory signals.
- Reports novel signal processing and time-frequency methods for cardio-respiratory signals.
- Presents the theoretical basis of cardio-respiratory analysis and state-of-the-art applications.
- Explains new and improved techniques and theories related to cardio-respiratory signal analysis.
- Combines the primary knowledge of cardio-respiratory signal analysis and processing, from theory and applications.

This book is aimed at researchers and graduate students in biomedical signal processing, signal processing, and electrical engineering.

Biomedical Signal and Image Processing

Series Editor: Ganesh Naik, *MARCS Institute for Brain, Behaviour, and Development, Western Sydney University, Sydney, Australia*

Biomedical signal and image processing involve the analysis of physiological measurements to provide useful information upon which clinicians can make decisions. Working with traditional bio-measurement tools, the signals and images can be computed by software to provide physicians with real-time data and greater insights to aid in clinical assessments. These challenges motivate the further study of biomedical signal and image analysis, and this book series intends to report the new results of these efforts. Topic coverage aims to include Neurological signal processing, Pathological speech signal analysis, Electromyography (EMG) signal processing, EEG, ECG, BCI and all associated analytical techniques. This book series is intended for both biomedical Engineers and clinicians (researchers and graduate students) who wish to get novel research ideas and some training in theory and recent advances of Clinical, Neural engineering and Biomedical signal/image processing applications.

Biomedical Signal Processing
A Modern Approach
Edited by Ganesh Naik and Wellington Pinheiro dos Santos

Advanced Electroencephalography Analytical Methods
Fundamentals, Acquisition, and Applications
Edited by Ganesh Naik, Wellington Pinheiro dos Santos, and Gaetano Gargiulo

Cardio-Respiratory Signal Processing and Classification
Trends, Applications, and Future Directions
Edited by Ganesh R. Naik

For more information about this series, please visit: www.routledge.com/Biomedical-Signal-and-Image-Processing/book-series/BSIP

Cardio-Respiratory Signal Processing and Classification

Trends, Applications, and Future Directions

Edited by Ganesh R. Naik

CRC Press
Taylor & Francis Group
Boca Raton London New York

CRC Press is an imprint of the
Taylor & Francis Group, an **informa** business

Designed cover image: ©Shutterstock Images

First edition published 2027
by CRC Press
2385 NW Executive Center Drive, Suite 320, Boca Raton FL 33431

and by CRC Press
4 Park Square, Milton Park, Abingdon, Oxon, OX14 4RN

CRC Press is an imprint of Taylor & Francis Group, LLC

ISBN: 978-1-032-79703-8 (hbk)
ISBN: 978-1-041-35395-9 (pbk)
ISBN: 978-1-003-79752-4 (ebk)

DOI: 10.1201/ 9781003797524

Typeset in Times New Roman
by Deanta Global Publishing Services, Chennai, India

Contents

Preface vii
Contributors ix
About the Editor xii

Chapter 1 Time-Frequency Analysis of ECG Signals 1
Sudestna Nahak and Goutam Saha

Chapter 2 Detection of Cardiac Signals Abnormalities Using MUSIC and Random Subspace Methods 28
Muhammed Enes Subasi, Saeed Mian Qaisar, and Abdulhamit Subasi

Chapter 3 ECG Signal Analysis Using Dual-Tree Complex Wavelet Transform and Bagging Ensemble Machine Learning 48
Abdulhamit Subasi, Tuba Nur Subasi, and Saeed Mian Qaisar

Chapter 4 Heart and Respiratory Sound Expert 69
Rahul Lalwani, Akshada Telang, and Vibha Tiwari

Chapter 5 Individual Discriminating Power Assessment of ECG Multi-Scale Entropies for Cardiovascular Disease Detection 87
Pedro Ribeiro, João Alexandre Marques Lobo, and Pedro Miguel Rodrigues

Chapter 6 Development of a Far Infrared Thermal Sensor-Based Contactless Breath Rate Measuring System with a Constraint on Resources 108
Sukesh Rao, Roopa B Hegde, and Sanith Bangera

Chapter 7 Electrocardiographic Signature Assessment of Post-COVID-19 Syndrome via Machine Learning Algorithms in Patients with Comorbid Cardiovascular Conditions 126
Pedro Ribeiro, João Alexandre Marques Lobo, Maria Inês Barbosa, Clarice Cristina Cunha de Souza, Cristine Mayara Cavalcante Camerino, Daniel Pordeus, Camila Ferreira Leite, João Paulo Madeiro, and Pedro Miguel Rodrigues

Chapter 8 Real-Time Deep Learning Pipeline for ECG Anomaly Detection 146

Yamini Niharika, Akhila, Ganesh R Naik, and Tripty Singh

Chapter 9 Analysis of Ballistocardiography for Cardiac and Respiratory Monitoring in Sleep 167

Lalitha Vaddadi, Yashas Nallathambi, Manju Khanna, T. V. Smitha, and K.V. Nagaraja

Chapter 10 PhysioBot: A Deep Learning Chatbot for ECG–PPG Anomaly Detection 180

Bandi Harshitha Reddy, Gopa Pulastya, Ganesh R Naik, and Tripty Singh

Chapter 11 LLM-Facilitated Differential Diagnosis of Cardiovascular Conditions from ECG and PPG 197

Okesh Reddy, Mouhitha Arella, Ganesh R Naik, and Tripty Singh

Index 217

Preface

The cardio-respiratory system plays a central role in sustaining human life by continuously coordinating cardiac and respiratory functions. With the growing availability of non-invasive physiological measurements such as electrocardiogram (ECG), respiratory signals, photoplethysmography (PPG), and wearable-sensor data, researchers now have unprecedented opportunities to explore the complex dynamics of this system. These signals provide important insights into autonomic regulation, physiological modulation, and the pathophysiology of a wide range of acute and chronic diseases.

Advances in biomedical engineering, machine learning, and computational modeling have accelerated the development of innovative methods for analyzing cardiovascular and respiratory signals. Through heart rate variability (HRV), airflow dynamics, and other time-series features, the changing patterns of these signals reveal biological responses to stress, disease, and therapeutic interventions. As data from clinical environments and consumer wearables continue to expand, the need for robust processing techniques, intelligent algorithms, and clinically relevant interpretation becomes increasingly important.

This edited volume, *Cardio-Respiratory Signal Processing and Classification: Trends, Applications, and Future Directions*, brings together contributions from researchers and practitioners, addressing contemporary challenges and future directions in the field. The book integrates theoretical advances, practical methodologies, and real-world applications, offering a comprehensive view of emerging innovations in cardio-respiratory signal analysis. The book consists of 11 chapters.

OVERVIEW OF CHAPTERS

- **Chapter 1** introduces time-frequency analysis techniques for ECG signals, capturing transient and nonstationary cardiac features.
- **Chapter 2** presents advanced detection of cardiac abnormalities using MUSIC and random subspace methods for improved diagnostic accuracy.
- **Chapter 3** explores ECG signal analysis through Dual-Tree Complex Wavelet Transform combined with bagging ensemble machine-learning models.
- **Chapter 4** discusses expert systems for heart and respiratory sound analysis, including segmentation and classification of cardiopulmonary acoustics.
- **Chapter 5** evaluates the discriminative power of multi-scale entropy measures derived from ECG signals for cardiovascular disease detection.
- **Chapter 6** describes the development of a resource-constrained, contactless respiratory-rate monitoring system using far-infrared thermal sensing.
- **Chapter 7** investigates ECG signatures associated with post-COVID-19 syndrome, applying machine-learning techniques to patients with comorbid cardiovascular conditions.

- **Chapter 8** presents a real-time deep learning pipeline for ECG anomaly detection, emphasizing robust and scalable solutions.
- **Chapter 9** examines ballistocardiograph-based analysis for unobtrusive monitoring of cardiac and respiratory activity during sleep.
- **Chapter 10** introduces PhysioBot, a deep learning chatbot designed for ECG–PPG anomaly detection, bridging AI and clinical decision support.
- **Chapter 11** explores the use of large language models (LLMs) for differential diagnosis of cardiovascular conditions from ECG and PPG signals.

I extend our sincere gratitude to all contributing authors for their dedication, expertise, and high-quality scholarship. Their collective efforts have shaped this volume into a valuable resource for the cardio-respiratory research community. I also appreciate their commitment to advancing knowledge in this evolving field and for sharing their innovative ideas, methodologies, and applications.

Together, the contributions in this book reflect the rapid evolution of cardio-respiratory signal processing and its potential to transform clinical practice, remote monitoring, and personalized healthcare. I hope that this book will serve as a timely reference and inspire continued progress and innovation in this important and growing discipline.

Ganesh R. Naik
December 2025

Contributors

Akhila
Department of Computer Science
School of Engineering
Amrita University
Bengaluru, Karnataka, India

Mouhitha Arella
Department of Computer Science
School of Engineering
Amrita University
Bengaluru, Karnataka, India

Sanith Bangera
Department of Electronics and Communication Engineering
NMAM Institute of Technology
Nitte, Udupi, India

Maria Inês Barbosa
UCP-School of Biotechnology
Catholic University of Portugal
Porto, Portugal

Cristine Mayara Cavalcante Camerino
Universidade Federal do Ceará (UFC)
Fortaleza, Brazil

Clarice Cristina Cunha de Souza
Federal University of Ceara
Fortaleza, Brazil

Roopa B Hegde
Department of Electronics and Communication Engineering
NMAM Institute of Technology
Nitte, Udupi, India

Manju Khanna
Department of Computer Science
School of Engineering
Amrita University
Bengaluru, Karnataka, India

Rahul Lalwani
Centre for Artificial Intelligence
Madhav Institute of Technology and Science
Gwalior, India

Camila Ferreira Leite
Universidade Federal do Ceará
Presidente Kennedy
Fortaleza, Brazil

João Alexandre Lobo Marques
Laboratory of Applied Neurosciences
University of Saint Joseph
Macau SAR, China

João Paulo Madeiro
Universidade Federal do Ceará
Presidente Kennedy
Fortaleza, Brazil

Sudestna Nahak
SRM IST, IIT Kharagpur
Kharagpur, India

Ganesh R Naik
School of Technology, Business Vertical
Torrens University
Adelaide, Australia

Yashas Nallathambi
Department of Computer Science
School of Engineering
Amrita University
Bengaluru, Karnataka, India

Yamini Niharika
Department of Computer Science
School of Engineering
Amrita University
Bengaluru, Karnataka, India

Daniel Pordeus
Petrobras: Brazilian Energy
Brazil

Gopa Pulastya
Department of Computer Science
School of Engineering
Amrita University
Bengaluru, Karnataka, India

Saeed Mian Qaisar
School of Computer Engineering
American University of the Middle East
Kuwait

Sukesh Rao
Department of Electronics and Communication Engineering
NMAM Institute of Technology
Nitte, Udupi, India

Bandi Harshitha Reddy
Department of Computer Science
School of Engineering
Amrita University
Bengaluru, Karnataka, India

Okesh Reddy
Department of Computer Science
School of Engineering
Amrita University
Bengaluru, Karnataka, India

Pedro Ribeiro
Faculty of Biotechnology
Universidade Católica Portuguesa
Porto, Portugal

Pedro Miguel Rodrigues
Faculty of Biotechnology
Universidade Católica Portuguesa
Porto, Portugal

Goutam Saha
SRM IST, IIT Kharagpur
Kharagpur, India

Tripty Singh
Department of Computer Science
School of Engineering
Amrita University
Bengaluru, Karnataka, India

Abdulhamit Subasi
Institute of Biomedicine
Faculty of Medicine
University of Turku
Turku, Finland

Muhammed Enes Subasi
Faculty of Medicine
Izmir Katip Celebi University
Izmir Turkey

Tuba Nur Subasi
Faculty of Medicine
Trakya University
Edirne, Turkey

Akshada Telang
Centre for Artificial Intelligence
Madhav Institute of Technology and Science
Gwalior, India

Vibha Tiwari
Centre for Artificial Intelligence
Madhav Institute of Technology and Science
Gwalior, India

Nagaraja K. V.
Department of Mathematics
School of Engineering
Amrita University
Bengaluru, Karnataka, India

Smitha T. V.
Department of Mathematics
School of Engineering
Amrita University
Bengaluru, Karnataka, India

Lalitha Vaddadi
Department of Computer Science
School of Engineering
Amrita University
Bengaluru, Karnataka, India

About the Editor

Ganesh R. Naik is a globally recognized biomedical engineer and signal processing expert, ranked among the top 2% of researchers worldwide by Stanford University. He holds a PhD from RMIT University and currently serves as an Associate Professor at Torrens University Australia. A highly prolific researcher, he has edited 16 books, authored 2 books, and published more than 175 scientific papers. Dr. Naik is an associate editor for several prestigious journals, including *IEEE Access*. His career spans influential research roles at Flinders University, Western Sydney University, and the University of Technology Sydney, where he made significant contributions to sleep health and wearable technologies. His achievements have been recognized through numerous competitive fellowships, including those awarded by the Royal Academy of Engineering (UK), the Australian government, and Germany's Baden–Württemberg Scholarship program.

1 Time-Frequency Analysis of ECG Signals

Sudestna Nahak and Goutam Saha

Signs are small measurable things, but interpretations are illimitable.

George Eliot, **Middlemarch**

1.1 INTRODUCTION

Cardiovascular dynamics describes the mechanical and electrical processes that enable the heart to function as a highly efficient pump, which is responsible for circulating blood throughout the body. The rhythmic contraction of the heart is governed by a precisely coordinated electrical conduction system that begins at the sinoatrial (SA) node, which generates spontaneous impulses that propagate through the atria, the atrioventricular (AV) node, His bundle, and the Purkinje fibers to activate the ventricles. These electrical events regulate mechanical systole and diastole, ensuring uninterrupted blood flow to vital organs of the human body (Weinhaus and Roberts, 2005). Any disturbance in this finely balanced electrical–mechanical cycle can affect cardiac performance and cause conditions such as arrhythmias, ischemia, or heart failure. Understanding these physiological principles provides the foundation for analyzing cardiac signals and enables the development of computational tools capable of interpreting complex dynamics of the heart.

Since the heart plays a vital role in overall health, it is important to understand the disorders that can affect its function. Cardiovascular diseases (CVDs) remain the leading cause of death worldwide, responsible for more than 17 million deaths each year and projected to rise significantly in the coming decades (Kaptoge et al., 2019). Conditions such as atrial fibrillation, ventricular arrhythmias, coronary artery disease, and heart failure contribute heavily to premature mortality and disability, particularly in low- and middle-income countries where access to early diagnosis and treatment is limited. Aging populations and growing lifestyle-related risks such as hypertension, diabetes, obesity, and smoking are contributing to the growing global burden of CVD. Early identification of cardiac abnormalities is therefore vital for preventing life-threatening complications such as stroke, myocardial infarction, and sudden cardiac death. This growing health challenge highlights the need for reliable and efficient diagnostic techniques capable of capturing subtle variations in cardiac function. To identify these conditions accurately, clinicians rely on a range

DOI: 10.1201/9781003797524-1

of diagnostic methods, among which electrocardiography (ECG) remains the most widely used and clinically informative. This makes ECG analysis a foundation for understanding and detecting early signs of cardiovascular abnormalities.

1.2 ELECTROCARDIOGRAPHY

ECG records the electrical activity of the heart by placing electrodes at specific positions on the limbs and chest, allowing clinicians to capture the electrical behavior of the heart from multiple positions. The standard 12-lead ECG traces the propagation of electrical impulses during each heartbeat, generating characteristic waveforms such as the P wave, QRS complex, and T wave, along with clinically important intervals. Figure 1.1 presents an overview of the fundamentals of electrocardiography. The 12-lead placement in (a) shows how electrodes on the chest and limbs capture the electrical activity of the heart from multiple angles, forming the basis of clinical

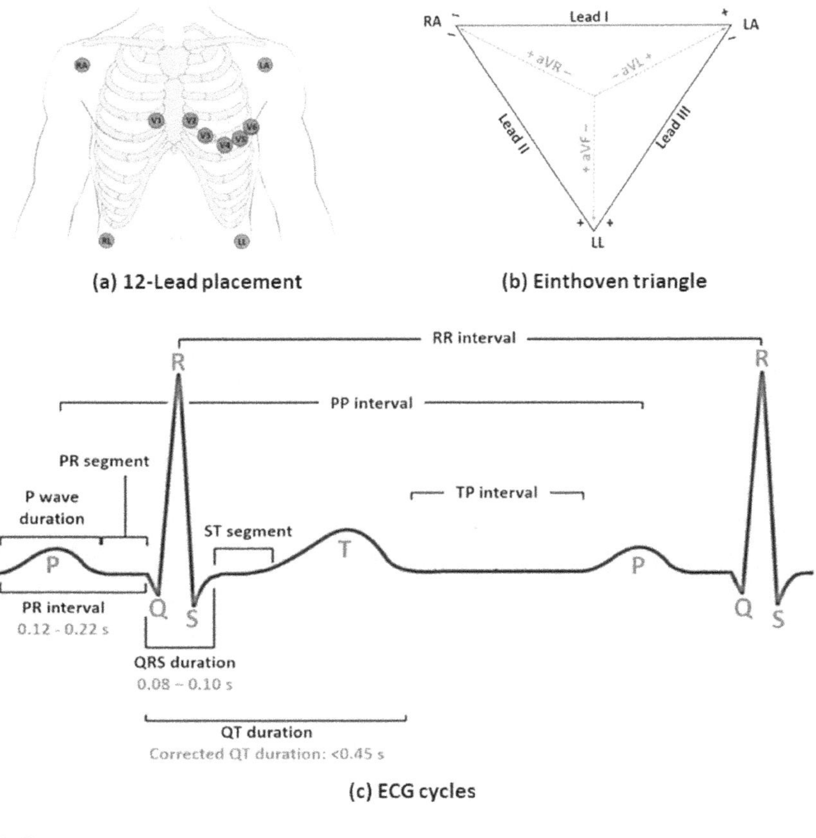

FIGURE 1.1 (a) Standard ECG electrode placement. (b) Einthoven triangle to measure limb lead (I, II, and III) and chest lead (V1, V2, V3, V4, V5, V6) potential. aVR, aVL, and aVF: Augmented lead right, left, and foot. (c) ECG cycle components.

ECG recording. In (b), the Einthoven triangle illustrates the relationship between the limb leads and how they measure voltage differences across the heart to create Leads I, II, and III. Finally, (c) depicts a typical ECG cycle, highlighting the waveforms and key intervals such as PR, QT, and RR, each representing different phases of atrial and ventricular activity. Together, these figures offer a better visual understanding of how ECG signals are recorded and how their main components correspond to the electrical behavior of the heart. Each component of the ECG reflects important aspects of atrial and ventricular depolarization and repolarization, enabling the detection of arrhythmias, conduction defects, myocardial ischemia, electrolyte disturbances, and other cardiac conditions (Rangayyan 2015). Long-term monitoring tools, such as Holter recordings, extend ECG analysis to daily activities that help in identifying intermittent or transient abnormalities that may not be captured during short clinical examinations. As the ECG provides detailed insights into cardiac physiology, its accurate interpretation is important for better cardiovascular diagnosis. However, interpreting ECG signals requires analytical methods capable of capturing the complex and time-varying behavior of the heart.

1.3 TRADITIONAL ECG ANALYSIS

The human heartbeat is far from a monotonous rhythm; it is a living symphony whose tempo and tone constantly shift with every breath, emotion, and physiological change. Such variability reflects the complex interaction between the heart's electrical and physiological systems and carries related diagnostic information for clinical use. Traditional time-domain analysis shows how the ECG waveform changes over time, while frequency-domain analysis identifies the dominant spectral components present throughout the length of the signal (Worley et al., 1988; Kinoshita et al., 1995). However, both perspectives fail to capture how components evolve during different cardiac events. Since ECG signals are inherently nonstationary, abnormalities such as arrhythmias, HRV, ischemic episodes, or autonomic fluctuations go undetected in classical time-domain or frequency-domain analysis. Time-frequency analysis overcomes this limitation by jointly mapping temporal and spectral features, offering a detailed picture of cardiac dynamics (Mahmoud et al., 2006). This representation enables clinicians and researchers to detect subtle energy variations and transient frequency shifts associated with early pathological changes, thus improving diagnostic accuracy and prompt intervention.

1.4 WHY TIME-FREQUENCY ANALYSIS (TFA) MATTERS?

Imagine being a detective examining a complex mystery, and the ECG is your evidence. Time-domain clues reveal when something happened, frequency clues tell what kind of event it was, but only a time-frequency lens shows how the events unfolded over time. Through this integrated representation, one can trace the temporal evolution of cardiac oscillations and uncover fleeting abnormalities that would otherwise go unnoticed. Biomedical signals are reflections of the body's internal state, and even minor abnormal fluctuations can indicate significant physiological or pathological transitions. In the era of intelligent healthcare and automated diagnostic systems, the ability to represent and analyze these subtle time-varying characteristics is important. Thus, time-frequency analysis serves as a bridge between raw signal interpretation and meaningful clinical insight, transforming ECG signal analysis into a powerful tool for medical diagnosis and advanced signal processing research (Pradhan et al., 2023).

1.4.1 Limitations of Time-Domain Analysis

The ECG waveform is often viewed as a series of familiar peaks and valleys, the P wave, the QRS complex, and the T wave, painting a rhythmic portrait of the electrical activity of the heart. Time-domain analysis examines these shapes, measuring their amplitude, duration, and intervals to reveal conduction delays or rhythm disorders. However, this is comparable to observing only the visible waveform while missing the hidden frequency dynamics that lie beneath. Many cardiac phenomena manifest themselves not through obvious shape changes but through subtle oscillations hidden within the frequency content of the signal. Early ischemic changes, stress-induced modulations, or minute changes in heart rate variability can pass unnoticed when viewed only in time. Also, overlapping events within the ECG, such as fused beats or superimposed noise, can mask important details, limiting diagnostic accuracy. Thus, while time-domain features form the foundation of classical ECG interpretation, they are insufficient to characterize the full range of nonstationary cardiac activity.

1.4.2 Limitations of Frequency-domain Analysis

Although the most common frequency-domain analysis technique, the Fourier transform, provides a powerful view of the spectral composition of ECG signals, it captures only the frequency part. This approach reveals dominant frequencies corresponding to cardiac rhythms, respiratory cycles, or autonomic modulations such as low- and high-frequency components of HRV. However, it does so under a critical assumption: that the signal remains stationary, with its frequency content constant over time. In reality, the ECG is far different. The heart's rhythm accelerates during stress, decelerates during sleep, and can abruptly shift during arrhythmic or ischemic events. For example, a premature ventricular contraction introduces a sudden burst of high-frequency energy, while ischemia gradually alters the ST segment over a few seconds. Such transient or evolving patterns become blurred or completely lost in a purely spectral representation. The Fourier spectrum, though mathematically elegant, collapses all temporal details, making it impossible to tell when a particular frequency occurred. Thus, while frequency-domain methods beautifully summarize "what" frequencies exist, they remain blind to "when" those frequencies arise (Polikar et al., 1996), leading to an incomplete and sometimes misleading picture of the dynamic behavior of the heart. Hence, purely spectral methods fail to capture these dynamics, emphasizing the need for time-frequency approaches.

1.5 TFA USING SHORT-TIME FOURIER TRANSFORM (STFT)

The limitations of classical Fourier analysis gave rise to methods that could reveal how spectral content evolves. Among them, the Short-Time Fourier Transform (STFT) stands as one of the earliest and most intuitive solutions. The STFT works by slicing the ECG signal into short, overlapping segments, applying the Fourier transform to each slice, and assembling the results into a time-frequency map. This process captures what frequencies are present and when they occur, allowing dynamic events to be visualized in real time (Durak and Arikan, 2003; Huang et al., 2019).

In the context of ECG analysis, STFT provides a practical "window" into cardiac behavior. For example, it can reveal the temporal evolution of high-frequency bursts during ventricular arrhythmias, gradual shifts in spectral energy during ischemic episodes, or modulations in respiratory sinus arrhythmia across sleep–wake cycles. Clinically, these insights help distinguish between transient and persistent abnormalities, which is important for early diagnosis and intervention. However, the choice of window length introduces a trade-off: a narrow window offers better time resolution but poorer frequency detail, while a wider window does the reverse. This balance between time and frequency components makes STFT an invaluable yet carefully tuned tool in biomedical signal analysis.

1.5.1 Fundamentals of STFT

At its core, the STFT extends the classical Fourier approach by introducing localization in time. Instead of analyzing the entire ECG signal at once, STFT applies a sliding window function, often Gaussian or Hamming, across the signal to capture short, overlapping time segments. Within each window, the signal is assumed to be approximately stationary, allowing the Fourier transform to extract its local frequency content. As the window moves forward in time, these local spectra combine to form a time-frequency representation, effectively revealing how the signal's frequency components evolve. The STFT of a signal $x(t)$ is mathematically defined as:

$$x(t,f)_{\text{STFT}} = \int_{-\infty}^{\infty} x(\tau)\, w(\tau - t)\, e^{-j2\pi f\tau}\, d\tau \tag{1.1}$$

where $w(\tau - t)$ is the window function centered at time t, and f denotes frequency. This formulation provides a localized spectrum that varies with time, capturing transient behaviors that traditional Fourier analysis misses.

Figure 1.2 shows a time-domain arrhythmic ECG signal and its STFT spectrogram. The STFT provides a joint time-frequency view by applying the Fourier transform over sliding windows that allows periodic bursts of high-frequency energy to be observed during each arrhythmic beat. However, fixed window size results in blurred frequency boundaries, which indicates the time-frequency resolution trade-off inherent in STFT.

The STFT of the ECG signal can be viewed as a "spectral movie" of cardiac activity. During a normal heartbeat, spectral energy remains concentrated around

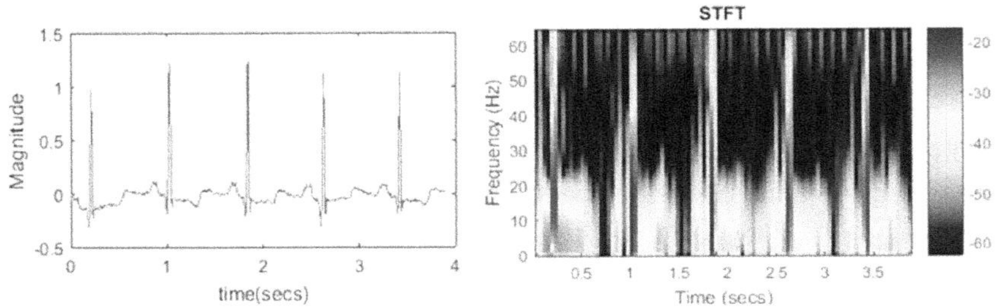

FIGURE 1.2 Time-domain ECG signal and its STFT representation.

characteristic frequencies associated with depolarization and repolarization (Hussein et al., 2018; Nahak and Saha, 2023). It has found extensive use in biomedical research and clinical ECG analysis due to its ability to uncover transient, frequency-varying cardiac phenomena that time-domain and frequency-domain analyses often overlook (Durak and Arikan, 2003). Despite its strengths, the STFT is constrained by the Heisenberg uncertainty principle, which limits simultaneous precision in both time and frequency domains. Selecting an appropriate window size is therefore important; short windows are ideal for transient events such as ectopic beats, while longer windows are better suited for slower physiological modulations like heart rate variability. Owing to this tunable balance, the STFT serves as a foundational tool for analyzing nonstationary biomedical signals and often acts as a bridge to more advanced time-frequency techniques, including the Continuous Wavelet Transform (CWT), Stockwell Transform (ST), Synchrosqueezing Transform (SST), and Wigner–Ville Distribution (WVD) (Hussein et al., 2018).

1.6 WAVELET TRANSFORM (WT)

While the STFT provides a compromise between time and frequency resolution, its fixed window size limits adaptability for signals whose frequency characteristics vary widely over time. The Wavelet Transform (WT) overcomes this limitation by using scalable and translatable basis functions called *wavelets*. Unlike the fixed window in STFT, wavelets stretch and compress dynamically, offering fine time resolution for high frequencies and fine frequency resolution for low frequencies. This adaptability makes WT particularly effective for analyzing nonstationary and transient features in ECG signals (Gutiérrez-Gnecchi et al., 2017). Mathematically, the wavelet transform decomposes a signal into components that are localized in both time and frequency, allowing multi-resolution analysis for a detailed view of cardiac dynamics.

1.6.1 Continuous Wavelet Transform (CWT)

The Continuous Wavelet Transform (CWT) provides a detailed, continuous mapping of a signal across time and scale (Polikar et al., 1996; Addison, 2017). It is defined as:

$$x(a,b)_{\mathrm{CWT}} = \frac{1}{\sqrt{|a|}} \int_{-\infty}^{\infty} x(t)\psi^*\left(\frac{t-b}{a}\right) dt \tag{1.2}$$

where $x(t)$ is the signal, $\psi(t)$ is the mother wavelet, a is the scale parameter controlling frequency (large a for low frequencies and small a for high frequencies), b is the translation parameter determining time localization, and $\psi^*(\cdot)$ denotes the complex conjugate of the wavelet function.

In ECG analysis, CWT acts like a time-frequency microscope. For example, high-frequency wavelets can highlight QRS complexes with sharp transitions, while lower-frequency scales can capture broader components such as P and T waves. Such analysis enables clinicians and researchers to visualize subtle variations in ECG morphology, making it invaluable for detecting transient abnormalities like premature ventricular contractions, ischemic shifts, or fibrillatory waves.

Figure 1.3 compares how different signal analysis methods capture information in time and frequency. The time series shows variations over time but lacks frequency information, while the Fourier transform captures frequency content but loses timing details. The STFT adds time localization using fixed windows but suffers from a resolution trade-off. The WT overcomes this by using variable window sizes, offering multi-resolution analysis ideal for nonstationary signals like ECG.

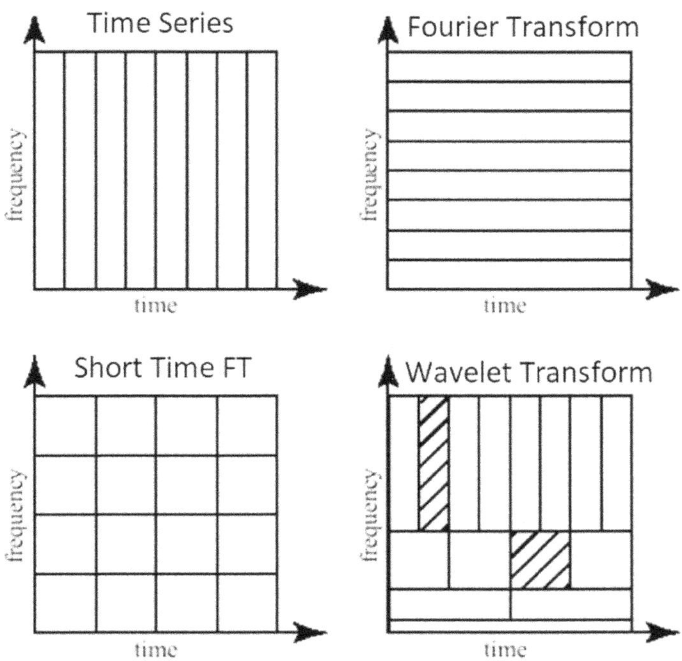

FIGURE 1.3 Schematics of different time-frequency representations.

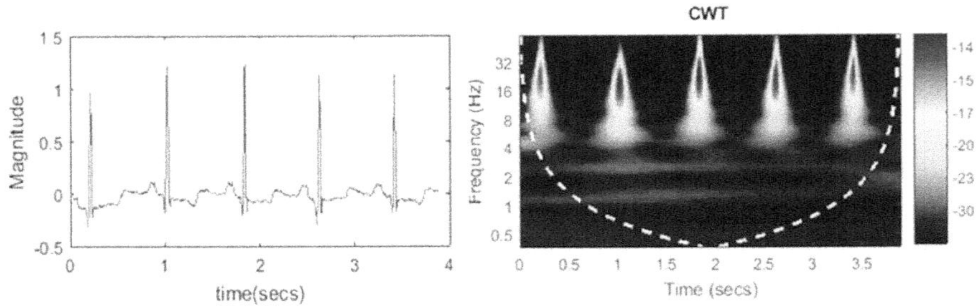

FIGURE 1.4 Time-domain ECG signal and its CWT representation.

Figure 1.4 shows an arrhythmic ECG signal and its CWT representation. The CWT provides a detailed time-frequency view, capturing both transient and sustained frequency components. The irregular spacing and varying intensity of the high-frequency bursts correspond to abnormal cardiac activity. This demonstrates how CWT effectively detects and localizes nonstationary features in arrhythmic ECG.

1.6.2 Discrete Wavelet Transform (DWT)

While CWT offers rich detail, it produces redundant data that can be computationally intensive. The Discrete Wavelet Transform (DWT) provides a more compact and efficient alternative by discretizing the scale and translation parameters, typically using dyadic scales ($a = 2^j$) and translations ($b = k2^j$).

The DWT is mathematically expressed as:

$$x(j,k)_{\text{DWT}} = \begin{cases} \dfrac{1}{\sqrt{2^j}} \displaystyle\int_{-\infty}^{\infty} x(t)\psi^*\left(\frac{t-k2^j}{2^j}\right)dt, & \text{(continuous-time form)} \\ \displaystyle\sum_{n=-\infty}^{\infty} x[n]\psi_{j,k}(n), & \text{(discrete-time form)} \end{cases} \tag{1.3}$$

with the discrete wavelet basis function defined as

$$\psi_{j,k}(n) = 2^{-j/2}\psi\left(2^{-j}n-k\right) \tag{1.4}$$

where j and k denote the scale (or level) and translation indices, respectively. The signal is recursively decomposed into *approximation coefficients* (low-frequency components) and *detail coefficients* (high-frequency components). This hierarchical representation is highly effective for feature extraction, noise reduction, and data compression.

In ECG processing, DWT enables multilevel decomposition of the waveform, allowing identification of characteristic components (Alickovic and Subasi, 2016):

1. Approximation coefficients (A): capture slow, baseline variations such as ST segments and T waves.
2. Detail coefficients (D): highlight fast transients like QRS complexes and noise artifacts.

The combination of these multi-resolution details forms a robust foundation for automated ECG interpretation.

Although the wavelet transform is widely used for ECG and other biomedical signals because of its multi-resolution ability, it has certain practical limitations. Its performance depends strongly on the choice of the mother wavelet, and there is no single wavelet that works best for all signal types or clinical conditions. The time-frequency tiling is fixed by design, so the transform cannot fully adapt to rapid or irregular changes in the signal, and closely spaced frequency components may still overlap, especially at higher frequencies. Wavelet analysis can also introduce edge effects near the start and end of the signal, and the computational cost of the Continuous Wavelet Transform makes real-time implementation more challenging. For these reasons, wavelets often need to be combined with other methods when high accuracy, adaptive resolution, and instantaneous frequency tracking are required in ECG (Addison, 2005; Tary et al., 2018).

1.7 EMPIRICAL MODE DECOMPOSITION (EMD)

Empirical Mode Decomposition (EMD) is a fully data-driven, adaptive time-frequency technique introduced by Huang et al. (1998) to analyze nonlinear and non-stationary signals such as the ECG. Unlike Fourier or wavelet methods, which rely on predefined basis functions, EMD decomposes the signal into a finite set of oscillatory components called *Intrinsic Mode Functions* (IMFs), derived directly from the data itself. This makes EMD particularly suited for biomedical signals, where oscillatory patterns vary dynamically due to physiological processes, artifacts, or disease conditions.

Mathematically, EMD acts as a sifting process that separates the signal $x(t)$ into IMFs based on local time scales determined by the signal's own extrema. The decomposition can be expressed as:

$$x(t) = \sum_{i=1}^{n} c_i(t) + r_n(t) \tag{1.5}$$

where $c_i(t)$ represents the ith IMF and $r_n(t)$ is the final residual or trend. Each IMF captures oscillations within a specific frequency band, offering a multi-scale representation without requiring any prior basis selection.

1.7.1 Intrinsic Mode Functions

An IMF is defined by two essential conditions:

1. The number of extrema and the number of zero crossings must either be equal or differ at most by one.
2. At any point, the mean value of the upper and lower envelopes (formed by local maxima and minima) is zero.

The EMD algorithm extracts IMFs iteratively through a process known as *sifting* and includes the following steps:

1. Identify all local maxima and minima of the signal $x(t)$.
2. Interpolate the maxima and minima to form the upper ($e_{\max}(t)$) and lower ($e_{\min}(t)$) envelopes.
3. Compute the mean envelope $m(t) = \frac{e_{\max}(t) + e_{\min}(t)}{2}$.
4. Subtract this mean from the signal: $h_1(t) = x(t) - m(t)$.
5. Repeat the process on $h_1(t)$ until it satisfies IMF conditions, yielding $c_1(t)$.
6. Subtract $c_1(t)$ from the original signal to obtain the residual $r_1(t) = x(t) - c_1(t)$, and apply the same process to $r_1(t)$.

In ECG analysis, IMFs correspond to different physiological oscillations. High-frequency IMFs often represent QRS complexes, while lower-frequency IMFs capture P and T waves or baseline wander (Anas et al., 2011). This adaptive decomposition makes EMD robust against nonstationarity, noise, and amplitude modulation commonly seen in real-world ECG recordings.

1.7.2 Hilbert–Huang Transform

Once the IMFs are extracted, the Hilbert–Huang Transform (HHT) (Huang 2014) provides a high-resolution time-frequency representation by applying the Hilbert transform to each IMF. The Hilbert transform $\mathcal{H}\{c_i(t)\}$ of the ith IMF is defined as:

$$\mathcal{H}\{c_i(t)\} = \frac{1}{\pi} P.V. \int_{-\infty}^{\infty} \frac{c_i(\tau)}{t - \tau} d\tau \tag{1.6}$$

where $P.V.$ denotes the Cauchy principal value. This allows construction of the analytic signal:

$$z_i(t) = c_i(t) + j\mathcal{H}\{c_i(t)\} = A_i(t) e^{j\theta_i(t)} \tag{1.7}$$

Here, $A_i(t)$ is the instantaneous amplitude and $\theta_i(t)$ is the instantaneous phase. The instantaneous frequency $\omega_i(t)$ is then given by:

$$\omega_i(t) = \frac{d\theta_i(t)}{dt} \tag{1.8}$$

The combination of EMD and Hilbert analysis yields the Hilbert spectrum, $H(\omega,t)$, representing the amplitude (or energy) of each IMF as a function of time and frequency:

$$H(\omega,t) = \mathrm{Re}\left\{\sum_{i=1}^{n} A_i(t)e^{j\int \omega_i(t)dt}\right\} \tag{1.9}$$

This spectrum effectively captures how different frequency components evolve. In ECG studies, HHT reveals instantaneous frequency modulations linked to arrhythmias, autonomic regulation, or ischemic changes, enabling detailed characterization of cardiac dynamics beyond traditional spectral methods. The EMD-HHT framework thus provides a powerful and fully adaptive alternative to fixed-basis transforms. It decomposes the ECG into intrinsic oscillations and reveals their instantaneous energy and frequency dynamics, an important step toward data-driven and interpretable cardiovascular diagnostics.

1.8 ADVANCED APPROACHES

As biomedical signals such as ECG or respiratory signals exhibit complex, nonlinear, and highly nonstationary behavior, advanced time-frequency approaches are helpful in uncovering subtle physiological dynamics. While classical techniques like the Short-Time Fourier Transform (STFT) and Continuous Wavelet Transform (CWT) offer valuable insights, they suffer from trade-offs between time and frequency resolution. Advanced methods such as the Wigner–Ville Distribution (WVD), Stockwell Transform (ST), Constant-Q Transform (CQT), Synchrosqueezing Transform (SST), and Wavelet Scattering Transform (WST) extend these classical frameworks to achieve higher resolution, interpretability, and robustness against noise.

1.8.1 Wigner–Ville Distribution (WVD)

The Wigner–Ville Distribution (WVD) provides a quadratic time-frequency representation with superior energy concentration compared to linear methods such as STFT and CWT (Boashash and Black 1987). It is defined as:

$$x(t,f)_{\mathrm{WVD}} = \int_{-\infty}^{\infty} x\left(t+\frac{\tau}{2}\right)x^*\left(t-\frac{\tau}{2}\right)e^{-j2\pi f\tau}\,d\tau \tag{1.10}$$

where $x(t)$ is the analytic form of the ECG signal and $x(t,f)_{\mathrm{WVD}}$ provides highly localized energy information in both time and frequency. Because of its strong concentration properties, WVD is well-suited for detecting short-duration cardiac events such as premature beats, sudden QRS morphology changes, and rapid frequency bursts linked to arrhythmias.

1.8.1.1 Overcoming Cross-Term Interference: Smoothed and Pseudo-WVD

A major drawback of WVD is the presence of cross-term interference components that appear when a signal contains multiple oscillatory modes. These artifacts can mask clinically relevant features and complicate interpretation in multicomponent ECG signals. To reduce such interference, smoothed extensions of WVD apply windowing in time and/or frequency. A commonly used variant is the *Pseudo Wigner–Ville Distribution (PWVD)*, defined as:

$$x(t,f)_{\text{PWVD}} = \int_{-\infty}^{\infty} h(\tau)\, x\left(t+\frac{\tau}{2}\right) x^*\left(t-\frac{\tau}{2}\right) e^{-j2\pi f\tau}\, d\tau \tag{1.11}$$

where $h(\tau)$ is a smoothing kernel that attenuates cross-term energy while retaining the high-resolution auto-terms. Further variants, including the Choi Williams Distribution and general Cohen-class distributions, provide adaptive smoothing strategies, making WVD-based representations more suitable for biomedical applications where readability and accuracy must be balanced (Dliou et al., 2014; Hussein et al., 2018).

1.8.2 Stockwell Transform (ST)

The Stockwell Transform, also known as the S-transform (Stockwell et al., 1996), merges the localization property of the wavelet transform with the phase-preserving characteristics of the STFT. It is expressed as:

$$S(t,f) = \int_{-\infty}^{\infty} x(\tau) \frac{|f|}{\sqrt{2\pi}} e^{-\frac{(t-\tau)^2 f^2}{2}} e^{-j2\pi f\tau} d\tau \tag{1.12}$$

ST is a special case of the CWT using a Morlet-type wavelet, with a phase and amplitude correction. It emphasizes higher frequency content due to the factor $|f|$. This transform provides frequency-dependent resolution, high temporal resolution at high frequencies, and fine spectral resolution at low frequencies, making it particularly suitable for analyzing ECG segments with varying heart rates or arrhythmic episodes (Das and Ari, 2013; Allam et al., 2020). Figure 1.5 presents the ST representation of the ECG signal taken as an example.

1.8.3 Constant-Q Transform (CQT)

The Constant-Q Transform (CQT) (Holighaus et al., 2012; Singh et al., 2021) offers logarithmic frequency resolution, maintaining a constant ratio of frequency to bandwidth. Its mathematical form is given by:

$$X(k,n) = \sum_{m=0}^{N-1} x[m]\, w_k[m-n]\, e^{-j2\pi Qm/k} \tag{1.13}$$

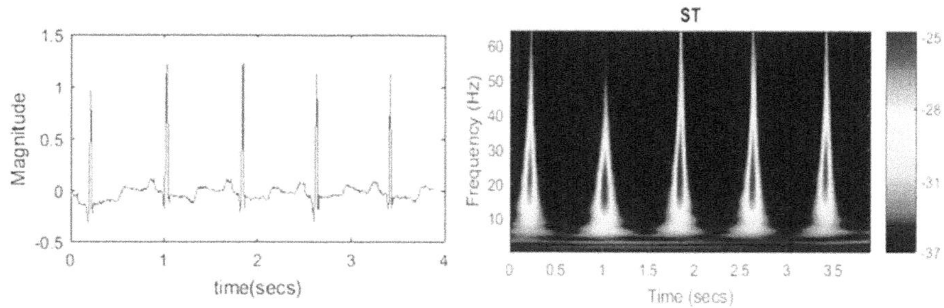

FIGURE 1.5 Time-domain ECG signal and its ST representation.

where Q is the quality factor determining the trade-off between time and frequency resolution. CQT's design aligns with human auditory perception, making it highly effective in ECG denoising and spectral pattern extraction where low-frequency components dominate.

Constant-Q Nonstationary Gabor Transform (CQNSGT): The Constant-Q Nonstationary Gabor Transform (CQNSGT) is a modern extension of CQT that achieves a fully invertible, nonstationary, and adaptive time-frequency representation. Unlike the traditional CQT, which uses fixed filter banks, CQNSGT employs frequency-dependent nonstationary Gabor frames that adjust window lengths dynamically across frequency bands (Eltrass et al., 2021). This approach preserves the constant-Q property while ensuring perfect reconstruction. The CQNSGT representation of a signal $x(t)$ can be expressed as:

$$X(k,n) = \sum_{m=0}^{N-1} x[m] g_k[m-n] e^{-j2\pi f_k m} \tag{1.14}$$

where $g_k(\cdot)$ is the nonstationary Gabor window for the kth frequency channel, and f_k denotes the corresponding center frequency. Its adaptability enables finer time resolution at high frequencies and enhanced frequency localization at lower bands. This makes CQNSGT particularly suitable for nonstationary biomedical signals such as ECG and respiratory recordings, providing improved temporal and spectral discrimination for transient cardiac events. Figure 1.6 is referred to as an example of CQNGST representation of the example ECG signal.

1.8.4 Synchrosqueezing Transform (SST)

The Synchrosqueezing Transform (SST) is an advanced time-frequency reassignment technique that refines the representation obtained from the CWT. Originally proposed by Daubechies et al. (2011), SST aims to improve frequency localization by redistributing smeared spectral energy to its true instantaneous frequencies. This makes it particularly useful for analyzing nonstationary biomedical signals such as ECG, where dynamic spectral changes are often subtle yet clinically significant.

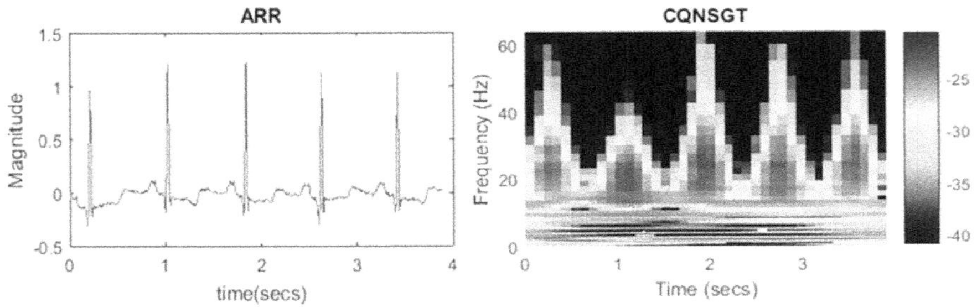

FIGURE 1.6 Time-domain ECG signal and its CQNSGT representation.

However, due to convolution in the time-scale domain, CWT often suffers from *spectral smearing*, resulting in reduced precision in frequency localization.

To counter this, SST performs a *frequency reassignment* by calculating the instantaneous frequency (IF) at each point (a,b) in the CWT plane as:

$$\omega_x(a,b) = \frac{-j}{2\pi\, x(a,b)_{CWT}} \frac{\partial x(a,b)_{CWT}}{\partial b} \tag{1.15}$$

This IF estimation provides a way to track how the frequency content of the signal evolves over time. The synchrosqueezing operation then reallocates the smeared spectral energy of the CWT along these instantaneous frequencies, effectively mapping the time–scale plane (b,a) into the time-frequency plane $(b,\omega_f(a,b))$. The SST representation is thus defined as:

$$T_f(b,\omega) = \int_A x(a,b)_{CWT}\, \delta(\omega - \omega_x(a,b))\, a^{-3/2}\, da \tag{1.16}$$

By compressing redundant spectral information into more compact frequency bands, SST yields a sharper and more interpretable time-frequency map. In ECG analysis, this improved readability helps identify subtle frequency modulations associated with arrhythmias, ischemic drifts, or other transient cardiac abnormalities, which may not be evident using conventional CWT or STFT representations. Figure 1.7 shows an

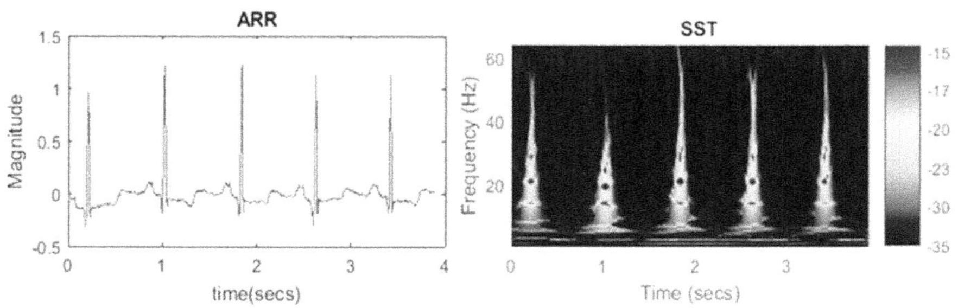

FIGURE 1.7 Time-domain ECG signal and its SST representation.

arrhythmic ECG signal and its time-frequency representation using SST. Unlike standard wavelet maps, SST sharpens the energy concentration along frequency ridges, allowing clearer visualization of transient high-frequency components associated with arrhythmic beats. This makes it easier to track frequency changes over time and detect subtle abnormalities that may not be visible in the raw ECG signal.

1.8.5 Wavelet Scattering Transform (WST)

While time-frequency methods such as STFT, CWT, ST, and SST provide rich representations of nonstationary signals, they still require manual feature extraction and expert-defined descriptors when used for classification and diagnosis. In contrast, deep learning models such as convolutional neural networks (CNNs) can learn discriminative features directly from data (Yildirim et al., 2019; Pławiak and Acharya, 2020; Eltrass et al., 2021; Singh and Mahapatra, 2024; Islam et al., 2024), but they lack the mathematical guarantees of stability, invariance, and interpretability that classical signal processing methods offer. The Wavelet Scattering Transform (WST) was introduced as a hybrid solution, combining the mathematical structure of wavelet theory with the layered architecture of CNNs. As a result, WST produces compact, translation-invariant, and deformation-stable feature representations while avoiding the need for learned filters, making it especially suitable for ECG signals. It offers a stable and mathematically grounded framework that bridges classical wavelet analysis and modern deep learning. WST inherits the interpretability of wavelets while mimicking the layered architecture of CNN, but with predefined (non-learned) filters based on principles of scale and frequency decomposition (Andén and Mallat 2014).

Let $X(t)$ denote the input ECG signal to be analyzed. A family of complex wavelet filters ψ and a low-pass filter ϕ are employed to cover the entire frequency spectrum. The low-pass filter $\phi_j(t)$ at scale j captures coarse, slowly varying signal components, ensuring local translation invariance over a scale T. The wavelet functions ψ_{λ_k}, parameterized by index λ_k and octave resolution Q_k, form a multi-scale high-pass filter bank for extracting detailed frequency information.

WST constructs representations through an iterative cascade of three key operations: convolution, complex modulus, and averaging. The zeroth-order scattering coefficient captures the global low-frequency envelope of the signal:

$$|W_1|X = \{X*\phi, |X*\psi_{\lambda_1}|\}_{\lambda_1 \in \Lambda_1} \tag{1.17}$$

However, the local averaging $X*\phi$ smooths out rapid variations, leading to the loss of high-frequency information. To recover this, the first-order scattering coefficients are computed by averaging the modulus of the wavelet coefficients:

$$|S_1|X = |X*\psi_{\lambda_1}|*\phi_j \tag{1.18}$$

This averaging provides invariance to local translations but again attenuates finer temporal details. Therefore, the wavelet modulus transform is recursively applied to restore the lost high-frequency components:

$$|W_2||X*\psi_{\lambda_1}| = \left\{|X*\psi_{\lambda_1}|*\phi, ||X*\psi_{\lambda_1}|*\psi_{\lambda_2}|\right\}_{\lambda_2 \in \Lambda_2} \quad (1.19)$$

yielding the second-order scattering coefficients:

$$|S_2|X = ||X*\psi_{\lambda_1}|*\psi_{\lambda_2}|*\phi_j \quad (1.20)$$

By continuing this process, higher-order scattering paths are constructed iteratively:

$$|U_m|X = |||X*\psi_{\lambda_1}|*\cdots|*\psi_{\lambda_m}| \quad (1.21)$$

and the corresponding m^{th}-order scattering coefficients are obtained through averaging:

$$|S_m|X = |||X*\psi_{\lambda_1}|*\cdots|*\psi_{\lambda_m}|*\phi \quad (1.22)$$

All scattering coefficients up to a maximum order l are concatenated to form the final scattering representation:

$$|S|X = \{|S_m|X\}_{0 \le m \le l} \quad (1.23)$$

Because of the low-pass averaging with ϕ_j, WST representations become invariant to translations within the scale T. The coefficients are also stable to small temporal deformations, a property inherited from the wavelet transform. These features make WST particularly suitable for ECG analysis, where minor variations in amplitude, duration, or morphology can indicate underlying cardiac conditions. By capturing both global and localized frequency patterns, the scattering network yields compact and discriminative features for arrhythmia or ischemia classification.

Although WST and CNNs share architectural similarities, two important differences exist: (1) the filters in WST are mathematically defined rather than learned from data, and (2) features are aggregated across all layers rather than extracted solely from the final layer.

As reported in Bruna and Mallat (2011), the first two scattering layers capture nearly 99% of the total signal energy, making them sufficient for most biomedical applications. Therefore, a second-order scattering network is typically employed for ECG feature extraction, as illustrated in Figure 1.8. This configuration achieves a balance between discriminative capacity and computational efficiency.

To demonstrate the potential and practical applicability of the WST, we conducted an extensive 17-class arrhythmia classification experiment, as presented in Nahak and Saha (2023). In this study, WST-based features enabled highly accurate

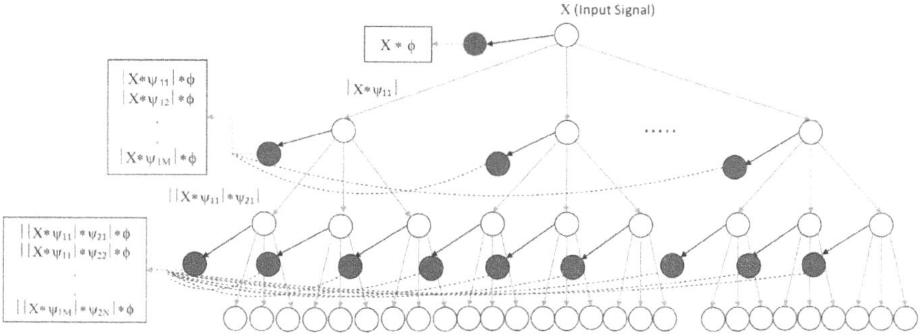

FIGURE 1.8 Wavelet scattering transform architecture: $X(t)$ denotes the input ECG signal; ψ and ϕ represent the wavelet and low-pass filters, respectively. Zeroth-, first-, and second-order scattering coefficients are illustrated in Nahak et al. (2023).

separation of ECG fragments across multiple arrhythmia types without requiring QRS detection or complex preprocessing. The method achieved a classification accuracy of 98.90% using an SVM classifier, with several arrhythmia classes reaching 100% detection accuracy. Further evaluations on reduced 15- and 13-class datasets also confirmed the strength of the WST feature representation, outperforming state-of-the-art deep learning and handcrafted feature-based approaches (Pławiak, 2018; Yıldırım et al., 2018; Tuncer et al., 2019). Beyond accuracy, the method offers lower computational complexity and reduced feature extraction time, making it well-suited for real-time and mobile healthcare applications. These results make WST a powerful and efficient signal representation technique for automated arrhythmia detection.

The above advanced approaches balance interpretability, resolution, and computational efficiency, offering deeper insights into cardiac signal dynamics. They serve as a bridge between classical signal analysis and modern machine learning frameworks for biomedical diagnostics.

1.9 A COMPARISON OF VARIOUS TFA

Figure 1.9 presents how various linear TFA methods capture the evolving spectral characteristics of ECG signals under different cardiac conditions like normal sinus rhythm (NSR), arrhythmia (ARR), and congestive heart failure (CHF). In the NSR case (top row), all transforms show well-defined and periodic frequency bursts corresponding to regular heartbeats. The CWT and SST provide smoother and better localized representations of these events compared to the STFT, which shows slight spectral smearing due to fixed windowing. For the ARR (middle row), irregular heartbeat intervals cause uneven spacing and fluctuating frequency components. The SST and CQNSGT highlight these variations more clearly, offering improved localization of transient features and frequency shifts associated with abnormal depolarizations. In the CHF condition (bottom row), the ECG shows broader low-frequency energy and reduced periodicity. The CWT and ST capture gradual spectral drifts, while

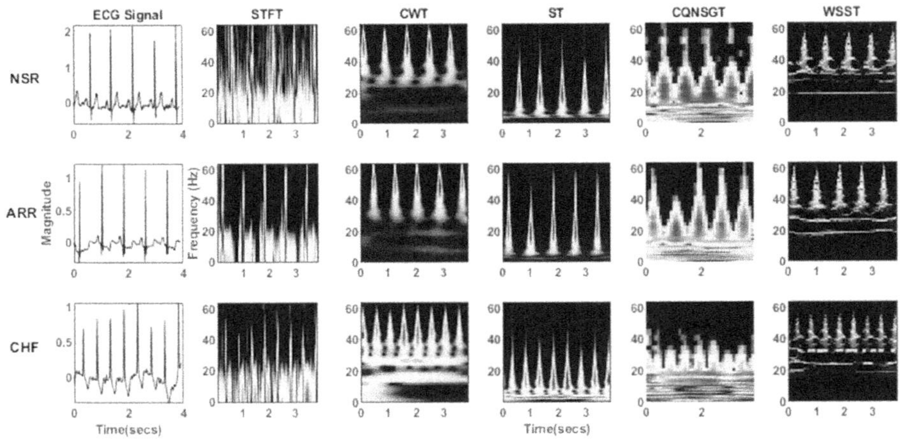

FIGURE 1.9 Different time-frequency representations of ECG signals (Nahak et al., 2023).

SST enhances the fine-scale representation of oscillatory components, revealing hidden sub-band variations. Overall, the comparison shows that advanced adaptive transforms such as CQNSGT and SST provide superior resolution and interpretability for nonstationary cardiac signals, making them valuable for automated diagnosis and signal characterization.

Table 1.1 summarizes the classification performance achieved using different time-frequency representations of ECG signals for separating NSR, ARR, and CHF conditions with an AlexNet-based transfer learning approach. The experiments were conducted using data from the PhysioNet database, which includes recordings from

TABLE 1.1
Performance Comparison of Different TFA for ECG Arrhythmia Classification

TFA Method	Acc. ± Std (%)	Sensitivity (%)	Specificity (%)	Precision (%)	F1-Score (%)
STFT	92.13 ± 0.35	94.32	95.00	92.62	91.06
CWT	93.04 ± 0.42	94.98	95.30	94.16	92.15
S-Transform (ST)	94.60 ± 0.34	95.63	96.48	95.98	93.41
CQNSGT	96.56 ± 0.47	95.72	97.78	96.29	95.45
SST	**97.35 ± 0.29**	**96.25**	**98.15**	**97.64**	**96.83**

Acc. – Accuracy; Std – Standard deviation.
Source: Nahak et al. (2023)

18 NSR, 47 ARR, and 14 CHF subjects. A total of 1280 ECG fragments were generated (288 NSR, 752 ARR, and 240 CHF), and a pretrained AlexNet model was fine-tuned using 5-fold cross-validation to evaluate the performance of each TFR method. Further methodological details and analysis are provided in Nahak et al. (2023). The results clearly indicate that the choice of TFR has a substantial impact on diagnostic performance. Conventional representations, such as STFT and CWT, achieve competitive but comparatively lower accuracy, while more adaptive transforms like the ST and CQNSGT show noticeable improvements across all evaluation metrics. SST yields the highest performance, achieving 97.35% accuracy with the best sensitivity, specificity, precision, and F1-score, reflecting its ability to sharpen energy localization and preserve transient cardiac dynamics. These findings demonstrate that advanced TFRs with improved time-frequency resolution provide more discriminative signal representations, enabling deep learning models to better capture subtle morphological and spectral variations associated with cardiac pathology.

To support reproducibility and further experimentation, Table 1.2 lists the major open-source and hands-on toolboxes used for TFA evaluated in this study. MATLAB toolboxes such as the Wavelet Toolbox and Time-Frequency Toolbox were used for classical transforms, including STFT and CWT, while advanced adaptive methods such as SST and CQNSGT were implemented using Python libraries like ssqueezepy, librosa, and nsgt. The WST was generated using the kymatio framework, which integrates seamlessly with deep learning backends such as PyTorch. These tools enable researchers to reproduce the TFRs, benchmark deep learning models, and extend the analysis to other ECG datasets or physiological signals.

These toolboxes provide opportunities for generating, visualizing, and experimenting with time-frequency representations, enabling both signal processing and deep-learning related studies in cardiovascular research.

1.10 APPLICATIONS OF TFA

TFA has emerged as a cornerstone in biomedical signal interpretation, particularly for nonstationary and multicomponent signals such as the ECG signal. Its ability to capture both temporal and spectral dynamics enables clinicians and researchers to uncover subtle physiological variations that traditional analyses often overlook. The following subsections outline key application areas of TFA in cardiovascular diagnostics and monitoring.

1.10.1 Arrhythmia Classification

Arrhythmias often manifest as transient changes in the ECG waveform, involving variations in QRS morphology, beat interval irregularities, or frequency modulation. TFA methods such as the STFT, WT, WVD, CQT, SST, and WST allow simultaneous examination of temporal and frequency components, enhancing discrimination between normal and pathological rhythms. For example, ventricular tachycardia may exhibit high-frequency bursts localized within short time intervals, whereas atrial fibrillation reveals low-frequency, irregular oscillations distributed over longer

TABLE 1.2
Software Tools and Libraries for Time-Frequency Analysis of ECG Signals

Tool/Library	Platform and Purpose	TFA Methods Supported	Link
MATLAB Wavelet Toolbox	Commercial MATLAB toolbox for biomedical signal analysis	STFT, CWT, DWT, WSST, Reassigned STFT	wavelet[1]
MATLAB Time-Frequency Toolbox (TFTB)	Free MATLAB add-on for Cohen-class and quadratic TFRs	WVD, PWVD, Choi-Williams, Spectrograms	TFTB[2]
S-Transform Toolkit (Python)	Implementation of Stockwell Transform for nonstationary biomedical signals	S-Transform (ST) for ECG and EEG analysis	S-Transform[3]
SST Toolkit (ssqueezepy)	Advanced synchrosqueezing transform and ridge extraction	CWT, STFT, SST, instantaneous frequency estimation	ssqueezepy[4]
librosa (Python)	Audio TFR library usable for ECG CQT/CQNSGT image generation	STFT, CQT, Mel-spectrogram, CQNSGT	librosa[5]
nsgt (Python)	Nonstationary Gabor and constant-Q decomposition	CQNSGT, time-varying filterbanks	nsgt[6]
kymatio (Python / PyTorch)	Deep-learning compatible scattering networks	1D/2D Wavelet Scattering Transform (WST)	kymatio[7]
PyWavelets (pywt)	General-purpose wavelet transform and denoising	DWT, IDWT, multi-resolution filtering	pywt[8]
tftb (Python)	Python version of Time-Frequency Toolbox	WVD, Gabor, Choi-Williams, Scalograms	tftb[9]
PyEMD / PyHHT	Adaptive decomposition for nonstationary ECG analysis	EMD, IMF extraction, Hilbert–Huang Transform	PyEMD[10]
GhostiPy (Python DSP)	High-speed TFA for long signals/edge devices	STFT, CWT, SST, CQT, multitaper TFRs	ghostipy[11]

(*Continued*)

TABLE 1.2 CONTINUED
Software Tools and Libraries for Time-Frequency Analysis of ECG Signals

Tool/Library	Platform and Purpose	TFA Methods Supported	Link
BioSPPy (Python)	Biomedical signal processing toolkit for ECG and PPG	Preprocessing, feature extraction, TFA	BioSPPy[12]

[1] https://www.mathworks.com/products/wavelet.html (Accessed: 20/11/2025)
[2] https://tftb.nongnu.org/ (Accessed: 20/11/2025)
[3] https://github.com/xli2522/S-Transform (Accessed: 20/11/2025)
[4] https://github.com/OverLordGoldDragon/ssqueezepy (Accessed: 20/11/2025)
[5] https://librosa.org (Accessed: 20/11/2025)
[6] https://github.com/grrrr/nsgt (Accessed: 20/11/2025)
[7] https://www.kymat.io (Accessed: 20/11/2025)
[8] https://pywavelets.readthedocs.io (Accessed: 20/11/2025)
[9] https://github.com/scikit-signal/tftb (Accessed: 20/11/2025)
[10] https://github.com/laszukdawid/PyEMD (Accessed: 20/11/2025)
[11] https://github.com/DrKrar/ghostipy (Accessed: 20/11/2025)
[12] https://github.com/PIA-Group/BioSPPy (Accessed: 20/11/2025)

durations (Gutiérrez-Gnecchi et al., 2017; Sultan Qurraie and Ghorbani Afkhami, 2017; Huang et al., 2019; Nahak and Saha, 2023; Daydulo et al., 2023). When coupled with machine learning or deep learning models, TFA-derived features significantly improve classification accuracy, providing robust biomarkers for automated ECG interpretation and arrhythmia screening (Allam et al., 2020; Eltrass et al., 2021; Bing et al., 2022; Daydulo et al., 2023). Figure 1.10 presents the block diagram of the WST-based ECG arrhythmia classification framework, and Figure 1.11 shows the overall pipeline in which raw ECG signals are preprocessed, converted into time-frequency representations, and used to train and evaluate deep learning models for automated arrhythmia classification.

1.10.2 Detection of Myocardial Ischemia and Infarction

Myocardial ischemic episodes cause transient ST-segment deviations and subtle spectral shifts that are often missed in conventional time-domain analysis. TFA techniques, especially the CWT, ST, and SST, offer high sensitivity to such short-lived changes by tracking the evolution of low-frequency energy in the ECG. These methods can isolate ischemic signatures in both resting and stress-test recordings, aiding in early myocardial ischemia detection (Pławiak, 2018; Fernández Biscay et al., 2020; Hussein et al., 2021; Gupta et al., 2025). Other adaptive approaches, such as EMD

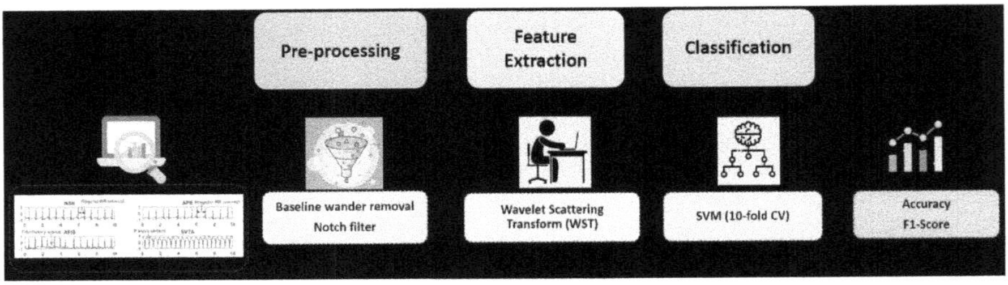

FIGURE 1.10 Block diagram of WST-based ECG arrhythmia classification framework (Nahak and Saha, 2023).

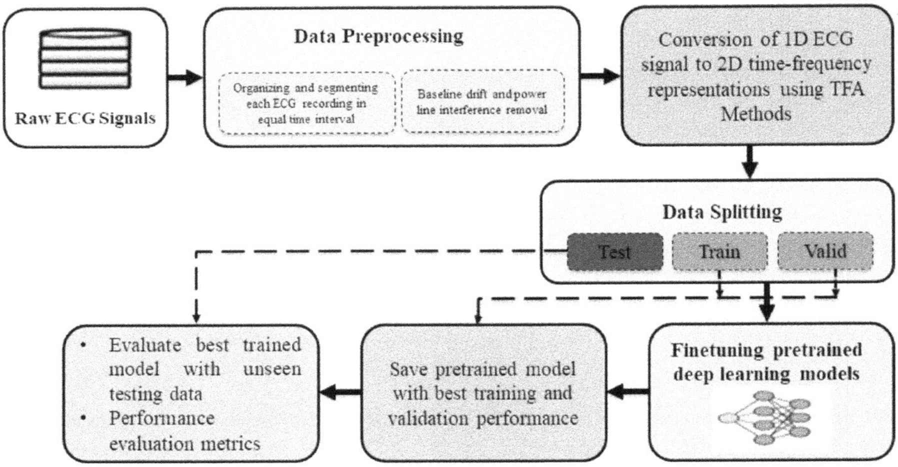

FIGURE 1.11 Block diagram of the ECG arrhythmia classification pipeline using time-frequency analysis.

combined with HHT, allow time-localized analysis of the ST segment and T-wave alterations, improving diagnostic accuracy in ECG signals (Wang et al., 2023).

1.10.3 Heart Rate Variability Analysis

Heart Rate Variability (HRV) reflects autonomic regulation of cardiac rhythm and is influenced by both sympathetic and parasympathetic activities. Traditional frequency-domain methods provide global spectral measures of HRV, but they fail to account for dynamic fluctuations. TFA methods, including the DWT, EMD, SST, and WVD, enable high-resolution tracking of instantaneous frequency variations, revealing transient autonomic modulations under stress, exercise, or disease conditions (Mainardi, 2009; Alickovic and Subasi, 2016; Herry et al., 2017; Huang et al., 2019). Such analyses have been particularly valuable in assessing cardiac health, predicting sudden cardiac death risk, and monitoring recovery following myocardial infarction.

1.10.4 Real-Time Monitoring in Wearable Devices

With the advent of smart wearable technologies, TFA has become important for continuous and real-time ECG monitoring. Algorithms based on short-window STFT, discrete WT, or adaptive EMD variants can be efficiently implemented on embedded processors, balancing computational efficiency and diagnostic accuracy (Shoughi et al., 2024; Song and Lee, 2024). These methods allow real-time detection of abnormal heart rhythms, ischemic changes, or HRV variations directly on wearable platforms. Recent studies also demonstrate that hybrid deep models incorporating Wavelet Scattering features can enable energy-efficient inference for mobile health applications, supporting personalized cardiovascular care and early warning systems. Different transforms offer different strengths: linear methods such as STFT and CWT provide intuitive joint time-frequency views, while advanced approaches such as SST, WVD, and WST improve resolution, interpretability, or machine-learning readiness (Gong and Ding, 2019; Smital et al., 2020). As shown in Table 1.3, the choice of TFA method depends on the clinical objective, the signal

TABLE 1.3
Applications of TFA in ECG Signal Processing

Applications	Purpose	TFA Methods and Outcomes
Arrhythmia detection and classification (Gutiérrez-Gnecchi et al., 2017; Farag, 2022; Nahak et al., 2023; Nahak and Saha, 2023)	Identify abnormal beats and rhythms (PVC, AF, VT)	STFT, CWT, HHT, WST, SST – detects bursts of high-frequency energy during ventricular arrhythmia
Myocardial ischemia detection (Sahu and Ray, 2021; Hussein et al., 2021)	Track ST-segment shifts and low-frequency spectral drift	CWT, WVD, PWVD – ridge tracking reveals ischemic frequency shifts over time
Heart rate variability (HRV) analysis (Herry et al., 2017; Huang et al., 2019)	Assess autonomic balance via LF/HF spectral bands	SST, CWT, ST – instantaneous frequency tracks RR-interval fluctuations
Fetal ECG extraction and monitoring (Krupa et al., 2022)	Separate overlapping maternal–fetal ECG components	WT, WVD – resolves nonstationary sources with high resolution
Wearable/real-time ECG monitoring (Smital et al., 2020)	Low-power TFA feature extraction for edge devices	CWT, WST, CQNSGT – enables TF-based analytics in smartwatches and patches
ECG denoising and artifact removal (Chatterjee et al., 2020)	Suppress muscle noise, motion artifacts, and baseline wander	WT, EMD, SST – TF-domain thresholding for improved signal quality

characteristics, and whether the goal is visual diagnosis, feature extraction, or automated classification.

1.10.5 Challenges: Noise, Computational Complexity, and Interpretability

Even though time-frequency analysis is a powerful tool for ECG processing, several challenges still limit its use in real-world systems. ECG signals collected from wearable devices or clinical settings often contain noise from motion, muscle activity, baseline drift, or power-line interference, which can blur the time-frequency representation and lead to incorrect interpretation (Chatterjee et al., 2020). Denoising methods such as wavelet filtering or EMD-based decomposition can help, but they also increase the processing load. Some high-resolution TFA methods, like WVD, CQT, and SST, produce very detailed outputs but require heavy computation, making them difficult to use in real-time or low-power devices (Smital et al., 2020). Another challenge is interpretability; many advanced TFRs look like complex images or coefficient maps that clinicians may find difficult to read without automated support (Ayano et al., 2022). Finding the right balance between accuracy, speed, and clinical usability remains an important goal for future TFA-based ECG systems.

BIBLIOGRAPHY

Addison, P. S. (2005). Wavelet transforms and the ECG: A review. *Physiological Measurement*, 26(5):R155.

Addison, P. S. (2017). *The illustrated wavelet transform handbook: Introductory theory and applications in science, engineering, medicine and finance.* CRC Press.

Alickovic, E. and Subasi, A. (2016). Medical decision support system for diagnosis of heart arrhythmia using DWT and random forests classifier. *Journal of Medical Systems*, 40(4):108.

Allam, J. P., Samantray, S., and Ari, S. (2020). SpEC: A system for patient specific ECG beat classification using deep residual network. *Biocybernetics and Biomedical Engineering*, 40(4):1446–1457.

Anas, E. M. A., Lee, S. Y., and Hasan, M. K. (2011). Exploiting correlation of ECG with certain EMD functions for discrimination of ventricular fibrillation. *Computers in Biology and Medicine*, 41(2):110–114.

Andén, J. and Mallat, S. (2014). Deep scattering spectrum. *IEEE Transactions on Signal Processing*, 62(16):4114–4128.

Ayano, Y. M., Schwenker, F., Dufera, B. D., and Debelee, T. G. (2022). Interpretable machine learning techniques in ECG-based heart disease classification: A systematic review. *Diagnostics*, 13(1):111.

Bing, P., Liu, Y., Liu, W., Zhou, J., and Zhu, L. (2022). Electrocardiogram classification using tsst-based spectrogram and convit. *Frontiers in Cardiovascular Medicine*, 9:983543.

Boashash, B. and Black, P. (1987). An efficient real-time implementation of the Wigner-Ville distribution. *IEEE Transactions on Acoustics, Speech, and Signal Processing*, 35(11):1611–1618.

Bruna, J. and Mallat, S. (2011). Classification with scattering operators. In *CVPR 2011*, pages 1561–1566. IEEE.

Chatterjee, S., Thakur, R. S., Yadav, R. N., Gupta, L., and Raghuvanshi, D. K. (2020). Review of noise removal techniques in ECG signals. *IET Signal Processing*, 14(9):569–590.

Das, M. and Ari, S. (2013). Analysis of ECG signal denoising method based on S-transform. *Irbm*, 34(6):362–370.

Daubechies, I., Lu, J., and Wu, H.-T. (2011). Synchrosqueezed wavelet transforms: An empirical mode decomposition-like tool. *Applied and Computational Harmonic Analysis*, 30(2):243–261.

Daydulo, Y. D., Thamineni, B. L., and Dawud, A. A. (2023). Cardiac arrhythmia detection using deep learning approach and time frequency representation of ECG signals. *BMC Medical Informatics and Decision Making*, 23(1):232.

Dliou, A., Latif, R., Laaboubi, M., and Maoulainine, F. (2014). Abnormal ECG signals analysis using non-parametric time–frequency techniques. *Arabian Journal for Science and Engineering*, 39(2):913–921.

Durak, L. and Arikan, O. (2003). Short-time fourier transform: Two fundamental properties and an optimal implementation. *IEEE Transactions on Signal Processing*, 51(5):1231–1242.

Eltrass, A. S., Tayel, M. B., and Ammar, A. I. (2021). A new automated CNN deep learning approach for identification of ECG congestive heart failure and arrhythmia using constant-Q non-stationary Gabor transform. *Biomedical Signal Processing and Control*, 65:102326.

Farag, M. M. (2022). A self-contained STFT CNN for ECG classification and arrhythmia detection at the edge. *IEEE Access*, 10:94469–94486.

Fernández Biscay, C., Arini, P. D., Rincón Soler, A. I., and Bonomini, M. P. (2020). Classification of ischemic and non-ischemic cardiac events in holter recordings based on the continuous wavelet transform. *Medical & Biological Engineering & Computing*, 58(5):1069–1078.

Gong, Z. and Ding, Y. (2019). Design and implementation of wearable dynamic electrocardiograph real-time monitoring terminal. *IEEE Access*, 8:6575–6582.

Gupta, K., Bajaj, V., and Ansari, I. A. (2025). CardioNet: A lightweight deep learning framework for screening of myocardial infarction using ECG sensor data. *IEEE Sensors Journal*, 25(4):6794–6800.

Gutiérrez-Gnecchi, J. A., Morfin-Magaña, R., Lorias-Espinoza, D., del Carmen Tellez-Anguiano, A., Reyes-Archundia, E., Méndez-Patiño, A., and Castañeda-Miranda, R. (2017). DSP-based arrhythmia classification using wavelet transform and probabilistic neural network. *Biomedical Signal Processing and Control*, 32:44–56.

Herry, C. L., Frasch, M., Seely, A. J., and Wu, H.-T. (2017). Heart beat classification from single-lead ECG using the synchrosqueezing transform. *Physiological Measurement*, 38(2):171.

Holighaus, N., Dörfler, M., Velasco, G. A., and Grill, T. (2012). A framework for invertible, real-time constant-Q transforms. *IEEE Transactions on Audio, Speech, and Language Processing*, 21(4):775–785.

Huang, J., Chen, B., Yao, B., and He, W. (2019). ECG arrhythmia classification using STFT-based spectrogram and convolutional neural network. *IEEE Access*, 7:92871–92880.

Huang, N. E. (2014). *Hilbert-Huang transform and its applications*, volume 16. World Scientific.

Huang, N. E., Shen, Z., Long, S. R., Wu, M. C., Shih, H. H., Zheng, Q., Yen, N.-C., Tung, C. C., and Liu, H. H. (1998). The empirical mode decomposition and the Hilbert spectrum for nonlinear and non-stationary time series analysis. *Proceedings of the Royal Society of London. Series A: Mathematical, Physical and Engineering Sciences*, 454(1971):903–995.

Hussein, A. F., Hashim, S. J., Aziz, A. F. A., Rokhani, F. Z., and Adnan, W. A. W. (2018). Performance evaluation of time-frequency distributions for ECG signal analysis. *Journal of Medical Systems*, 42(1):15.

Hussein, A. F., Hashim, S. J., Rokhani, F. Z., and Wan Adnan, W. A. (2021). An automated high-accuracy detection scheme for myocardial ischemia based on multi-lead long-interval ECG and Choi-Williams time-frequency analysis incorporating a multi-class SVM classifier. *Sensors*, 21(7):2311.

Islam, M. R., Qaraqe, M., Qaraqe, K., and Serpedin, E. (2024). Cat-net: Convolution, attention, and transformer based network for single-lead ECG arrhythmia classification. *Biomedical Signal Processing and Control*, 93:106211.

Kaptoge, S., Pennells, L., De Bacquer, D., Cooney, M. T., Kavousi, M., Stevens, G., Riley, L. M., Savin, S., Khan, T., Altay, S., et al. (2019). World health organization cardiovascular disease risk charts: Revised models to estimate risk in 21 global regions. *The Lancet Global Health*, 7(10):e1332–e1345.

Kinoshita, O., Fontaine, G., Rosas, F., Elias, J., Iwa, T., Tonet, J., Lascault, G., and Frank, R. (1995). Time-and frequency-domain analyses of the signal-averaged ECG in patients with arrhythmogenic right ventricular dysplasia. *Circulation*, 91(3):715–721.

Krupa, A. J. D., Dhanalakshmi, S., and Kumar, R. (2022). Joint time-frequency analysis and non-linear estimation for fetal ECG extraction. *Biomedical Signal Processing and Control*, 75:103569.

Mahmoud, S. S., Hussain, Z. M., Cosic, I., and Fang, Q. (2006). Time-frequency analysis of normal and abnormal biological signals. *Biomedical Signal Processing and Control*, 1(1):33–43.

Mainardi, L. T. (2009). On the quantification of heart rate variability spectral parameters using time–frequency and time-varying methods. *Philosophical Transactions of the Royal Society A: Mathematical, Physical and Engineering Sciences*, 367(1887):255–275.

Nahak, S., Pathak, A., and Saha, G. (2023). Evaluation of handcrafted features and learned representations for the classification of arrhythmia and congestive heart failure in ECG. *Biomedical Signal Processing and Control*, 79:104230.

Nahak, S. and Saha, G. (2023). Ensembled feature based multi-label ECG arrhythmia classification. In *2023 45th Annual International Conference of the IEEE Engineering in Medicine & Biology Society (EMBC)*, pages 1–4. IEEE.

Pławiak, P. (2018). Novel genetic ensembles of classifiers applied to myocardium dysfunction recognition based on ECG signals. *Swarm and Evolutionary Computation*, 39:192–208.

Pławiak, P. and Acharya, U. R. (2020). Novel deep genetic ensemble of classifiers for arrhythmia detection using ECG signals. *Neural Computing and Applications*, 32(15):11137–11161.

Polikar, R. et al. (1996). *The wavelet tutorial: Second edition, part I—Fundamental concepts and an overview of wavelet theory.* Rowan University.

Pradhan, B. K., Neelappu, B. C., Sivaraman, J., Kim, D., and Pal, K. (2023). A review on the applications of time-frequency methods in ECG analysis. *Journal of Healthcare Engineering*, 2023(1):3145483.

Rangayyan, R. M. (2015). *Biomedical signal analysis*, volume 33. John Wiley & Sons.

Sahu, G. and Ray, K. C. (2021). An efficient method for detection and localization of myocardial infarction. *IEEE Transactions on Instrumentation and Measurement*, 71:1–12.

Shoughi, A., Dowlatshahi, M. B., Amiri, A., Kuchaki Rafsanjani, M., and Batth, R. S. (2024). Automatic ECG classification using discrete wavelet transform and one-dimensional convolutional neural network. *Computing*, 106(4):1227–1248.

Singh, P., Saha, G., and Sahidullah, M. (2021). Non-linear frequency warping using constant-Q transformation for speech emotion recognition. In *2021 International Conference on Computer Communication and Informatics (ICCCI)*, pages 1–6. IEEE.

Singh, P. N. and Mahapatra, R. P. (2024). A novel deep learning approach for arrhythmia prediction on ECG classification using recurrent CNN with GWO. *International Journal of Information Technology*, 16(1):577–585.

Smital, L., Haider, C. R., Vitek, M., Leinveber, P., Jurak, P., Nemcova, A., Smisek, R., Marsanova, L., Provaznik, I., Felton, C. L., et al. (2020). Real-time quality assessment of long-term ECG signals recorded by wearables in free-living conditions. *IEEE Transactions on Biomedical Engineering*, 67(10):2721–2734.

Song, M.-S. and Lee, S.-B. (2024). Comparative study of time-frequency transformation methods for ECG signal classification. *Frontiers in Signal Processing*, 4:1322334.

Stockwell, R. G., Mansinha, L., and Lowe, R. (1996). Localization of the complex spectrum: The S transform. *IEEE Transactions on Signal Processing*, 44(4):998–1001.

Sultan Qurraie, S. and Ghorbani Afkhami, R. (2017). ECG arrhythmia classification using time frequency distribution techniques. *Biomedical Engineering Letters*, 7(4):325–332.

Tary, J. B., Herrera, R. H., and van der Baan, M. (2018). Analysis of time-varying signals using continuous wavelet and synchrosqueezed transforms. *Philosophical Transactions of the Royal Society A: Mathematical, Physical and Engineering Sciences*, 376(2126):20170254.

Tuncer, T., Dogan, S., Pławiak, P., and Acharya, U. R. (2019). Automated arrhythmia detection using novel hexadecimal local pattern and multilevel wavelet transform with ECG signals. *Knowledge-Based Systems*, 186:104923.

Wang, C.-L., Wei, C.-C., Tsai, C.-T., Lee, Y.-H., Liu, L. Y.-M., Chen, K.-Y., Lin, Y.-J., and Lin, P.-L. (2023). Early detection of myocardial ischemia in resting ECG: Analysis by HHT. *BioMedical Engineering OnLine*, 22(1):23.

Weinhaus, A. J. and Roberts, K. P. (2005). Anatomy of the human heart. In *Handbook of cardiac anatomy, physiology, and devices*, pages 55–85. Humana Press.

Worley, S. J., Mark, D. B., Smith, W. M., Wolf, P., Califf, R. M., Strauss, H. C., Manwaring, M. G., and Ideker, R. E. (1988). Comparison of time domain and frequency domain variables from the signal-averaged electrocardiogram: A multivariable analysis. *Journal of the American College of Cardiology*, 11(5):1041–1051.

Yildirim, O., Baloglu, U. B., Tan, R.-S., Ciaccio, E. J., and Acharya, U. R. (2019). A new approach for arrhythmia classification using deep coded features and LSTM networks. *Computer Methods and Programs in Biomedicine*, 176:121–133.

Yıldırım, Ö., Pławiak, P., Tan, R.-S., and Acharya, U. R. (2018). Arrhythmia detection using deep convolutional neural network with long duration ECG signals. *Computers in Biology and Medicine*, 102:411–420.

2 Detection of Cardiac Signals Abnormalities Using MUSIC and Random Subspace Methods

Muhammed Enes Subasi, Saeed Mian Qaisar, and Abdulhamit Subasi

2.1 INTRODUCTION

The heart is crucial for pumping blood through the body's vast network of vessels, beating approximately 100,000 times daily to supply oxygen and nutrients while removing waste. Its electrical activity, which drives these beats, is measured using an electrocardiogram (ECG)—electrodes on the skin record this activity, displaying the heart's function through the PQRST waves. Analyzing the ECG signal's morphology and heart rate variability (HRV) gives insights into cardiac health. Irregularities in the ECG, such as abnormal rates or patterns, can indicate cardiac arrhythmias, which pose serious risks, including immediate conditions like ventricular fibrillation or tachycardia and long-term dangers. Premature beats, or ectopic beats, disrupt the normal rhythm; they are classified as premature atrial contractions (PACs) if they originate above the ventricles or premature ventricular contractions (PVCs) if they arise in the ventricles. PACs feature an abnormal P wave but a QRS complex similar to a normal beat, with a compensatory pause shorter than two normal RR intervals. PVCs can cause a compensatory pause due to tissue refractory periods, resulting in a distorted and prolonged QRS complex. PACs and PVCs can be detected during physical exams and confirmed with ECG recordings. Holter monitors and stress tests may be used for a more thorough assessment. Manual ECG analysis, especially from Holter recordings, is labor-intensive and complex, necessitating specialist interpretation. Computer-aided diagnosis (CAD) systems assist cardiologists by streamlining the diagnostic process and improving patient outcomes through automated ECG analysis for early arrhythmia detection (Sraitih et al., 2021).

DOI: 10.1201/9781003797524-2

Cardiovascular disorders (CVDs) are a leading cause of death globally. Developing accurate and efficient techniques for automatically classifying electrocardiogram (ECG) heartbeat signals is essential for diagnosing various CVDs, such as arrhythmia. Arrhythmia, which involves irregular electrical activities in the heart depicted by ECG beats or patterns, can be effectively detected using ECG—a simple, non-invasive diagnostic tool. Medical professionals analyze the characteristics of ECG waveforms (e.g., amplitude and polarity) to diagnose and treat heart diseases (Alickovic & Subasi, 2016).

The World Health Organization reports that cardiovascular diseases (CVDs) account for 17.7 million deaths each year, with around 31% of these fatalities occurring in low- and middle-income countries, where 75% of all CVD deaths happen. Arrhythmias, a type of CVD marked by irregular heartbeats, can cause the heart to beat too quickly or slowly. Common arrhythmias include atrial fibrillation (AF), premature ventricular contraction (PVC), ventricular fibrillation (VF), and tachycardia. While occasional arrhythmias may have little effect on health, persistent arrhythmias can be deadly. For example, extended PVCs can lead to ventricular tachycardia (VT) or ventricular fibrillation, potentially resulting in immediate heart failure. Ventricular arrhythmias are responsible for nearly 80% of sudden cardiac deaths and are among the most prevalent types of arrhythmias. Early identification of these conditions through ECG signal analysis can enhance the detection of cardiac arrest risk factors. Thus, regular monitoring of heart rhythms is vital for preventing CVDs. Medical professionals use electrocardiographs to detect arrhythmias by analyzing the heart's electrical activity. An ECG machine typically employs ten electrodes to record 12 leads (signals) from the body, providing a detailed view of heart function. Overall, CVDs, especially arrhythmias, are a leading global cause of death, with regular monitoring and early detection via ECG analysis being crucial for identifying risks and preventing serious conditions (Madan et al., 2022).

Early diagnosis and treatment of cardiovascular diseases can significantly increase life expectancy. Biomedical signals, image analysis, and medical assessments are essential for diagnosing and managing these conditions. Cardiovascular changes such as reduced blood vessel elasticity and thickening of the left ventricular muscle wall contribute to diastolic dysfunction as people age. Common arrhythmias in older adults include atrial premature beats (APB), premature ventricular contractions (PVC), left bundle branch block (LBBB), and right bundle branch block (RBBB). Diagnosing arrhythmias often involves detailed analysis of ECG signals by experienced cardiologists, which is labor-intensive and time-consuming. This has increased interest in developing computer-aided diagnosis (CAD) systems to automate arrhythmia detection, enhancing diagnostic accuracy and efficiency. ECG signals are crucial for assessing various heart conditions, including conduction disorders, heart wall thickening, pacemaker effects, medication impacts, non-cardiac diseases, coronary failure, and myocardial infarction (Tuncer et al., 2022).

Several key issues must be addressed when developing an automatic ECG signal classification system. The first concern is pre-processing, for which this study used multi-scale principal component analysis (MSPCA). The second issue is selecting suitable feature extraction methods to ensure high performance. The third challenge is the classification approach itself. Although many studies aim to design automatic arrhythmia diagnostic systems, classification accuracy, sensitivity, and specificity improvements are still necessary for large databases. Additionally, many techniques reported in the literature involve complex mathematical features that require significant computational power (Alickovic & Subasi, 2016).

This study seeks to develop a straightforward automatic system for detecting and classifying arrhythmias with high accuracy, even when dealing with large datasets. A key challenge in creating automatic ECG signal classification systems is the pre-processing stage, where various types of noise during signal recording can significantly distort the data. Typically, denoising the ECG signal is part of this pre-processing phase. In a prior study (Alickovic & Subasi, 2016), MSPCA enhanced the signal-to-noise ratio (SNR) of ECG heartbeat signals before classification. In this study, MSPCA is applied during pre-processing to eliminate noise and adapt to the morphological features of ECG waveforms. After pre-processing and detecting ECG heartbeats, selecting an effective classifier to identify different arrhythmia types accurately remains a challenge. The trend is toward implementing automatic ECG signal classification systems, which are increasingly common in medical settings. Accurate feature extraction is essential for classifying ECG heartbeats and other electrocardiograph applications (Alickovic & Subasi, 2016). For this purpose, MUSIC was utilized in this study.

2.2 LITERATURE REVIEW

Recent advancements in devices and machine learning models have made it feasible to implement practical automatic computer-aided diagnosis (CAD) systems for ECG classification in real clinical environments. These developments call for ECG arrhythmia classification methods that can be generalized across patients. Sraitih et al. (2021) explored an automatic classification system utilizing a comprehensive ECG database with an inter-patient paradigm to improve the detection of rare arrhythmia types without feature extraction. They evaluated four supervised machine learning models: support vector machine (SVM), k-nearest neighbors (KNN), Random Forest (RF), and an ensemble of these methods. The performance of these models was assessed for classifying normal beats (NOR), left bundle branch block beats (LBBB), right bundle branch block beats (RBBB), premature atrial contractions (PAC), and premature ventricular contractions (PVC) using inter-patient ECG records from the MIT-DB after segmentation and normalization. Four metrics were analyzed: accuracy, precision, recall, and F1-score. The results indicated that, without complex data pre-processing or feature engineering, the SVM classifier outperformed the other methods, achieving an accuracy of 0.83 with the proposed inter-patient paradigm. This approach is well-suited for clinical settings where ECG signals from various patients are collected and is also computationally efficient, which is essential for deploying classification models for ECG arrhythmias.

Alfaras et al. (2019) developed a fully automatic and rapid ECG arrhythmia classifier using Echo State Networks, a simple brain-inspired machine learning approach. This classifier, requiring minimal feature processing and only a single ECG lead, is trained and validated with an inter-patient procedure. It supports online classification, making it suitable for modern health-monitoring devices and wearables. The classifier benefits from parallel processing for speedier training by employing ensemble methods. Tested on the MIT-BIH AR and AHA ECG databases, the method achieved a sensitivity of 92.7% and a positive predictive value of 86.1% for ventricular ectopic beats with lead II and 95.7% sensitivity with a 75.1% positive predictive value using lead V1. These results are comparable to or exceed those of more complex ECG classifiers.

Alickovic and Subasi (2016) developed a Random Forests (RF) classifier for ECG heartbeat signal classification to diagnose heart arrhythmias. Their approach uses Discrete Wavelet Transform (DWT) to decompose ECG signals into various frequency bands, from which statistical features are extracted. The RF classifier, tested with 10-fold cross-validation, performed better than other decision tree methods. Evaluations on the MIT-BIH and St. Petersburg Institute of Cardiological Technics 12-lead Arrhythmia Databases revealed overall accuracies of 99.33% and 99.95%, respectively, outperforming C4.5 and CART classifiers. Incorporating multi-scale principal component analysis (MSPCA) denoising, DWT, and RF into a combined model enhanced performance, achieving a high area under the ROC curve (AUC) and F-measure values. These results highlight the classifier's effectiveness in accurately detecting arrhythmias and supporting clinical diagnoses of cardiovascular disorders.

Mian Qaisar and Subasi (2020) developed an intelligent event-driven system for detecting chronic heart disorders using ECG signals. This system focuses on real-time compression and efficient processing and transmission of ECG signals. Their approach demonstrated a 2.6-fold improvement in compression and bandwidth utilization compared to traditional methods, significantly reducing the complexity and time required for post-denoising, feature extraction, and classification. The system achieved an overall classification accuracy of 94.07% and strong performance metrics, including the F-measure, area under the ROC curve (AUC), and Kappa Statistics. This method offers a computationally efficient solution for automatic cardiac arrhythmia diagnosis and high-precision decision support in cloud-based mobile health monitoring.

Tuncer et al. (2022) developed a new ECG signal recognition method combining Discrete Wavelet Concatenated Mesh Tree (DW-CMT) and ternary chess pattern (TCP). The technique involves four stages: pre-processing with DW-CMT to segment ECG signals into 15 sub-bands, feature extraction using TCP, feature selection via neighborhood component analysis (NCA) to identify 128 key features, and classification. The approach was tested with traditional classifiers such as Linear Discriminant Analysis (LDA), k-nearest neighbor (k-NN), and support vector machine (SVM). The method achieved a maximum classification accuracy of 96.60% with k-NN on the MIT-BIH dataset and 97.80% with SVM on the St. Petersburg dataset, demonstrating its effectiveness in accurately recognizing ECG signals for arrhythmia diagnosis.

Dhyani et al. (2023) developed a method for analyzing and classifying ECG signals using 3D Discrete Wavelet Transform (DWT) combined with a Support Vector

Machine (SVM). The approach involves three stages: pre-processing of ECG signals, feature extraction through 3D wavelet transform for denoising and coefficient extraction, and classification of the signals. The SVM classifier was used to identify nine different types of heartbeats from about 6400 ECG beats in the China Physiological Signal Challenge (CPSC) 2018 dataset. The method achieved a high accuracy of 99.02% using level 4 wavelet decomposition with Symlet-8 channels, outperforming other SVM variants such as CSVM and WSVM. This technique proves to be highly effective for classifying various arrhythmia conditions.

C. U. Kumari et al. (2020) developed a method for classifying heartbeat irregularities into three categories: Cardiac Arrhythmia (ARR), Normal Sinus Rhythm (NSR), and congestive heart failure (CHF). Their study used 162 ECG records, dividing them into training (70%) and testing (30%) sets. The method involved four main stages: collecting ARR and non-ARR signals from the MIT-BIH database, pre-processing these signals, extracting features using Discrete Wavelet Transform (DWT), and combining these features into a single vector. This vector was then classified using a support vector machine (SVM), achieving an accuracy of 95.92% based on performance metrics such as precision, recall, and F1 score.

ECG signals, which represent the heart's electrical activity, are characterized by waveforms (P, QRS, and T) whose durations, structures, and distances between their peaks are used to identify heart issues. Taloba et al. (2021) explored ECG signal analysis by employing autoregressive (AR) analysis to extract distinctive features from the electrical activity of the heart, focusing on waveforms (P, QRS, and T). Their method effectively differentiates AR characteristics for three types of ECG signals, facilitating accurate classification and diagnosis of heart conditions. They introduced a novel approach combining two-event-related moving averages (TERMAs) with fractional Fourier transform (FFT) algorithms for improved ECG signal evaluation. This technique is designed to enhance the assessment of current methods for arrhythmia detection by incorporating cross-database training and testing to bolster feature evaluation.

Ketu and Mishra (2022) reviewed advanced machine learning solutions for detecting heart diseases by analyzing ECG-based arrhythmia datasets. They evaluated eight algorithms—Support Vector Machine, K-Nearest Neighbors, Random Forest, Extra Tree, Bagging, Decision Tree, Linear Regression, and Adaptive Boosting—under both balanced and imbalanced class conditions. The performance of these algorithms was measured using precision, recall, accuracy, and F1-score. Their analysis revealed the challenges of imbalanced datasets, where the majority class can overshadow minority classes. To mitigate this, they used the Synthetic Minority Over-sampling Technique (SMOTE) to balance the data, which improved overall accuracy and ensured better performance for minority classes.

Mohanty et al. (2020) developed an automated system to predict ventricular arrhythmias (VAs) using machine learning techniques to reduce mortality rates. They introduced a novel method combining variational mode decomposition (VMD) for feature extraction from ECG signals with a C4.5 classifier for VA detection. The system was tested on ECG signals from PhysioNet databases, including CUDB and VFDB. Features extracted using VMD were evaluated and ranked, and then classified into normal, ventricular tachycardia (VT), and ventricular fibrillation (VF) using both support vector machine (SVM) and C4.5 classifiers. The C4.5 classifier outperformed SVM with a sensitivity of 97.97%, specificity of 99.15%, and accuracy of 99.18% for data within a 5-second window, demonstrating its effectiveness in detecting VAs and providing valuable support for clinicians.

Pham et al. (2021) developed a Computer-aided Decision Support System (CDSS) using machine learning to distinguish between normal rhythm and arrhythmias such as atrial fibrillation (Afib), atrial flutter (Afl), and ventricular fibrillation (Vfib). The system analyzes ECG segments of 2 and 5 seconds using predictive models and addresses class imbalance by generating synthetic samples with ADASYN. Third-order cumulant images from ECG segments were used to extract 18 nonlinear features. Significant features were selected through t-tests and used to train various classifiers. The Random Forest classifier outperformed others in both 2-second and 5-second datasets, achieving accuracy of 98.2% and 98.8%, sensitivity of 98.1% and 98.8%, and specificity of 99.4% and 99.6%, respectively. The CDSS's ability to analyze longer ECG segments improves arrhythmia detection accuracy, enhancing its clinical applicability for real-time monitoring.

Deep learning (DL) has become a pivotal research focus in various fields, including healthcare, where prompt detection of anomalies in electrocardiogram (ECG) signals is vital for patient monitoring. Ebrahimi et al. (2020) thoroughly reviewed recent DL techniques for ECG signal classification. Their review included various DL methods such as convolutional neural networks (CNN), Deep Belief Networks (DBN), Recurrent Neural Networks (RNN), Long Short-Term Memory (LSTM), and Gated Recurrent Units (GRU). Out of 75 studies reviewed from 2017 to 2018, CNNs were most commonly used for feature extraction, appearing in 52% of the studies. DL methods achieved high classification accuracy for conditions like atrial fibrillation (AF) (100%), Supraventricular Ectopic Beats (SVEB) (99.8%), and Ventricular Ectopic Beats (VEB) (99.7%), using combinations of GRU/LSTM, CNN, and LSTM architectures, respectively.

M. Hammad et al. (2021) developed a deep neural network (DNN) approach to improve classification accuracy by leveraging robust feature extraction methods and a genetic algorithm (GA) to find the optimal combination of techniques. Their model achieved an average accuracy increase of 0.94 and a 0.953 increase in F1 score compared to state-of-the-art methods, showing its potential as an effective tool for detecting anomalies. G et al. (2018) used deep learning methods, including convolutional neural networks (CNNs) and Recurrent Neural Networks (RNNs) like Long Short-Term Memory (LSTM) and Gated Recurrent Units (GRU), for diagnosing cardiac arrhythmia with minimal pre-processing. Their CNN-LSTM hybrid model achieved a five-fold cross-validation accuracy of 0.834 in distinguishing between normal and abnormal ECG signals. Other hybrid deep learning architectures demonstrated similar accuracies. S. Irfan et al. (2022) proposed a deep-learning framework that combines multiple networks by stacking similar layers to form a unified model. Evaluated on two datasets, their framework classified five types of arrhythmias with high-performance metrics: sensitivity of 98.37%, specificity of 99.59%, positive predictive value of 98.41%, and accuracy of 99.35%. This approach outperformed existing methods in sensitivity, specificity, positive predictive value, accuracy, and computational efficiency.

Advancing health-monitoring systems continues to be an active research area. Wearable and remote devices now allow continuous tracking of physiological and clinical metrics like heart rate, respiration rate, and temperature. These devices use cloud-based machine learning and decision support systems to predict critical health conditions. However, Scirè et al. (2019) propose a shift from a cloud-centric model to a decentralized approach, where data processing and analysis occur directly on the wearable devices. This method enables real-time analysis and alerts without depending on cloud services. Their supervised-learning system detects heartbeats and classifies arrhythmias using a window-based feature definition optimized for an asymmetric multicore embedded processor with a hardware-assisted pattern matching core. Performance comparisons show that this embedded system achieves high detection rates, sometimes equaling the accuracy of advanced algorithms on standard processors.

Rahman et al. (2022) compared various transfer learning methods for ECG classification to identify arrhythmias using real-time and augmented data from sources like the MIT-BIH dataset. They evaluated the effectiveness of transfer learning techniques such as ResNet50, AlexNet, and SqueezeNet, finding significant accuracy improvements over previous methods. The accuracies achieved were 98.8% for AlexNet, 90.08% for SqueezeNet, and 91% for ResNet50. Madan et al. (2022) introduced a hybrid deep learning model combining 2D convolutional neural networks (CNN) and Long Short-Term Memory (LSTM) networks, named 2D-CNN-LSTM, to automate arrhythmia detection. They transformed 1D ECG signals into 2D Scalogram images for enhanced noise filtering and feature extraction. The model, tested on the MIT-BIH database, achieved high accuracies of approximately 98.7% for Cardiac Arrhythmias, 99% for congestive heart failure, and 99% for Normal Sinus Rhythm. It also showed an average sensitivity of 98.33% and specificity of 98.35%, offering a promising approach for improving arrhythmia classification with reduced medical intervention. Bollepalli et al. (2021) aimed to improve life-threatening arrhythmia detection in ICUs by analyzing 953 alarms from 410 patients, focusing on ECG, arterial blood pressure, and photoplethysmograph signals. They developed a hybrid CNN classifier that combines handcrafted features with features learned by CNNs. This approach outperformed traditional CNN-only methods, achieving an accuracy of 87.5%±0.5% in cross-validation and 93.9% in the PhysioNet 2015 Challenge database. Their method enhances arrhythmia detection, reduces false alarms, and could improve ICU patient care and provider efficiency.

Kumar et al. (2023) employed AlexNet, VGG-16, and VGG-19 models for feature extraction, with these features fed into four popular classifiers: decision tree, k-nearest neighbors (kNN), linear discriminant analysis (LDA), and support vector machine (SVM) for detecting arrhythmias. They also explored combining the CNN model with the Minimum Redundancy Maximum Relevance (mRMR) feature selection method. Their experiments showed that LDA achieved the highest classification accuracy among the tested methods, with the proposed model reaching an accuracy of 99.46%, surpassing previous approaches in arrhythmia detection.

Chang et al. (2021) utilized a Long Short-Term Memory (LSTM) model to classify 12 distinct heart rhythm classes from a dataset of 65,932 12-lead ECG signals from 38,899 patients. Annotations by three board-certified electrophysiologists were used as the reference standard. The LSTM model achieved high classification accuracy for all 12 rhythms, with accuracies between 0.982 and 1.0 and AUC-ROC scores ranging from 0.987 to 1.0. Precision and recall ranged from 0.692 to 1 and 0.625 to 1, respectively, with F1 scores of 0.777 or higher. The model's overall accuracy of 0.90 exceeded the accuracy of internists (0.55), emergency physicians (0.73), and cardiologists (0.83). The study highlights the LSTM model's effectiveness in accurately interpreting 12-lead ECG signals for heart rhythm classification, which is significant for early cardiac rhythm disorder diagnosis.

2.3 MATERIALS AND METHODS

The block diagram of the devised method is shown in Figure 2.1. Details of different modules are presented below.

2.3.1 Data

This study used the MIT-BIH Arrhythmia Database, a well-known dataset established in 1980 for testing arrhythmia detectors and classifiers. The database comprises 24-hour ECG recordings from 47 subjects, including 25 men and 22 women aged between 23 and 89 years. The ECG data were initially captured using Del Mar Avionics model 445 Holter recorders and digitized at 360 samples per second per channel. Each recording includes two leads, typically the modified limb lead II (MLII) and V1, positioned on the chest to simplify the removal of 60 Hz interference with digital notch filters. The primary lead is mostly MLII, while the secondary precordial lead varies among V1, V2, V4, and V5. The dataset's original

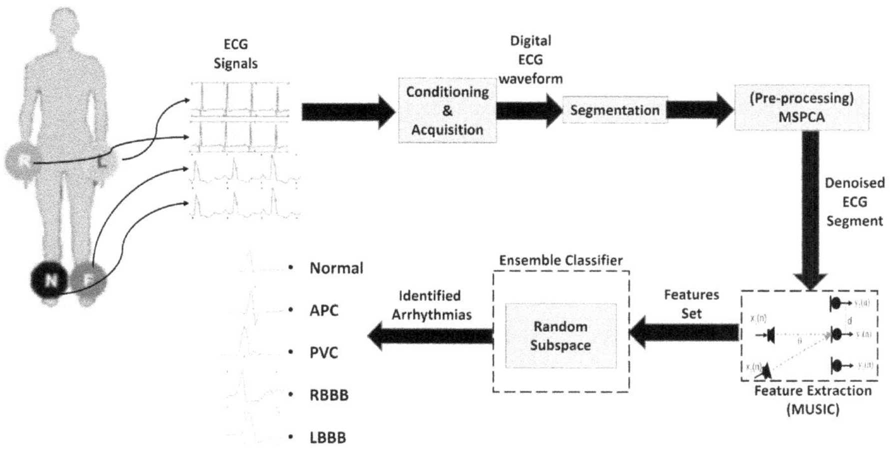

FIGURE 2.1 The proposed system block diagram.

annotations cover 16 rhythm classes, offering a comprehensive basis for analysis. The research targeted five types of arrhythmic beats: normal (NORMAL), left bundle branch block (LBBB), right bundle branch block (RBBB), atrial premature (APC), and premature ventricular contraction (PVC). Each 30-minute recording was segmented into 81-sample portions without pre-processing. These specific classes were extracted from 23 randomly selected recordings, totaling 7500 segments. The model's performance was assessed using 10-fold cross-validation, ensuring robust and reliable results.

2.3.2 Signal Denoising with MSPCA

Multi-scale principal component analysis (MSPCA) merges the functionalities of PCA and wavelet analysis to remove inter-variable relationships, identify deterministic features, and reduce correlations in autocorrelated measurements. By performing PCA on wavelet coefficients across multiple scales and consolidating outcomes from these scales, MSPCA is adept at handling data with events that exhibit different behaviors over time and frequency. This method enhances the detection of deterministic changes. It identifies abnormal operations during monitoring processes through adaptive filtering of scores and residuals and setting detection thresholds, all without needing matrix augmentation or time-series modeling (Bakshi, 1998).

For effective empirical modeling from multi-scale data, leveraging multi-scale representation is crucial as it significantly impacts the quality of models. This involves pre-processing variables through compression or filtering to enhance data quality by reducing less relevant signal features. Multi-scale methods capture contributions across multiple scales and are superior to current methods. These methods often pre-process each variable using wavelet thresholding before building empirical models from the filtered signals. Despite the benefits, this approach can require heuristic methods and trial-and-error to identify the most pertinent features. Integrating a multi-scale and multivariate approach improves noise removal efficacy since it fully utilizes the multivariate nature inherent in empirical modeling problems. While latent variable regression methods mitigate errors by retaining only latent variables that capture relationships between variables, PCA typically mitigates rather than entirely removes errors from the data matrix (Malinowski, 2002).

Enhancing noise removal and improving latent variable regression models' quality can be achieved by integrating wavelet thresholding, which discards noise dependent on variable relationships while removing less important latent variables. This method enhances noise reduction and the quality of empirical models by leveraging the synergy between wavelet thresholding and latent variable models. Multi-scale modeling approaches can benefit from representing input and output variables in the wavelet domain and employing effective strategies for selecting relevant coefficients. Multi-scale PCA improves noise removal and decorrelates relationships between variables by decomposing each variable using a chosen wavelet and applying PCA to the coefficient matrix. This approach establishes distinct PCA models for coefficients at each scale, improving noise removal, especially when dealing with non-white or scale-dependent noise. Criteria for selecting wavelet coefficients and principal components at each scale are based on application requirements, ensuring consistency across scales and maintaining relationships between variables (Bakshi, 1999).

2.3.3 Feature Extraction with MUSIC

This study uses the Multiple Signal Classification (MUSIC) algorithm to extract pertinent features from the considered ECG signals. The fundamental concept of the MUSIC algorithm is to use the orthogonality of two spaces to estimate the signal parameter after obtaining the signal subspace and noise subspace via eigenvalue decomposition of the signal covariance matrix. The spatial spectrum characterizes the orthogonality between signal and noise subspace. The procedure is further illustrated in Figure 2.2 using a flowchart. It shows that the correlation matrix is computed from the incoming arrays of the ECG signals. Onward, the Eigen decomposition of the correlation matrix is performed (Elbir, 2020). Onward, the findings of the Eigen decomposition are used to calculate the spatial spectrum (Chen et al.,

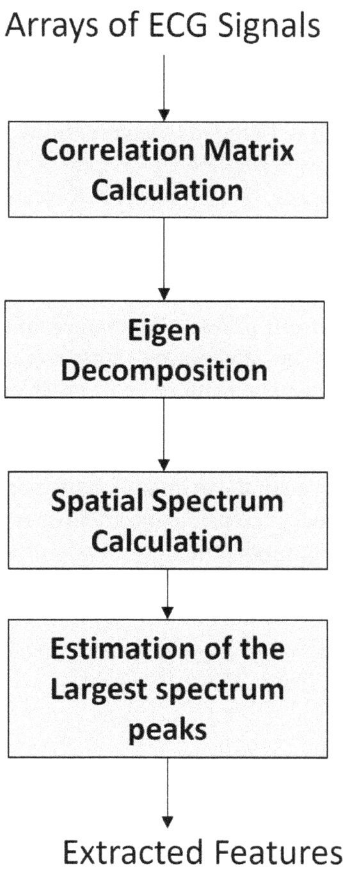

FIGURE 2.2 The flow chart of MUSIC algorithm.

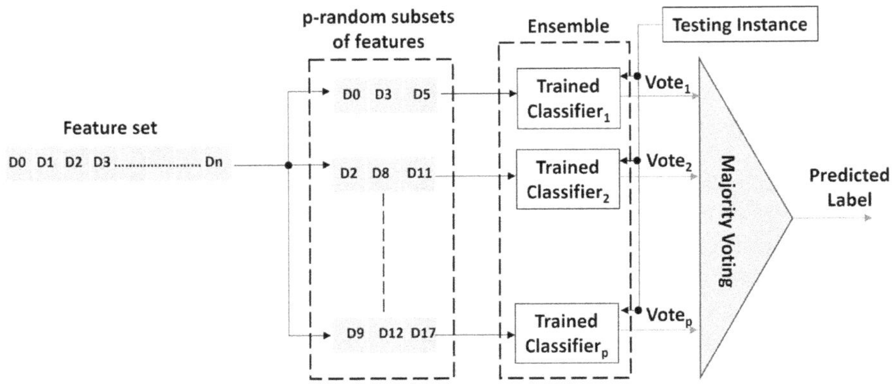

FIGURE 2.3 The principle of the Random Subspace algorithm.

2023). The next step identifies and extracts the largest spectrum peaks as pertinent attributes.

2.3.4 Random Subspace Ensemble Learning

The Random Subspace Method (RSM) is the combining technique proposed by Ho (1998). In the Random Subspace Method (RSM), the training data undergoes modification within the feature space. This process involves obtaining a p-dimensional random subspace from the original n-dimensional feature space. Consequently, the modified training set comprises p-dimensional training instances. The process is depicted with the help of Figure 2.3. It shows that the randomly generated p-subsets of features are used to train p-base classifiers. Utilizing random subspaces in both constructing classifiers and combining their outputs can provide advantages in the RSM. Particularly, when the number of training instances is relatively small compared to the data dimensionality, constructing classifiers within random subspaces can effectively address the issue of small sample sizes. Despite the subspace dimensionality being smaller than the original feature space, the number of training instances remains unchanged, increasing the relative training sample size. When the data contains numerous redundant features, classifiers built within random subspaces may yield superior results to those constructed directly within the original feature space. The collective decision made by such classifiers could potentially outperform a single classifier developed using the original training set within the full feature space (Skurichina & Duin, 2002).

2.4 RESULTS AND DISCUSSION

2.4.1 Performance Evaluation Measures

The evaluation measures are performed by analyzing the outcomes generated by the classification model and deriving a relationship between these findings and the ground truth. In real problems, the availability of datasets, particularly labeled ones, is limited. To overcome this limitation of dimensionality, the available dataset is tactfully divided into subsets by following the cross-validation strategy (Qaisar, Nisar, et al., 2023). One popular method for evaluating an artificial intelligence (AI) model's performance and generalizability is the *k*-fold cross-validation. The dataset is randomly divided into *k* equally sized sub-groups, also known as the folds. Given the scale of the intended application and the available dataset, care should be taken while selecting the value of this user-specified parameter, *k*. The *k*-fold cross-validation technique ensures the model performs consistently and dependably on various data subsets. In this study, $k = 10$ is selected.

The selection of an AI model for the intended application is based on the outcome of the considered evaluation measures. It helps identify the most suitable model from an available choice. Multiple evaluation measures lead to a correct choice (Cichosz, 2014; Sokolova et al., 2006). The evaluation measures used in this study are the Accuracy, F-measure, ROC, the Area Under the Curve (AUC), and the Kappa index. These are measurable using the confusion matrices obtained with experimentation. The confusion matrix is presented as a table, presenting the outcomes of binary or multi-class classification tasks (Qaisar, Nisar, et al., 2023). An example of a confusion matrix for a binary classification problem is shown in Figure 2.4. A model with high TP, TN, and low FP, FN is a good model with a high value in performance evaluation measures.

The following equations present the process of computing the evaluation measures considered, such as accuracy, F-measure, AUC, and Kappa index.

$$Accuracy = \frac{TP + TN}{TP + TN + FP + FN}. \tag{2.1}$$

$$F - measure = \frac{2.TP}{2.TP + FP + FN}. \tag{2.2}$$

$$Pe = \frac{(TP + FN)\times(TP + FP) + (FP + TN)\times(FN + TN)}{(TP + TN + FP + FN)^2}. \tag{2.3}$$

Actual Values

Predicted Values

	Positive	Negative
Positive	True Positive (TP)	False Positive (FP)
Negative	True Negative (TN)	False Negative (FN)

FIGURE 2.4 Confusion matrix for a binary classification problem.

$$Kappa = \frac{Po - Pe}{1 - Pe}. \tag{2.4}$$

In Equation (2.4), *Po* is the same as the Accuracy in Equation (2.1).

The area under the Receiver Operating Characteristic (ROC) curve is called the AUC. It is a graphical picture that shows the categorization capability of a classifier (Chawla et al., 2004). Here, the y-axis represents the True Positive Rate (TPR), and the x-axis represents the False Positive Rate (FPR). The TPR and FPR are defined using Equations (2.5) and (2.6).

$$TPR = \frac{TP}{TP + FN}. \tag{2.5}$$

$$FPR = \frac{FP}{FP + TN}. \tag{2.6}$$

2.4.2 Experimental Results

In this study, the Bagging-based ensemble classification configuration is used to process the ECG-based extracted features to precisely identify arrhythmia. Noise from the considered ECG signals is reduced using the MSPCA. In the next step, the MUSIC analyzes the pre-processed ECG signals. It permits an in-depth analysis and allows effective feature mining. These mined attributes define each instance in the prepared feature set. The prepared feature set is further processed by the devised RSM-based ensemble classifiers for automated arrhythmia identification. The classification performance is evaluated in terms of ROC area, F-measure, Accuracy, and Kappa Statistics.

The study's experimental findings show that applying the suggested classifier provides high accuracy for the considered dataset. The entire set of ECG data is split into training and test sets to determine each model's performance. The performance of classification is evaluated while following the 10-fold cross-validation strategy.

In arrhythmia identification systems, the primary objective revolves around classifying ECG signal patterns, as the subject's cardiac state elicits specific heartbeat patterns. Notable algorithms employed in the classification process include k-Nearest-Neighbor (k-NN), Support Vector Machine (SVM), Random Forest (RF), Artificial Neural Networks (ANN), Classification and Regression Trees (CART), C4.5 decision tree, REP Tree, Random Tree, and Linear Discriminant Analysis (LDA) Tree. MATLAB and WEKA are utilized to implement these algorithms in experiments.

A summary of the classification performance scores obtained using RSM-based ensemble configuration of the considered classifiers is outlined in Table 2.1.

First, let us look at the accuracy scores attained for the case of NORMAL class. In this case, the most momentous classification accuracy of 100% is achieved for all the machine learning-based classifiers with RSM-based ensemble configuration. The machine learning-based classifiers are the SVM, k-NN, ANN, RF, CART, C4.5, REPTree, RandomTree, and LADTree.

TABLE 2.1
Performance of RSM-Based Ensemble Classifier

	NORMAL	APC	PVC	RBBB	LBBB	AVERAGE	F-Measure	AUC	Kappa
SVM	1	0.957	0.98	0.97	0.977	0.977	0.977	0.997	0.971
k-NN	1	0.933	0.96	0.963	0.953	0.962	0.962	0.993	0.953
ANN	1	0.903	0.957	0.95	0.963	0.955	0.955	0.994	0.943
Random Forest	1	0.953	0.95	0.947	0.97	0.964	0.964	0.998	0.955
Simple CART	1	0.91	0.943	0.907	0.953	0.943	0.943	0.995	0.928
C4.5	1	0.94	0.95	0.957	0.963	0.962	0.962	0.997	0.953
REPTree	1	0.903	0.93	0.917	0.947	0.939	0.94	0.995	0.924
RandomTree	1	0.95	0.943	0.937	0.953	0.957	0.957	0.997	0.946
LADTree	1	0.9	0.91	0.92	0.937	0.933	0.934	0.993	0.917

In the APC class, the most significant classification accuracy of 95.70% is attained with SVM. The second highest accuracy score is 95.30%, achieved with the RF. Random Tree is the third-best performer, with an accuracy score of 95.00%. C4.5 follows the Random Tree with an accuracy score of 94.00%. LADTree attains the lowest accuracy score of 90.00%. In this case, the SVM with RSM achieves the most incredible accuracy score of 95.70%.

In the case of the PVC class, the most significant classification accuracy of 98.00% is attained with the SVM. The second highest accuracy score is 96.00%, achieved with the k-NN. ANN is the third-best performer, with an accuracy score of 95.70%. RF and C4.5 follow the ANN with an accuracy score of 95.00%. LADTree attains the lowest accuracy score of 91.00%. In this case, the SVM with RSM achieves the most remarkable accuracy score of 98.00%.

In the case of the RBBB class, the most significant classification accuracy of 97.00% is attained with SVM. The second highest accuracy score is 96.30%, attained with the k-NN. C4.5 is the third-best performer, with an accuracy score of 95.70%. ANN follows the C4.5 with an accuracy score of 95.00%. REPTree attains the lowest accuracy score of 90.70%. In this case, the SVM with RSM achieves the most implausible accuracy score of 97.00%.

In the case of the LBBB class, the most noteworthy classification accuracy of 97.70% is attained with SVM. The second highest accuracy score is 97.00%, achieved with the RF. ANN and C4.5 are the third-best performers, with an accuracy score of 96.50%. Random Tree, CART, and k-NN follow the ANN and C4.5 with an accuracy score of 95.30%. LADTree attains the lowest accuracy score of 93.70%. In this case, the SVM with RSM achieves the most noteworthy accuracy score of 97.70%.

The average accuracy scores obtained for the five classes show that the most significant classification accuracy of 97.70% is attained with SVM. The second highest accuracy score is 96.40%, attained with the RF. C4.5 and k-NN are the third-best performers, with an accuracy score of 96.20%. Random Tree follows the C4.5 and k-NN with an accuracy score of 95.70%. LDATree attains the lowest accuracy score of 93.30%. The SVM with RSM achieves an average accuracy score of 97.70% for the five-class problem studied.

The average F-measure scores obtained for the five classes show that the most significant F-measure value of 0.977 is attained with SVM. The second highest F-measure value is 0.964, attained with the RF. C4.5 and k-NN are the third-best performers, with a F-measure value of 0.962. Random Tree follows the C4.5 and k-NN with an F-measure value of 0.957. LADTree attains the lowest F-measure value of 0.934. The SVM with RSM achieves the most noteworthy average F-measure value of 0.977 for the studied five-class problem.

The average AUC values obtained for the five classes show that the most weighty AUC value of 0.998 is attained with RF. The second highest AUC value is 0.997, attained with the SVM, C4.5, and RandomTree. CART and REPTree are the third-best performers, with an AUC value of 0.995. ANN follows the CART and REPTree with an AUC value of 0.994. LADTree attains the lowest AUC value of 0.993. The RF with RSM achieves the most noteworthy average AUC value of 0.998 for the studied five-class problem.

The average Kappa values obtained for the five classes show that the most substantial Kappa value of 0.971 is attained with SVM. The second highest Kappa value is 0.955, achieved with the RF. C4.5 and k-NN are the third-best performers, with a Kappa value of 0.953. ANN follows the C4.5 and k-NN with a Kappa value of 0.943. LAD Tree attains the lowest Kappa value of 0.917. The SVM with RSM achieves the most remarkable average Kappa value of 0.971 for the studied five-class problem.

2.5 DISCUSSION

Various RSM-based ensemble learning classifiers are designed and evaluated in this study for automated classification of arrhythmia. Since the early days of computer-assisted diagnosis, alternative classification algorithms have also gained popularity and are appropriate in numerous circumstances. Performance is the most crucial factor when selecting an algorithm, followed by usability and interpretation. This study suggests that the most accurate arrhythmia diagnosis can be performed using one of the considered machine learning algorithms in an ensemble configuration.

From the findings presented in Section 2.4.2, it is clear that using RSM-based ensemble classification provides high accuracy in most situations. It is clear that for the considered ensemble classification configurations, the devised assembly of MSPCA-based noise removal, MUSIC-based features extraction, and SVM with RSM-based ensemble classification assembly is the best performer by securing the highest average accuracy score of 97.70% for the studied five-class problem.

It is evident that for the considered ensemble classification configurations, the SVM with RSM is the best performer because it also secures the highest average F-measure value of 0.977. Moreover, the highest Kappa value of 0.9708 is attained using the SVM with RSM. The RF with RSM secures the highest overall average AUC value of 0.998. The SVM with RSM stays very close to being the best performer in terms of AUC score. The AUC value of 0.997 is secured using the SVM with RSM, which is 0.1% less than the value secured using RF with RSM. However, the performance of SVM is superior to that of RF in terms of the average accuracy score, F-measure, and Kappa index. It shows the outperformance of SVM compared to the other considered counterparts for the five-class categorization problem.

Compared to other considered classifiers, the SVM with RSM is noticeably more accurate in this study. It is also superior in terms of ease of model creation. Using a random selection of the data and characteristics for training, RSM generates an ensemble of SVM classifiers. It decreases the possibilities of overfitting and bias, which are significant issues with individual SVM classifiers. The SVM can represent intricate, nonlinear decision boundaries. It can, therefore, be applied to a variety of classification issues. In contrast to LADTree or k-NN, SVM is robust and less biased when used in the RSM-based ensemble configuration. The experimental results confirm its robustness. Also, it exhibits an inherent maturity that facilitates its real-time application implementation.

The choice of input variable and classification method are the two unique considerations that determine the performance of the classifiers for ECG signal categorization. The signal processing methodology and feature selection strategy aim to identify and extract the most valuable parameters from the ECG data. The model's inputs must have parameters for classifying ECG signals. These classifiers were chosen because they provide insight into the evolution of the ECG's regularity and complexity and are suitable for classifying the nonlinear dynamics underpinning muscle activity. Accurate ECG signal identification is necessary for both diagnosis and treatment assessment. It is confirmed that the RF with Boosting is capable of much more accurate ECG signal classification than other considered classifiers.

The incorporation of event-driven tools can further enhance the performance of the devised method in terms of real-time compression and computational effectiveness (Mian Qaisar & Alsharif, 2020; Mian Qaisar, 2021; Qaisar, 2019). Moreover, the metaheuristics-based offline analysis can further augment the dimension reduction (Qaisar et al., 2022; Qaisar, Khan, et al., 2023). The feasibility of integrating these tools in the devised approach can be investigated in the future.

2.6 CONCLUSION

This chapter introduces the application of Random Subspace Method (RSM)-based ensemble learning models combined with the Multiple Signal Classification (MUSIC) algorithm in "Electrocardiogram" (ECG)-based arrhythmia identification. The "Multi Scale Principle Component Analysis" (MSPCA) method is used to remove the noise from the considered ECG signals, and signal decomposition employs MUSIC. The experimental investigation involves five-class ECG signals from the MIT-BIH dataset. A novel hybridization of the MSPCA, MUSIC, "Support Vector Machine" (SVM), and RSM-based ensemble learning approach is proposed specifically for ECG arrhythmia categorization. The suggested ensemble model demonstrates a lower susceptibility to overfitting than other classifiers. The devised assembly of MSPCA, MUSIC, SVM with RSM has secured the highest average classification accuracy of 97.70% for a five-class problem. Consequently, this method can potentially enhance the automated arrhythmia diagnosis by processing the ECG signals.

In conclusion, this study demonstrates the potential of integrating MUSIC and ensemble classifiers to enhance the performance of automated biomedical signal analysis, particularly the ECG-based arrhythmia categorization. The promising results from this study underscore the importance of continued research and innovation in the field, with the ultimate goal of facilitating individuals with cardiac diseases. As we move forward, further refinements and advancements in signal processing algorithms and "Artificial Intelligence" (AI)-based classification models hold the potential to unlock even greater capabilities and accessibility in healthcare technology, ultimately improving the quality of life for those in need.

REFERENCES

Alfaras, M., Soriano, M. C., & Ortín, S. (2019). A fast machine learning model for ECG-based heartbeat classification and arrhythmia detection. *Frontiers in Physics*, *7*. https://www.frontiersin.org/journals/physics/articles/10.3389/fphy.2019.00103

Alickovic, E., & Subasi, A. (2016). Medical decision support system for diagnosis of heart arrhythmia using dwt and random forests classifier. *Journal of Medical Systems*, *40*(4), Article 4.

Bakshi, B. R. (1998). Multiscale PCA with application to multivariate statistical process monitoring. *AIChE Journal*, *44*(7), 1596–1610.

Bakshi, B. R. (1999). Multiscale analysis and modeling using wavelets. *Journal of Chemometrics*, *13*(3–4), 415–434.

Bollepalli, S. C., Sevakula, R. K., Au-Yeung, W. M., Kassab, M. B., Merchant, F. M., Bazoukis, G., Boyer, R., Isselbacher, E. M., & Armoundas, A. A. (2021). Real-ime arrhythmia detection using hybrid convolutional neural networks. *Journal of the American Heart Association*, *10*(23), e023222. https://doi.org/10.1161/JAHA.121.023222

Chang, K.-C., Hsieh, P.-H., Wu, M.-Y., Wang, Y.-C., Chen, J.-Y., Tsai, F.-J., Shih, E. S. C., Hwang, M.-J., & Huang, T.-C. (2021). Usefulness of machine learning-based detection and classification of cardiac arrhythmias with 12-lead electrocardiograms. *Canadian Journal of Cardiology*, *37*(1), 94–104. https://doi.org/10.1016/j.cjca.2020.02.096

Chawla, N. V., Japkowicz, N., & Kotcz, A. (2004). Special issue on learning from imbalanced data sets. *ACM Sigkdd Explorations Newsletter*, *6*(1), 1–6.

Chen, X., Feng, Z., Wei, Z., Yuan, X., Zhang, P., Zhang, J. A., & Yang, H. (2023). Multiple signal classification based joint communication and sensing system. *IEEE Transactions on Wireless Communications*, *22*(10), 6504–6517.

Cichosz, P. (2014). *Data Mining Algorithms: Explained Using R*. John Wiley & Sons.

Dhyani, S., Kumar, A., & Choudhury, S. (2023). Analysis of ECG-based arrhythmia detection system using machine learning. *MethodsX*, *10*, 102195. https://doi.org/10.1016/j.mex.2023.102195

Ebrahimi, Z., Loni, M., Daneshtalab, M., & Gharehbaghi, A. (2020). A review on deep learning methods for ECG arrhythmia classification. *Expert Systems with Applications: X*, *7*, 100033. https://doi.org/10.1016/j.eswax.2020.100033

Elbir, A. M. (2020). DeepMUSIC: Multiple signal classification via deep learning. *IEEE Sensors Letters*, *4*(4), 1–4.

Hammad, M., Iliyasu, A. M., Subasi, A., Ho, E. S. L., & El-Latif, A. A. A. (2021). A multitier deep learning model for arrhythmia detection. *IEEE Transactions on Instrumentation and Measurement*, *70*, 1–9. https://doi.org/10.1109/TIM.2020.3033072

Ho, T. K. (1998). The random subspace method for constructing decision forests. *IEEE Transactions on Pattern Analysis and Machine Intelligence*, *20*(8), 832–844.

Irfan, S., Anjum, N., Althobaiti, T., Alotaibi, A. A., Siddiqui, A. B., & Ramzan, N. (2022). Heartbeat classification and arrhythmia detection using a multi-model deep-learning technique. *Sensors*, *22*(15). https://doi.org/10.3390/s22155606

Ketu, S., & Mishra, P. K. (2022). Empirical analysis of machine learning algorithms on imbalance electrocardiogram based arrhythmia dataset for heart disease detection. *Arabian Journal for Science and Engineering*, *47*(2), 1447–1469. https://doi.org/10.1007/s13369-021-05972-2

Kumari, C. U., Ankita, R., Pavani, T., Vignesh, N. A., Varma, N. T., Manzar, M. A., & Reethika, A. (2020). Heart rhythm abnormality detection and classification using machine learning technique. *2020 4th International Conference on Trends in Electronics and Informatics (ICOEI)(48184)*, 580–584. https://doi.org/10.1109/ICOEI48184.2020.9142914

Kumar, S., Bhushan, B., Bhambhu, L., Singh, D., & Choubey, D. K. (2023). A deep learning-based model for arrhythmia detection using feature selection and machine learning methods. In B. Pati, C. R. Panigrahi, P. Mohapatra, & K.-C. Li (Eds.), *Proceedings of the 6th International Conference on Advance Computing and Intelligent Engineering* (pp. 13–22). Springer Nature Singapore.

Madan, P., Singh, V., Singh, D. P., Diwakar, M., Pant, B., & Kishor, A. (2022). A hybrid deep learning approach for ECG-based arrhythmia classification. *Bioengineering*, *9*(4). https://doi.org/10.3390/bioengineering9040152

Malinowski, E. R. (2002). *Factor Analysis in Chemistry*. Wiley.

Mian Qaisar, S. (2021). Signal-piloted processing and machine learning based efficient power quality disturbances recognition. *PloS One*, *16*(5), e0252104.

Mian Qaisar, S., & Alsharif, F. (2020). Signal piloted processing of the smart meter data for effective appliances recognition. *Journal of Electrical Engineering & Technology*, *15*(5), 2279–2285.

Mian Qaisar, S., & Subasi, A. (2020). Cloud-based ECG monitoring using event-driven ECG acquisition and machine learning techniques. *Physical and Engineering Sciences in Medicine*, *43*(2), 623–634.

Mohanty, M., Biswal, P., & Sabut, S. (2020). Machine learning approach to recognize ventricular arrhythmias using VMD based features. *Multidimensional Systems and Signal Processing*, *31*(1), 49–71. https://doi.org/10.1007/s11045-019-00651-w

Pham, T.-H., Sree, V., Mapes, J., Dua, S., Lih, O. S., Koh, J. E. W., Ciaccio, E. J., & Acharya, U. R. (2021). A novel machine learning framework for automated detection of arrhythmias in ECG segments. *Journal of Ambient Intelligence and Humanized Computing*, *12*(11), 10145–10162. https://doi.org/10.1007/s12652-020-02779-1

Qaisar, S. M. (2019). Efficient mobile systems based on adaptive rate signal processing. *Computers & Electrical Engineering*, *79*, 106462.

Qaisar, S. M., Khan, S. I., Dallet, D., Tadeusiewicz, R., & Pławiak, P. (2022). Signal-piloted processing metaheuristic optimization and wavelet decomposition based elucidation of arrhythmia for mobile healthcare. *Biocybernetics and Biomedical Engineering*, *42*(2), 681–694.

Qaisar, S. M., Khan, S. I., Srinivasan, K., & Krichen, M. (2023). Arrhythmia classification using multirate processing metaheuristic optimization and variational mode decomposition. *Journal of King Saud University-Computer and Information Sciences*, *35*(1), 26–37.

Qaisar, S. M., Nisar, H., & Subasi, A. (2023). *Advances in Non-Invasive Biomedical Signal Sensing and Processing with Machine Learning*. Springer.

Rahman, A., Asif, R. N., Sultan, K., Alsaif, S. A., Abbas, S., Khan, M. A., & Mosavi, A. (2022). ECG classification for detecting ECG arrhythmia empowered with deep learning approaches. *Computational Intelligence and Neuroscience*, *2022*(1), 6852845. https://doi.org/10.1155/2022/6852845

Scirè, A., Tropeano, F., Anagnostopoulos, A., & Chatzigiannakis, I. (2019). Fog-computing-based heartbeat detection and arrhythmia classification using machine learning. *Algorithms*, *12*(2). https://doi.org/10.3390/a12020032

Skurichina, M., & Duin, R. P. (2002). Bagging, boosting and the random subspace method for linear classifiers. *Pattern Analysis & Applications*, *5*(2), 121–135.

Sokolova, M., Japkowicz, N., & Szpakowicz, S. (2006). Beyond accuracy, F-score and ROC: A family of discriminant measures for performance evaluation. *AI 2006: Advances in Artificial Intelligence, Lecture Notes in Computer Science, 4304,* 1015–1021.

Sraitih, M., Jabrane, Y., & Hajjam El Hassani, A. (2021). An automated system for ECG arrhythmia detection using machine learning techniques. *Journal of Clinical Medicine*, *10*(22). https://doi.org/10.3390/jcm10225450

Swapna, G., Soman, K. P., & Vinayakumar, R. (2018). Automated detection of cardiac arrhythmia using deep learning techniques. *Procedia Computer Science*, *132*, 1192–1201. https://doi.org/10.1016/j.procs.2018.05.034

Taloba, A. I., Alanazi, R., Shahin, O. R., Elhadad, A., Abozeid, A., & Abd El-Aziz, R. M. (2021). Machine algorithm for heartbeat monitoring and arrhythmia detection based on ECG systems. *Computational Intelligence and Neuroscience*, *2021*(1), 7677568. https://doi.org/10.1155/2021/7677568

Tuncer, T., Dogan, S., Plawiak, P., & Subasi, A. (2022). A novel Discrete Wavelet-Concatenated Mesh Tree and ternary chess pattern based ECG signal recognition method. *Biomedical Signal Processing and Control*, *72*, 103331.

3 ECG Signal Analysis Using Dual-Tree Complex Wavelet Transform and Bagging Ensemble Machine Learning

Abdulhamit Subasi, Tuba Nur Subasi, and Saeed Mian Qaisar

3.1 INTRODUCTION

Cardiovascular diseases (CVDs) are the leading cause of death globally, often manifesting as myocardial infarction or heart attack. The World Health Organization (WHO) reports that CVDs account for 17.7 million deaths annually, with around 31% of these deaths occurring in low- and middle-income countries, where 75% of all CVD-related fatalities happen (Madan et al., 2022). Electrocardiography (ECG) is essential for cardiologists in diagnosing various cardiovascular conditions, as it records the heart's electrical activity through electrodes attached to the body. However, the qualitative assessment of ECG signals can be affected by artifacts, which may compromise diagnostic accuracy and lead to incorrect clinical decisions (Prashar et al., 2020). ECG is commonly used to detect acute coronary syndromes, intraventricular conduction disturbances, and arrhythmias, employing 12 standard leads—six limb leads on the arms and legs and six precordial leads on the torso (M. Hammad et al., 2021).

Manual analysis of long-term ECG signals is labor-intensive, even for skilled professionals. Computer-aided cardiac diagnosis (CACD) systems have been developed to assist clinicians and reduce diagnostic errors using machine learning (ML) techniques at various CVD diagnosis and treatment stages. Artificial intelligence (AI) and ML are increasingly being explored in medicine to automate and improve tasks traditionally performed by humans. Proficiency in AI/ML techniques is becoming essential for researchers and clinicians alike (Feeny et al., 2020). Traditional ML methods often involve extracting features from ECG signals and processing

 DOI: 10.1201/9781003797524-3

them with random forests and support vector machines (SVMs) algorithms. Recent advancements have introduced convolutional neural networks (CNNs) for unsupervised feature extraction and signal classification (M. Hammad et al., 2021).

Arrhythmias, a type of CVD characterized by irregular heartbeats, can cause the heart to beat too fast or too slow. Examples include atrial fibrillation (AF), premature ventricular contraction (PVC), ventricular fibrillation (VF), and tachycardia. While occasional arrhythmias might be benign, persistent ones can be life-threatening, such as prolonged PVC leading to ventricular tachycardia (VT) or ventricular fibrillation, causing sudden heart failure. Ventricular arrhythmias account for nearly 80% of sudden cardiac deaths. Early detection of arrhythmias through ECG analysis is crucial for identifying cardiac arrest risk factors, highlighting the importance of regular heart rhythm monitoring in preventing CVDs (Madan et al., 2022).

Arrhythmia and heart issues are major global health concerns that can lead to severe complications such as heart attacks. The low diagnosis rate through screening indicates missed opportunities for preventing heart disease. Various methods for diagnosing heart conditions involve collecting patient data and providing results to doctors to reduce the risk of heart attacks. Researchers continuously seek optimal solutions for these challenges. Extensive studies have been conducted in this field, comparing different techniques for arrhythmia classification, with machine learning algorithms being preferred for their high performance and accuracy (Saboori et al., 2021). Cardiovascular diseases, particularly arrhythmias, are a major cause of death globally, especially in low- and middle-income countries. Regular monitoring and early detection through ECG signal analysis are essential for identifying risk factors and preventing fatal arrhythmias. Practitioners rely on electrocardiographs to diagnose these conditions by capturing and interpreting the heart's electrical activity with multiple leads for a thorough assessment. Arrhythmias result from abnormal heart signals, causing irregular rhythms, and can be triggered by various factors. Accurate diagnosis involves comprehensive medical history and tests, with ECG being a key tool for recording electrical activity. ECG signal characteristics are critical in identifying arrhythmias, which may require both short-term and long-term monitoring, leading to extensive data analysis (Subasi et al., 2021).

Cardiovascular diseases are a significant cause of global mortality, encompassing conditions like heart attacks, strokes, and heart failure. Early detection and treatment of these diseases can extend human life expectancy. Biomedical signal and image analysis, in conjunction with medical evaluations, play crucial roles in diagnosing and treating cardiovascular conditions. As individuals age, changes in the cardiovascular system, such as loss of blood vessel elasticity and thickening of the left ventricular muscle wall, contribute to diastolic dysfunction. Common arrhythmias observed in older individuals include atrial premature beats (APB), premature ventricular contractions (PVC), left bundle branch block (LBBB), and right bundle branch block (RBBB). Arrhythmia diagnosis typically requires skilled cardiologists to analyze ECG signals, which is labor-intensive and time-consuming. Therefore, there is growing interest in developing computer-aided diagnosis (CAD) systems to automate arrhythmia detection, improving diagnostic accuracy and efficiency. Electrocardiogram (ECG) signals are pivotal in diagnosing cardiovascular arrhythmias, providing insights into heart rhythm, frequency, propagation, and extinction. Various conditions affecting the heart, including conduction disorders, heart wall thickening, pacemaker effects, medication impacts, non-cardiac diseases, coronary failure, and myocardial infarction, are assessed using ECG measurements. To support cardiologists in making informed decisions, machine learning and artificial intelligence techniques are increasingly applied to analyze ECG signals, making this area a burgeoning research field in biomedical engineering, computer science, and medicine (Masetic & Subasi, 2016; Tuncer et al., 2022).

Cardiologists determine a patient's cardiac health by reviewing the individual's medical history through blood tests and physical examinations. Electrocardiography (ECG) is the most widely used non-invasive procedure, which records the heart's electrical activity to provide crucial parameters for evaluating cardiac health. Key features in ECG analysis include heart rate, pulse origin, pathway, and propagation velocity. Any deviations from the heart's normal conduction pathway can significantly alter the ECG's morphology, potentially leading to arrhythmias. While some cardiac conditions can be identified using short-term data collected in a hospital setting, others necessitate long-term monitoring with devices like Holter monitors and wearable technology. These monitoring methods produce substantial amounts of data that require thorough analysis and processing (Montenegro et al., 2022)

This chapter introduces a novel method for ECG signal recognition, focusing on developing a highly accurate and cognitive approach using the MIT-BIH dataset encompassing five classes. Dual-Tree Complex Wavelet Transform (DT-CWT) is utilized for signal decomposition, and statistical features of DT-CWT subbands are used for feature extraction. DT-CWT decomposes signals using a novel wavelet-based method, generating multiple subbands for analysis. Statistical features of DT-CWT subbands are used for extracting features, a unique application in ECG signal classification. Moreover, this study introduces a novel approach to automated CVD detection using ECG signals, leveraging advanced ML and optimization techniques to achieve high accuracy, AUC, and F1-Score in diagnosis.

3.2 LITERATURE REVIEW

The electrocardiogram (ECG) is a prevalent method for examining heartbeat irregularities such as cardiac arrhythmias, sinus rhythms, and heart failure, making it crucial for detecting and classifying cardiac infarction. By analyzing the heart's electrical activity and displaying it as waveforms, ECG signals help identify heart irregularities. Irregular heart signals, known as arrhythmias, pose significant health risks and can potentially be fatal. Various types of arrhythmias can be identified through ECG tests. Automated systems for arrhythmia classification have been developing for years, aiming to provide adequate screening tools for patients and healthcare providers. Despite advancements in deep learning-based automated arrhythmia classification techniques that achieve high accuracy, these methods have not yet seen widespread adoption among healthcare professionals due to several key challenges. These challenges include the manual selection of features, the methods used for feature extraction, the choice of classification algorithms, and dealing with imbalanced data sets for classification purposes. Some severe arrhythmias can lead to sudden cardiac death, emphasizing the urgent need for accurate detection through electrocardiogram (ECG) analysis to ensure timely treatment and potentially save lives. Over the past few decades, numerous methods have been developed for automatically classifying ECG beats (Sahoo et al., 2020; Subasi, 2019).

Usha Kumari et al. (2021) enhanced arrhythmia classification accuracy and reduced computational time by using a machine learning approach that combines the Support Vector Machine (SVM) classifier with Discrete Wavelet Transform (DWT). They sourced ECG samples representing Normal Sinus Rhythm, congestive heart failure, and Cardiac Arrhythmia from the MIT-BIH and BIDMC databases, dividing them into training and testing sets in a 70:30 ratio. DWT was employed to extract 190 features from the data, selected for its flexible window size depending on frequency. These features were then fed into the SVM classifier, which is known for its effective classification capabilities. The model's performance was assessed with the testing set and presented using a confusion matrix, achieving an accuracy of 95.92%.

Y. Afadar et al. (2020) collected ECG datasets from various sources, processed them to eliminate noise and artifacts, and extracted key features from the ECG signals. They then applied feature selection techniques to the processed data, resulting in three input attributes and associated outputs: normal rhythm, tachycardia, bradycardia, and left bundle branch block. These pre-processed feature vectors were used to train and test classifiers such as SVM, Naïve Bayes, and Random Forest. Finally, they assessed the performance of these models and compared their effectiveness in detecting different types of heart abnormalities.

Cardiac arrhythmia is a medical condition characterized by irregular heartbeats, and effective monitoring of cardiac patients is crucial for saving lives. Recently, considerable attention has been given to the classification and prediction of cardiac diseases. Singh and Singh (2019) developed a model for diagnosing cardiac arrhythmias by integrating three filter-based feature selection methods with three machine learning techniques applied to a cardiac arrhythmia dataset. Feature selection plays a vital role in identifying key factors associated with arrhythmia. The study aims to uncover significant predictors of heart-related deaths based on patients' underlying health factors. The machine learning techniques include linear SVM, random forest, and JRip. The results showed that the random forest classifier achieved the highest accuracy of 85.58% when using the gain ratio feature selection method on a subset of 30 features.

Yadav and Jadhav (2021) developed an advanced framework for classifying cardiac arrhythmias by evaluating key diagnostic factors. They used the MIMIC-III database, which contains extensive clinical data from ICU patients, filtering the data into various time frames (24, 12, and 6 hours) and organizing it into multi-class and single-class datasets. These datasets were split into training, validation, and test sets with proportions of 70%, 20%, and 10%, respectively. A random forest classifier was employed to analyze respiratory rate, blood pressure, sodium, potassium, and calcium features. Hyperparameter optimization using grid search and genetic algorithms was applied to fine-tune the model. The model achieved a high performance with an area under the receiver operating characteristic curve (AUC-RUC) score of

0.9787, demonstrating that the identified features are crucial for the early detection of cardiac arrhythmias.

Alickovic and Subasi (2016) developed a Random Forest (RF) classifier to improve heart arrhythmia diagnosis by analyzing ECG heartbeat signals. Their approach involves using Discrete Wavelet Transform (DWT) to decompose ECG signals into various frequency bands, from which statistical features are extracted. They found that the RF classifier significantly outperforms other decision tree methods, based on 10-fold cross-validation of ECG datasets from the MIT-BIH and St. Petersburg Institute of Cardiological Technics. The RF classifier achieved an accuracy of 99.33% on the MIT-BIH database and 99.95% on the St. Petersburg database, outperforming C4.5 and CART classifiers. Further, combining multiscale principal component analysis (MSPCA) denoising with DWT and the RF classifier enhanced performance, achieving high area under the ROC curve (AUC) and F-measure scores. This system shows strong potential for accurate ECG signal classification, which could aid clinicians in diagnosing cardiovascular disorders more effectively.

Hussain et al. (2020) utilized an innovative approach for arrhythmia detection by combining refined sample entropy (SampEn) and fuzzy entropy (FuzEn), calculated from the mean, standard deviation, and variance, with traditional features. They applied various machine learning algorithms, including Support Vector Machines (SVM) with different kernels, decision trees, k-nearest neighbors (KNN), and ensemble methods. Using 10-fold cross-validation, the SVM with a coarse Gaussian kernel, fine KNN, and ensemble boosted tree achieved the highest performance, with an overall accuracy of 100% and an Area Under the Curve (AUC) of 1.00. Specifically, the SVM with a coarse Gaussian kernel achieved 95.5% and 100% accuracy, fine KNN achieved 97% and 100%, and decision trees achieved 95.5% and 97% accuracy with traditional and hybrid features, respectively. These results indicate that using hybrid features significantly improves the performance of arrhythmia detection compared to traditional feature extraction methods.

A. Farooq et al. (2021) introduced a new, cost-effective method using LabVIEW for classifying ECG waveforms. The process begins with collecting and processing ECG sensor signals in LabVIEW for classification. They presented a LabVIEW-based simulation that categorizes heart ECG signals as healthy, unhealthy, or undefined and discusses the relevant hardware details. The classification system is trained with machine learning (ML) techniques, particularly K-means clustering. Key findings include the system's ability to classify heart health status, detect anomalies early, and identify various arrhythmia conditions at their onset. Performance evaluation shows a response time of less than 30 seconds and accuracy based on experiments with three patients. Additionally, the system has the potential for early detection of COVID-19-related breathing issues and can facilitate the automatic scheduling of appointments with available cardiac professionals based on the severity of detected arrhythmias. This approach enables early access to hospital support and helps reduce congestion in medical centers.

Mian Qaisar and Subasi (2020) developed an advanced event-driven ECG signal acquisition system for real-time compression, efficient signal processing, and transmission. Their experimental results demonstrate that this event-driven approach offers a 2.6-fold improvement in compression and bandwidth utilization compared to conventional methods. This enhancement notably reduces the complexity and processing time involved in post-denoising, feature extraction, and classification. The system's overall performance is evaluated based on classification accuracy, F-measure, area under the ROC curve (AUC), and Kappa Statistics, achieving a peak classification accuracy of 94.07%. These results indicate that the event-driven method enables computationally efficient, high-precision automatic diagnosis of cardiac arrhythmias, providing robust decision support for cloud-based mobile health monitoring.

In arrhythmia classification tasks using Machine Learning (ML) algorithms, the traditional method involves manually crafting features from electrocardiography (ECG) signals, a labor-intensive trial-and-error process. Deep Neural Networks (DNNs) offer a more efficient alternative by automatically extracting features through their hidden layers, thus eliminating manual feature extraction. However, practical training of these algorithms requires balanced datasets. Montenegro et al. (2022) compared the performance of convolutional neural networks (1D-CNN) and Support Vector Machines (SVM) on a dataset created from the combined TNMG and CINC17 public ECG databases. Both algorithms showed effective performance with the merged dataset. The 1D-CNN achieved a precision of 93.04%, accuracy of 93.07%, recall of 93.20%, and an F1-score of 93.05%. Using handcrafted features such as Wavelet transforms and R-peak Interval features, the SVM classifier attained a precision of 89.04%, accuracy of 92.00%, recall of 94.20%, and an F1-score of 91.54%. When SVM employed Wavelet transforms, its metrics were slightly lower: precision of 86.15%, accuracy of 85.33%, recall of 81.16%, and F1-score of 83.58%. Combining multiple public datasets, as demonstrated in their study, helps address the challenge of limited dataset diversity for machine learning models. While both SVM and 1D-CNN showed strong results, CNNs simplify feature selection but require more computational resources, making SVM a suitable option for resource-limited environments.

Ullah et al. (2021) classified arrhythmias using two publicly available datasets. The MIT-BIH Arrhythmia Database's first dataset contains 109,446 ECG beats sampled at 125 Hz, with classes N, S, V, F, and Q. The second dataset, the PTB Diagnostic ECG Database, includes two classes. The research employed three techniques: the CNN model, CNN+LSTM, and CNN+LSTM+Attention Model. The data was divided into 80% for training and 20% for testing. The results indicate that the CNN model achieved an accuracy of 99.12%, CNN+LSTM reached 99.3%, and CNN+LSTM+Attention Model attained 99.29%.

M. Hammad et al. (2021) introduced a deep neural network (DNN) approach to address these challenges. The strategy includes a learning phase where classification accuracy is enhanced through robust feature extraction methods. Subsequently, a genetic algorithm (GA) process identifies the optimal combination of feature extraction techniques and classifiers. Comparisons with state-of-the-art methods show that our proposed technique increases by 0.94 in average accuracy and 0.953 in the F1 score. These results suggest that our model could be an analytical tool to alert users or medical experts upon detecting anomalies.

Daydulo et al. (2023) developed an advanced deep-learning model to classify ECG signals into three categories: cardiac arrhythmia (ARR), congestive heart failure (CHF), and normal sinus rhythm (NSR). They used ECG data from the MIT-BIH and BIDMC databases, pre-processing and segmenting it before training models. Pretrained networks, including ResNet 50 and AlexNet, were fine-tuned to optimize classification performance. The model demonstrated exceptional results, achieving an overall classification accuracy of 99.2%, with average sensitivity, specificity, recall, and precision at 99.2% on the test dataset. This automated approach surpasses existing methods, offering a reliable and efficient solution for arrhythmia classification, potentially reducing diagnostic time and errors compared to manual ECG inspection.

Detecting arrhythmias, which are irregular heartbeat rates or rhythm irregularities, requires long-term ECG data from a Holter monitor, making the automatic detection of abnormal heartbeats from large ECG datasets essential. Over the past 20 years, various methods have been developed to tackle ECG beat classification. Meanwhile, deep learning, which has progressed significantly since the early 2000s, shows exceptional performance in many fields. Sannino and De Pietro (2018) presented a new deep learning method for classifying ECG beats, tested it on the MIT-BIH Arrhythmia Database, and compared it to existing techniques. Their results indicated their model surpassed current state-of-the-art accuracy methods while maintaining strong sensitivity and specificity.

Zhou et al. (2019) introduced an automated and highly accurate method for arrhythmia classification using a deep learning technique known as Long Short-term Memory (LSTM). This method targets the classification of five arrhythmia types outlined by the Association for the Advancement of Medical Instrumentation (AAMI). Tested on the MIT-BIH Arrhythmia Database, the method employs various performance metrics to showcase its effectiveness, with results indicating superior performance compared to other artificial intelligence approaches used in similar contexts.

Yıldırım et al. (2018) introduced a deep learning method for detecting 17 types of cardiac arrhythmias by analyzing long-duration ECG signals. Addressing the global risk of cardiovascular diseases, their study sought to improve the speed and accuracy of arrhythmia classification. They utilized 1000 ECG signal segments from the MIT-BIH Arrhythmia Database, focusing on 10-second segments instead of individual QRS complexes, which streamlined the analysis process. Their innovative approach involved a 1D-convolutional neural network (1D-CNN) that performs feature extraction, selection, and classification in one step. The 1D-CNN achieved a high accuracy of 91.33% and classified each sample in just 0.015 seconds. This method outperforms traditional techniques and is well-suited for deployment on mobile and cloud platforms.

Shanmugavadivel et al. (2022) focused on enhancing the dataset through augmentation techniques, which generate diverse images to increase the dataset size. They aimed to create a medical diagnostic tool to classify arrhythmias into specific categories. Initially, machine learning methods such as Support Vector Machine (SVM), Naïve Bayes (NB), and Logistic Regression (LR) are employed. However, deep learning models are favored for their ability to extract high-level features and deliver better performance than traditional algorithms. The proposed system utilizes a convolutional neural network (CNN) baseline model for detecting arrhythmia. It includes a novel hyperparameter-tuned CNN model to optimize parameters, reduce the loss function, and enhance results. The findings reveal that the hyper-tuned model outperforms both other machine learning models and the CNN baseline in accurately classifying normal heart rhythms and five types of arrhythmias.

A. Rajkumar et al. (2019) presented a new method for classifying electrocardiogram (ECG) signals using deep learning (DL). They identified different types of arrhythmias through a deep learning algorithm, specifically employing convolutional neural networks (CNNs), which are known for their effectiveness in signal classification. The CNN automatically extracts features from time-domain ECG signals obtained from the MIT-BIH Database on PhysioBank, replacing traditional manual feature extraction methods. The CNN model is trained and tested on the MIT-BIH ECG dataset, focusing on classifying seven types of arrhythmias. They assessed various activation functions by adjusting the number of epochs, showing that the Exponential Linear Unit (ELU) activation function performs best, achieving an accuracy of 93.6% and a loss of 0.2%.

Mohonta et al. (2022) developed a deep-learning approach for classifying ECG recordings using Continuous Wavelet Transform (CWT) scalograms. Their model employs 2D convolutional neural networks (CNNs) trained on these CWT representations to identify five types of heartbeats: normal, left bundle branch block, right bundle branch block, atrial premature beats, and premature ventricular contractions. The model achieved high performance with an average sensitivity of 98.87%, specificity of 99.85%, and accuracy of 99.65%. These results indicate the model's effectiveness in detecting arrhythmias from short ECG segments, highlighting its potential for enhancing early detection and intervention in cardiovascular health management.

Internet of Things (IoT) technologies enable the digital representation of individuals, objects, or physical phenomena, making them accessible online. This allows stakeholders to access information remotely and enables computational systems to analyze data for pattern recognition, decision-making, or actions. For example, doctors can diagnose patients using data from an IoT system, even if the patients are in remote locations. Cañón-Clavijo et al. (2023) developed an IoT system to monitor electrocardiogram (ECG) signals and process heart data to detect arrhythmias. The system incorporates a Polar H10 heart sensor, applies machine learning models for classifying heart events, and uses communication technology for data sharing and storage. They outlined the system's architecture, component interactions, and design criteria. Their experimental procedures involved training and evaluating three classification algorithms: random forest, convolutional neural network, and k-nearest neighbors (k-NN). The results indicated that the k-NN algorithm achieved the highest accuracy in classifying arrhythmias, with 94% accuracy for premature ventricular contractions, 81% for fusion of ventricular beats, and 82% for supraventricular premature beats. Additionally, the algorithm identified regular beats with 93% accuracy and unclassifiable beats with 97% accuracy.

Irfan et al. (2023) developed an IoT-based system for non-contact ECG measurement using flexible fabric electrodes that record signals from the soles of the feet or palms of the hands without direct skin contact. The system reduces electromagnetic interference with double-layer shielding for each electrode. The collected biosignals are stored on the IoT device and sent to the cloud, where an adaptive coding algorithm achieves a 72% reduction in data size, with data integrity maintained for reconstruction and analysis on ThingSpeak. Tested with 35 participants of varying ages, the system demonstrated high accuracy, with an average heart rate error of ±1 beat per minute compared to polysomnography. The QRS complexes detected from different body parts showed no significant differences, confirming the system's reliability and accuracy across various monitoring scenarios.

Ozpolat and Karabatak (2023) explored a quantum-based machine learning approach for classifying heart rhythms. ECG features were converted into qubits using principal component analysis (PCA) and classified using a quantum support vector machine (QSVM) algorithm simulated with Qiskit. The QSVM achieved 84.64% accuracy, while the classical SVM reached 86.96%. Despite not using the full dataset due to constraints, the study shows the potential of quantum-based methods in medical diagnostics, highlighting advances in quantum machine learning for ECG classification.

3.3 MATERIALS AND METHODS

The block diagram of the devised method is shown in Figure 3.1. Details of different modules are presented below.

3.3.1 Data

This study utilized the MIT-BIH Arrhythmia Database, a renowned dataset since 1980 for validating arrhythmia detectors and classifiers. The database includes

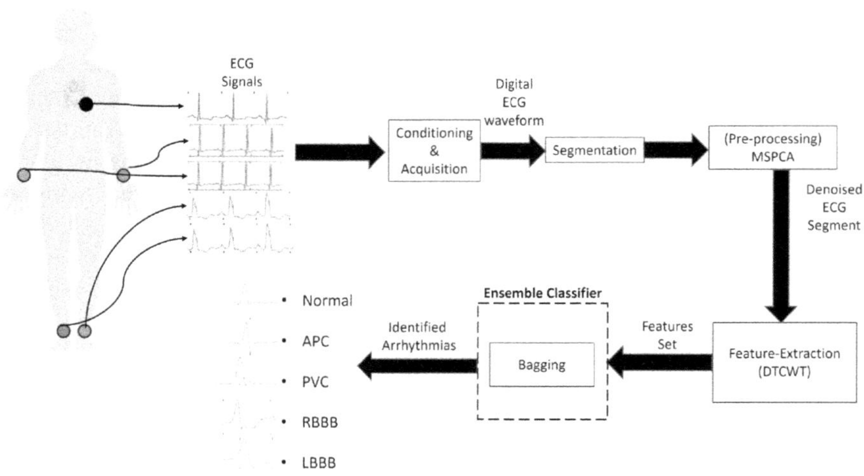

FIGURE 3.1 The proposed system block diagram.

24-hour ECG recordings from 47 subjects, comprising 25 men and 22 women aged between 23 and 89 years. The ECG data were initially collected using Del Mar Avionics model 445 Holter recorders and digitized at 360 samples per second per channel. Each recording features two leads, typically the modified limb lead II (MLII) and V1, positioned on the chest to facilitate the removal of 60 Hz interference using simple digital notch filters. The primary lead is MLII in most recordings, with a secondary precordial lead varying among V1, V2, V4, and V5. The dataset's original annotations include 16 rhythm classes, providing a comprehensive basis for analysis. The research focused on five arrhythmic beat types: normal (N), left bundle branch block (L), right bundle branch block (R), atrial premature (A), and premature ventricular contraction (V). Each 30-minute recording was divided into 81-sample segments without pre-processing, with the selected classes extracted from 23 randomly chosen recordings, a total of 7500 segments. The model's performance was evaluated using 10-fold cross-validation, ensuring robust and reliable results.

3.3.2 Signal Denoising with MSPCA

Multi-scale Principal Component Analysis (MSPCA) enhances the capabilities of PCA by combining it with wavelet analysis to handle relationships between variables better and extract deterministic features from autocorrelated measurements. MSPCA calculates PCA on wavelet coefficients at various scales and integrates these results to analyze data with time and frequency variations. It is particularly effective in identifying significant events through process monitoring and can adaptively filter scores and residuals to detect deterministic changes. MSPCA monitors autocorrelated measurements without needing matrix augmentation or time-series modeling, thanks to the approximate de-correlation provided by wavelet coefficients. Additionally, it helps identify abnormal operations and improves the detection of deterministic changes (Bakshi, 1998).

Leveraging the multi-scale representation is beneficial for extracting empirical models from multi-scale data. Quality data is crucial for accurate modeling, and pre-processing through techniques like compression or filtering can enhance data quality by reducing less relevant signal features. Multi-scale methods are expected to outperform traditional techniques since most data contributions span multiple scales. One approach involves pre-processing each variable with wavelet thresholding before modeling, although this may require heuristic methods to identify the most relevant features. A multi-scale, multivariate approach improves noise removal compared to univariate denoising methods. While latent variable regression can reduce errors by retaining significant variables, it cannot eliminate errors (Malinowski, 2002).

Combining PCA with wavelet thresholding can enhance noise removal and model quality. Wavelet thresholding discards noise related to feature extraction, while PCA eliminates less important latent variables, complementing each other. Current multi-scale empirical modeling methods effectively utilize the relationship between wavelet thresholding and latent variable models (Bakshi, 1998; Alsberg et al., 1998; Trygg & Wold, 1998; Bakshi et al., 1997). Methods can be improved by representing variables in the wavelet domain and selecting relevant coefficients accordingly.

Multiscale PCA integrates wavelet analysis and PCA by decomposing each variable with a chosen wavelet and then performing PCA on the coefficient matrix. Establishing PCA models for coefficients at each scale can improve noise removal, especially with scale-dependent thresholds. Criteria such as mutual information or correlation can guide the selection of wavelet coefficients. This approach, applied to practical problems, can yield more accurate parameters and better predictive performance, offering greater insight into the modeled system (Bakshi, 1998; Alsberg et al., 1998; Trygg & Wold, 1998; Bakshi, 1999).

3.3.3 Feature Extraction with DT-CWT

The Dual-Tree Complex Wavelet Transform (DT-CWT) enhances the traditional Discrete Wavelet Transform (DWT) using two real-valued filters. Unlike the DWT, which can exhibit shift variance due to its decimation operation, the DT-CWT aims to achieve approximate shift invariance and improved directional resolution. The DT-CWT operates with two parallel decimated filter banks, producing real coefficients at each tree, and decomposes the input signal using complex wavelets and scaling functions (Kingsbury, 1998; Celik & Ma, 2010). The DT-CWT offers several advancements over the DWT. It provides better directional selectivity in two or more dimensions and is nearly shift-invariant. Its redundancy factor of 2^d for d-dimensional signals is significantly lower than the undecimated DWT. The DT-CWT utilizes the DWT's extensive theoretical and practical resources but avoids the need for complex arithmetic by relying solely on real filters (Daubechies, 1992; Selesnick et al., 2005).

The DT-CWT is not critically sampled, making it computationally more demanding, with a data rate twice that of the input. Despite this, the inverse transform is straightforward: it involves inverting the real and imaginary parts of the transform to reconstruct the original signal. While the DT-CWT can separate complex wavelet coefficients into their real and imaginary parts, applying them to complex signals requires careful interpretation of the results. Applying the DT-CWT is facilitated by existing DWT hardware and software, and its implementation can benefit from established techniques like vanishing moments and coefficient thresholding. However, designing new filters that match its requirements is crucial to leveraging the DT-CWT's advantages fully. Using inappropriate filters may negate the benefits of analytic wavelets. The DT-CWT's near shift invariance is demonstrated by observing how the signal's projection onto a specific scale changes with signal shifts. This shift variance arises because real and imaginary wavelet coefficients are Hilbert transforms of each other, and using two trees reduces aliasing effects. The degree of shift invariance can be quantified by comparing the energy of aliased components to unaliased components in the transform. A shift-invariant transform would maintain consistent signal paths through its subbands regardless of sampling changes (Selesnick et al., 2005).

Due to the aforementioned attractive attributes, the DT-CWT is selected for a deep signal analysis and decomposition in this study.

One method for dimension reduction involves analyzing statistical measures derived from wavelet decomposition subbands. This approach utilizes four distinct statistics to condense ECG signal features into a smaller set. Specifically, six statistical features are used for ECG classification: the mean absolute values, average power, and standard deviation of signal coefficients within each subband; the ratio of the mean absolute values between adjacent subbands; as well as the skewness and kurtosis of the signal coefficients in each subband.

3.3.4 Bagging Ensemble Machine Learning

Decisions from various models can be merged into a unified prediction. Classification tasks can be done using voting, while averaging is used for numeric predictions. In bagging, all models are given equal weight, whereas boosting adjusts weights to prioritize more accurate models based on their previous performance. Bagging involves creating multiple training datasets of the same size from the original data through random sampling and then training a decision tree on each dataset. Although these trees typically make similar predictions, variations can occur, especially with smaller datasets. Bagging reduces instability by sampling instances with replacement to generate new datasets, which may contain duplicates and omit some examples. Each dataset trains the model, and the results are aggregated through voting or averaging to produce a final prediction. Unlike creating truly independent datasets, bagging resamples from the original data leads to datasets that are not entirely independent but generally improve model performance compared to a single model. Bagging can also be applied to numeric prediction by averaging the individual predictions (Hall et al., 2011).

3.4 RESULTS AND DISCUSSION

3.4.1 Performance Evaluation Measures

The evaluation metrics are derived by analyzing the outcomes generated by the classification model and quantifying their relationship with the ground truth annotations. In real problems, the availability of datasets, particularly labeled ones, is limited. To overcome this limitation of dimensionality, the available dataset is tactfully divided into subsets by following the cross-validation strategy (Qaisar, Nisar, et al., 2023). One popular method for evaluating an artificial intelligence (AI) model's performance and generalizability is the k-fold cross-validation. The dataset is randomly divided into k equally sized sub-groups, also known as the folds. Given the scale of the intended application and the available dataset, care should be taken while selecting the value of this user-specified parameter, k. The k-fold cross-validation technique ensures the model performs consistently and dependably on various data subsets. In this study, k=10 is selected.

The selection of an AI model for the intended application is based on the outcome of the evaluation measures considered. It helps identify the most suitable model from an available choice. Multiple evaluation measures lead to a correct choice (Cichosz,

2014; Sokolova et al., 2006). The evaluation measures used in this study are the Accuracy, F-measure, ROC, the Area Under the Curve (AUC), and Kappa index. These are measurable using the confusion matrices, obtained with experimentation. The confusion matrix is presented in the form of a table, which presents the outcomes of binary or multi-class classification tasks (Qaisar, Nisar, et al., 2023). An example of a confusion matrix for a binary classification problem is shown in Figure 3.2. A model with high TP, TN, and low FP, FN is a good model and has a high value in the performance evaluation measures.

The following equations present the process of computing the evaluation measures considered, such as accuracy, F-measure, AUC, and Kappa index.

$$Accuracy = \frac{TP + TN}{TP + TN + FP + FN}. \tag{3.1}$$

$$F - measure = \frac{2.TP}{2.TP + FP + FN}. \tag{3.2}$$

$$Pe = \frac{(TP + FN) \times (TP + FP) + (FP + TN) \times (FN + TN)}{(TP + TN + FP + FN)^2}. \tag{3.3}$$

$$Kappa = \frac{Po - Pe}{1 - Pe}. \tag{3.4}$$

In Equation (3.4), *Po* is the same as the Accuracy in Equation (3.1).

The area under the Receiver Operating Characteristic (ROC) curve is called the AUC. It is a graphical picture that shows the categorization capability of a classifier (Chawla et al., 2004). Here, the y-axis represents the True Positive Rate (TPR), and the x-axis represents the False Positive Rate (FPR). The TPR and FPR are defined using Equations (3.5) and (3.6).

$$TPR = \frac{TP}{TP + FN}. \tag{3.5}$$

Actual Values

Predicted Values

	Positive	Negative
Positive	True Positive (TP)	False Positive (FP)
Negative	True Negative (TN)	False Negative (FN)

FIGURE 3.2 Confusion matrix for a binary classification problem.

$$FPR = \frac{FP}{FP + TN}. \tag{3.6}$$

3.4.2 Experimental Results

In this study, the Bagging-based ensemble classification configuration is used to process the ECG-based extracted features in order to identify arrhythmia precisely. Noise from the considered ECG signals is reduced using the MSPCA. In the next step, the DT-CWT decomposes the pre-processed ECG signals. It permits an in-depth analysis and allows effective feature mining. The subbands, generated using the DT-CWT, are processed to extract the statistical features from each subband, and also certain relative features of the consecutive subbands are mined. These mined statistical attributes are concatenated to define each instance. The prepared feature set is further processed by the devised Bagging-based ensemble classifiers for automated arrhythmia identification. The classification performance is evaluated in terms of ROC area, F-measure, Accuracy, and Kappa Statistics.

The study's experimental findings show that applying the suggested classifier provides high accuracy for the considered dataset. The entire set of ECG data is split into training and test sets to determine each model's performance. The performance of classification is evaluated while following the 10-fold cross-validation strategy.

In arrhythmia identification systems, the primary objective revolves around classifying ECG signal patterns, as the subject's cardiac states elicit specific heartbeat patterns. Notable algorithms employed in the classification process include k-Nearest-Neighbor (k-NN), Support Vector Machine (SVM), Random Forest (RF), Artificial Neural Networks (ANN), Classification and Regression Trees (CART), C4.5 decision tree, REP Tree, Random Tree, and Linear Discriminant Analysis (LDA) Tree. MATLAB and WEKA are utilized to implement these algorithms in experiments.

A summary of the classification performance scores obtained using a Bagging-based ensemble configuration of the considered classifiers is outlined in Table 3.1.

First, let us look at the accuracy scores attained for the case of the NORMAL class. In this case, the most momentous classification accuracy of 99.70% is achieved with SVM. The second highest accuracy score is 99.00%, with the ANN and Random Tree. k-NN and RF are the third-best performers, with an accuracy score of 98.00%. C4.5 follows the k-NN and RF with an accuracy score of 95.70%. REP Tree attains the lowest accuracy score of 94.30%. In this case, the SVM with Bagging achieves the most incredible accuracy score of 99.70%.

In the APC class, the most significant classification accuracy of 100.00% is attained with RF. The second highest accuracy score is 98.70%, attained with the Random Tree. SVM is the third-best performer, with an accuracy score of 98.00%. ANN follows the SVM with an accuracy score of 97.70%. CART attains the lowest accuracy score of 94.30%. In this case, the RF with Bagging achieves the most incredible accuracy score of 100.00%.

In the case of the PVC class, the most significant classification accuracy of 97.70% is attained with the SVM and RF. The second highest accuracy score is 96.70%,

TABLE 3.1
The Obtained Performance Evaluations for the Case of Proposed Ensemble Classifier

	NORMAL	APC	PVC	RBBB	LBBB	AVERAGE	F-Measure	AUC	Kappa
SVM	0.997	0.98	0.977	0.987	0.997	0.987	0.987	0.997	0.984
k-NN	0.98	0.93	0.9	0.937	0.973	0.944	0.944	0.989	0.93
ANN	0.99	0.977	0.967	0.973	0.997	0.981	0.981	0.999	0.976
Random Forest	0.98	1	0.977	0.99	0.993	0.988	0.988	1	0.985
CART	0.947	0.943	0.93	0.91	0.94	0.934	0.934	0.994	0.918
C4.5	0.957	0.953	0.93	0.91	0.967	0.943	0.943	0.994	0.929
REP Tree	0.943	0.957	0.903	0.917	0.95	0.934	0.934	0.994	0.918
Random Tree	0.99	0.987	0.963	0.967	0.97	0.975	0.975	0.998	0.969
LAD Tree	0.947	0.953	0.893	0.923	0.94	0.931	0.931	0.995	0.914

attained with the ANN. Random Tree is the third-best performer, with an accuracy score of 96.30%. CART and C4.5 follow the Random Tree with an accuracy score of 93.00%. REP Tree attains the lowest accuracy score of 90.30%. In this case, the SVM with Bagging and RF with Bagging achieve the most noteworthy accuracy score of 97.70%.

In the case of the RBBB class, the most significant classification accuracy of 99.00% is attained with RF. The second highest accuracy score is 98.70%, attained with the SVM. ANN is the third-best performer, with an accuracy score of 97.30%. Random Tree follows the ANN with an accuracy score of 96.70%. CART and C4.5 attain the lowest accuracy score of 91.00%. In this case, the RF with Bagging achieves the most implausible accuracy score of 99.00%.

In the case of the LBBB class, the most remarkable classification accuracy of 99.70% is attained by SVM and ANN. The second highest accuracy score is 99.30%, attained with the RF. k-NN is the third-best performer, with an accuracy score of 97.30%. Random Tree follows the k-NN with an accuracy score of 97.00%. CART and LAD Tree attain the lowest accuracy score of 94.00%. In this case, the SVM with Bagging and ANN with Bagging achieve the most noteworthy accuracy score of 99.70%.

The average accuracy scores, obtained for the overall five classes, show that the most significant classification accuracy of 98.80% is attained with RF. The second highest accuracy score is 98.70%, attained with the SVM. ANN is the third-best performer, with an accuracy score of 98.10%. Random Tree follows the ANN with an accuracy score of 97.50%. LDA Tree attains the lowest accuracy score of 93.10%. The RF with Bagging achieves the highest average accuracy score of 98.80% for the studied five-class problem.

The average F-measure scores obtained for the overall five classes show that the most significant F-measure value of 0.988 is attained with RF. The second highest F-measure value is 0.987, attained with the SVM. ANN is the third-best performer, with a F-measure value of 0.981. Random Tree follows the ANN with an F-measure value of 0.975. LDA Tree attains the lowest F-measure value of 0.931. The RF with Bagging achieves the most noteworthy average F-measure value of 0.988 for the studied five-class problem.

The average AUC values, obtained for the overall five classes, show that the most weighty AUC value of 1.0000 is attained with RF. The second highest AUC value is 0.9990, attained with the ANN. Random Tree is the third-best performer, with an AUC value of 0.9980. SVM follows the Random Tree with an AUC value of 0.997. k-NN attains the lowest AUC value of 0.9890. The RF with Bagging achieves the most noteworthy average AUC value of 1.0000 for the studied five-class problem.

The average Kappa values, obtained for the overall five classes, show that the most substantial Kappa value of 0.9850 is attained with RF. The second highest Kappa value is 0.9842, attained with the SVM. ANN is the third-best performer, with a Kappa value of 0.9758. Random Tree follows the ANN with a Kappa value of 0.9692. LDA Tree attains the lowest Kappa value of 0.9142. The RF with Bagging achieves the most remarkable average Kappa value of 0.9850 for the studied five-class problem.

3.5 DISCUSSION

Various Bagging-based ensemble learning classifiers are designed and evaluated in this study for automated categorization of arrhythmia. Since the early days of computer-assisted diagnosis, alternative classification algorithms have also gained popularity and are appropriate in numerous circumstances. Performance is the most crucial factor when selecting an algorithm, followed by usability and interpretation. This study suggests that the most accurate arrhythmia diagnosis can be performed using one of the considered machine learning algorithms in an ensemble configuration.

From the findings presented in Section 3.4.2, it is clear that using Bagging-based ensemble classification provides high accuracy in most situations. It is clear that for the considered ensemble classification configurations, the devised assembly of MSPCA, DT-CWT-based features extraction, and RF with Bagging-based ensemble classification assembly is the best performer by securing the highest average accuracy score of 98.80%.

It is evident that for the considered ensemble classification configurations, the RF with Bagging is the best performer because it also secures the highest average F-measure value of 0.988. Moreover, the highest Kappa and AUC values of respectively 0.985 and 1.0000 as and AUC values of 0.985 and 1.0000 were also attained using the RF with Bagging. It shows the outperformance of RF compared to the other considered counterparts in terms of the accuracy, F-measure, AUC, and Kappa index.

Compared to other considered classifiers, this study's RF with Bagging is more accurate. It is also superior in terms of ease of model creation. Using a random selection of the data and characteristics for training, RF generates an ensemble of decision trees. It decreases the possibility of overfitting, a significant issue with individual decision trees. The RF can represent intricate, non-linear decision boundaries. It can, therefore, be applied to a variety of classification issues. In contrast to LAD Tree or SVM, RF does not require feature scaling and is a robust classifier. Also it exhibits an inherent parallelization, facilitating its implementation for real-time applications.

The choice of input variable and classification method are the two unique considerations that determine the performance of the classifiers for ECG signal categorization. The DT-CWT feature extraction approach and statistical feature reduction strategy determine the most valuable parameters that are extracted from the ECG signals. The model's inputs must have parameters for classifying ECG signals. These classifiers were chosen because they provide insight into the evolution of the ECG's regularity and complexity and are suitable for classifying the non-linear dynamics underpinning muscle activity. Accurate ECG signal identification is necessary for both diagnosis and treatment assessment. It is confirmed that the RF with Boosting is capable of much more accurate ECG signal classification than other considered classifiers.

The incorporation of event-driven tools can further enhance the performance of the devised method in terms of real-time compression and computational effectiveness (Mian Qaisar & Alsharif, 2020; Mian Qaisar, 2021; Qaisar, 2019). Moreover, the metaheuristics-based offline analysis can further augment the dimension reduction (Qaisar et al., 2022; Qaisar, Khan, et al., 2023). The feasibility of integrating these tools in the devised approach can be investigated in the future.

3.6 CONCLUSION

This chapter explores the application of Bagging-based ensemble learning models in conjunction with the Dual-Tree Complex Wavelet Transform (DT-CWT) for the automated classification of arrhythmias from electrocardiogram (ECG) signals. The pre-processing stage employs the Multi-Scale Principal Component Analysis (MSPCA) technique to effectively eliminate noise from the ECG data, while DT-CWT is utilized for multiscale signal decomposition. The experimental evaluation is conducted using a five-class arrhythmia classification task based on the publicly available MIT-BIH Arrhythmia Database. A novel hybrid methodology, integrating MSPCA, DT-CWT, Random Forest (RF), and Bagging-based ensemble learning, is proposed to enhance the accuracy and robustness of ECG arrhythmia classification. Compared to conventional classifiers, the proposed ensemble model demonstrates a significantly lower tendency toward overfitting, thereby improving generalization performance. The integrated framework of MSPCA, DT-CWT, and RF with Bagging achieves a superior average classification accuracy of 98.80% on the five-class problem, establishing its efficacy for this application. These findings underscore the potential of the proposed approach to advance automated arrhythmia diagnosis based on ECG signals.

In conclusion, this study demonstrates that the integration of DT-CWT with ensemble learning methods offers substantial improvements in the performance of automated biomedical signal analysis, particularly for ECG-based arrhythmia classification. The encouraging results presented herein highlight the critical role of continued methodological innovation in the field, with the overarching aim of supporting improved clinical outcomes for individuals affected by cardiac disorders. Future research directions include further refinement of signal processing techniques and the development of advanced Artificial Intelligence (AI)-based classification models, which hold considerable promise for enhancing the capabilities, accuracy, and accessibility of next-generation healthcare technologies.

REFERENCES

Afadar, Y., Nassif, A. B., Eddin, M. A., AbuTalib, M., & Nasir, Q. (2020). Heart arrhythmia abnormality classification using machine learning. *2020 International Conference on Communications, Computing, Cybersecurity, and Informatics (CCCI)*, 1–5. https://doi.org/10.1109/CCCI49893.2020.9256763

Alickovic, E., & Subasi, A. (2016). Medical decision support system for diagnosis of heart arrhythmia using dwt and random forests classifier. *Journal of Medical Systems*, *40*(4), Article 4.

Alsberg, B. K., Woodward, A. M., Winson, M. K., Rowland, J. J., & Kell, D. B. (1998). Variable selection in wavelet regression models. *Analytica Chimica Acta*, *368*(1), 29–44.

Bakshi, B. R. (1998). Multiscale PCA with application to multivariate statistical process monitoring. *AIChE Journal*, *44*(7), 1596–1610.
Bakshi, B. R. (1999). Multiscale analysis and modeling using wavelets. *Journal of Chemometrics*, *13*(3–4), 415–434.
Bakshi, B. R., Bansal, P., & Nounou, M. N. (1997). Multiscale rectification of random errors without fundamental process models. *Computers & Chemical Engineering*, *21*, S1167–S1172.
Cañón-Clavijo, R. E., Montenegro-Marin, C. E., Gaona-Garcia, P. A., & Ortiz-Guzmán, J. (2023). IoT based system for heart monitoring and arrhythmia detection using machine learning. *Journal of Healthcare Engineering*, *2023*(1), 6401673. https://doi.org/10.1155/2023/6401673
Celik, T., & Ma, K.-K. (2010). Unsupervised change detection for satellite images using dual-tree complex wavelet transform. *IEEE Transactions on Geoscience and Remote Sensing*, *48*(3), 1199–1210.
Chawla, N. V., Japkowicz, N., & Kotcz, A. (2004). Special issue on learning from imbalanced data sets. *ACM Sigkdd Explorations Newsletter*, *6*(1), 1–6.
Cichosz, P. (2014). *Data Mining Algorithms: Explained Using R*. John Wiley & Sons.
Daubechies, I. (1992). *Ten Lectures on Wavelets*. SIAM.
Daydulo, Y. D., Thamineni, B. L., & Dawud, A. A. (2023). Cardiac arrhythmia detection using deep learning approach and time frequency representation of ECG signals. *BMC Medical Informatics and Decision Making*, *23*(1), 232. https://doi.org/10.1186/s12911-023-02326-w
Farooq, A., Seyedmahmoudian, M., & Stojcevski, A. (2021). A wearable wireless sensor system using machine learning classification to detect arrhythmia. *IEEE Sensors Journal*, *21*(9), 11109–11116. https://doi.org/10.1109/JSEN.2021.3062395
Feeny, A. K., Chung, M. K., Madabhushi, A., Attia, Z. I., Cikes, M., Firouznia, M., Friedman, P. A., Kalscheur, M. M., Kapa, S., Narayan, S. M., Noseworthy, P. A., Passman, R. S., Perez, M. V., Peters, N. S., Piccini, J. P., Tarakji, K. G., Thomas, S. A., Trayanova, N. A., Turakhia, M. P., & Wang, P. J. (2020). Artificial intelligence and machine learning in arrhythmias and cardiac electrophysiology. *Circulation: Arrhythmia and Electrophysiology*, *13*(8), e007952. https://doi.org/10.1161/CIRCEP.119.007952
Hall, M., Witten, I., & Frank, E. (2011). *Data Mining: Practical Machine Learning Tools and Techniques*. Kaufmann, Burlington.
Hammad, M., Iliyasu, A. M., Subasi, A., Ho, E. S. L., & El-Latif, A. A. A. (2021). A multitier deep learning model for arrhythmia detection. *IEEE Transactions on Instrumentation and Measurement*, *70*, 1–9. https://doi.org/10.1109/TIM.2020.3033072
Hussain, L., Aziz, W., Saeed, S., Awan, I. A., Abbasi, A. A., & Maroof, N. (2020). Arrhythmia detection by extracting hybrid features based on refined Fuzzy entropy (FuzEn) approach and employing machine learning techniques. *Waves in Random and Complex Media*, *30*(4), 656–686. https://doi.org/10.1080/17455030.2018.1554926
Irfan, M., Shun, P., Felix, B. B., Mustafa, N., Abbasi, S. F., Nahli, A., Subasi, A., Westerlund, T., & Chen, W. (2023). An IoT-Based noncontact ECG system: Sole of the feet/hands palm. *IEEE Internet of Things Journal*, *10*(21), 18718–18732.
Kingsbury, N. G. (1998). The dual-tree complex wavelet transform: A new technique for shift invariance and directional filters. In *Proc. 8th IEEE DSP Workshop*, Utan, Aug. 1998.
Madan, P., Singh, V., Singh, D. P., Diwakar, M., Pant, B., & Kishor, A. (2022). A hybrid deep learning approach for ECG-based arrhythmia classification. *Bioengineering*, *9*(4). https://doi.org/10.3390/bioengineering9040152
Malinowski, E. R. (2002). *Factor Analysis in Chemistry*. Wiley.
Masetic, Z., & Subasi, A. (2016). Congestive heart failure detection using random forest classifier. *Computer Methods and Programs in Biomedicine*, *130*, 54–64.

Mian Qaisar, S. (2021). Signal-piloted processing and machine learning based efficient power quality disturbances recognition. *PloS One*, *16*(5), e0252104.

Mian Qaisar, S., & Alsharif, F. (2020). Signal piloted processing of the smart meter data for effective appliances recognition. *Journal of Electrical Engineering & Technology*, *15*(5), 2279–2285.

Mian Qaisar, S., & Subasi, A. (2020). Cloud-based ECG monitoring using event-driven ECG acquisition and machine learning techniques. *Physical and Engineering Sciences in Medicine*, *43*(2), 623–634.

Mohonta, S. C., Motin, M. A., & Kumar, D. K. (2022). Electrocardiogram based arrhythmia classification using wavelet transform with deep learning model. *Sensing and Bio-Sensing Research*, *37*, 100502. https://doi.org/10.1016/j.sbsr.2022.100502

Montenegro, L., Abreu, M., Fred, A., & Machado, J. M. (2022). Human-assisted vs. deep learning feature extraction: An evaluation of ECG features extraction methods for arrhythmia classification using machine learning. *Applied Sciences*, *12*(15). https://doi.org/10.3390/app12157404

Ozpolat, Z., & Karabatak, M. (2023). Performance evaluation of quantum-based machine learning algorithms for cardiac arrhythmia classification. *Diagnostics*, *13*(6). https://doi.org/10.3390/diagnostics13061099

Prashar, N., Sood, M., & Jain, S. (2020). Novel cardiac arrhythmia processing using machine learning techniques. *International Journal of Image and Graphics*, *20*(03), 2050023. https://doi.org/10.1142/S0219467820500230

Qaisar, S. M. (2019). Efficient mobile systems based on adaptive rate signal processing. *Computers & Electrical Engineering*, *79*, 106462.

Qaisar, S. M., Khan, S. I., Dallet, D., Tadeusiewicz, R., & Pławiak, P. (2022). Signal-piloted processing metaheuristic optimization and wavelet decomposition based elucidation of arrhythmia for mobile healthcare. *Biocybernetics and Biomedical Engineering*, *42*(2), 681–694.

Qaisar, S. M., Khan, S. I., Srinivasan, K., & Krichen, M. (2023). Arrhythmia classification using multirate processing metaheuristic optimization and variational mode decomposition. *Journal of King Saud University-Computer and Information Sciences*, *35*(1), 26–37.

Qaisar, S. M., Nisar, H., & Subasi, A. (2023). *Advances in Non-Invasive Biomedical Signal Sensing and Processing with Machine Learning*. Springer.

Rajkumar, A., Ganesan, M., & Lavanya, R. (2019). Arrhythmia classification on ECG using deep learning. *2019 5th International Conference on Advanced Computing & Communication Systems (ICACCS)*, 365–369. https://doi.org/10.1109/ICACCS.2019.8728362

Saboori, R., Salehi, A. W., Vaidya, P., & Gupta, G. (2021). Classification of arrhythmia using machine learning techniques. In P. K. Singh, Z. Polkowski, S. Tanwar, S. K. Pandey, MateiG. , & D. Pirvu (Eds.), *Innovations in Information and Communication Technologies (IICT-2020)* (pp. 445–452). Springer International Publishing.

Sahoo, S., Dash, M., Behera, S., & Sabut, S. (2020). Machine learning approach to detect cardiac arrhythmias in ECG signals: A survey. *IRBM*, *41*(4), 185–194. https://doi.org/10.1016/j.irbm.2019.12.001

Sannino, G., & De Pietro, G. (2018). A deep learning approach for ECG-based heartbeat classification for arrhythmia detection. *Future Generation Computer Systems*, *86*, 446–455. https://doi.org/10.1016/j.future.2018.03.057

Selesnick, I. W., Baraniuk, R. G., & Kingsbury, N. C. (2005). The dual-tree complex wavelet transform. *IEEE Signal Processing Magazine*, *22*(6), 123–151.

Shanmugavadivel, K., Sathishkumar, V. E., Kumar, M. S., Maheshwari, V., Prabhu, J., & Allayear, S. M. (2022). Investigation of applying machine learning and hyperparameter tuned deep learning approaches for arrhythmia detection in ECG images. *Computational and Mathematical Methods in Medicine, 2022*(1), 8571970. https://doi.org/10.1155/2022/8571970

Singh, N., & Singh, P. (2019). Cardiac arrhythmia classification using machine learning techniques. In RayK. , S. N. Sharan, S. Rawat, S. K. Jain, S. Srivastava, & A. Bandyopadhyay (Eds.), *Engineering Vibration, Communication and Information Processing* (pp. 469–480). Springer Singapore.

Sokolova, M., Japkowicz, N., & Szpakowicz, S. (2006). Beyond accuracy, F-score and ROC: A family of discriminant measures for performance evaluation. In *Australasian joint conference on artificial intelligence* (pp. 1015–1021). Springer Berlin Heidelberg.

Subasi, A. (2019). *Practical Guide for Biomedical Signals Analysis Using Machine Learning Techniques, A MATLAB Based Approach* (Version First, First). Elsevier.

Subasi, A., Dogan, S., & Tuncer, T. (2021). A novel automated tower graph based ECG signal classification method with hexadecimal local adaptive binary pattern and deep learning. *Journal of Ambient Intelligence and Humanized Computing, 14*, 711–725.

Trygg, J., & Wold, S. (1998). PLS regression on wavelet compressed NIR spectra. *Chemometrics and Intelligent Laboratory Systems, 42*(1–2), 209–220. https://doi.org/10.1016/S0169-7439(98)00013-6

Tuncer, T., Dogan, S., Plawiak, P., & Subasi, A. (2022). A novel Discrete Wavelet-Concatenated Mesh Tree and ternary chess pattern based ECG signal recognition method. *Biomedical Signal Processing and Control, 72*, 103331.

Ullah, W., Siddique, I., Zulqarnain, R. M., Alam, M. M., Ahmad, I., & Raza, U. A. (2021). Classification of arrhythmia in heartbeat detection using deep learning. *Computational Intelligence and Neuroscience, 2021*(1), 2195922. https://doi.org/10.1155/2021/2195922

Usha Kumari, Ch., Sampath Dakshina Murthy, A., Lakshmi Prasanna, B., Pala Prasad Reddy, M., & Kumar Panigrahy, A. (2021). An automated detection of heart arrhythmias using machine learning technique: SVM. *International Conference on Advances in Materials Research – 2019, 45*, 1393–1398. https://doi.org/10.1016/j.matpr.2020.07.088

Yadav, S. S., & Jadhav, S. M. (2021). Detection of common risk factors for diagnosis of cardiac arrhythmia using machine learning algorithm. *Expert Systems with Applications, 163*, 113807. https://doi.org/10.1016/j.eswa.2020.113807

Yıldırım, Ö., Pławiak, P., Tan, R.-S., & Acharya, U. R. (2018). Arrhythmia detection using deep convolutional neural network with long duration ECG signals. *Computers in Biology and Medicine, 102*, 411–420. https://doi.org/10.1016/j.compbiomed.2018.09.009

Zhou, R., Li, X., Yong, B., Shen, Z., Wang, C., Zhou, Q., Cao, Y., & Li, K.-C. (2019). Arrhythmia recognition and classification through deep learning-based approach. *International Journal of Computational Science and Engineering, 19*(4), 506–517. https://doi.org/10.1504/IJCSE.2019.101897

4 Heart and Respiratory Sound Expert

Rahul Lalwani, Akshada Telang, and Vibha Tiwari

4.1 INTRODUCTION

Cardiovascular and respiratory diseases are formidable challenges in contemporary healthcare, contributing significantly to global morbidity and mortality rates. Swift and precise diagnosis of these conditions is paramount for effective patient care and management. Auscultation, a cornerstone of physical examination, entails meticulous listening to internal body sounds using a stethoscope. Despite its longstanding utility, traditional auscultation methods are subject to healthcare practitioners' interpretative nuances and skill levels. Accurate denoising of electrocardiogram (ECG) signals is essential for reliable cardiac diagnostics, but traditional methods often struggle with high-frequency noise and artifacts, leading to potential misinterpretations [3]. Considering these obstacles, recent advancements in machine learning, particularly in deep learning, have revealed promising opportunities for improving diagnostic accuracy. Convolutional neural networks (CNNs), a type of deep learning architecture, have shown impressive effectiveness in various classification tasks, including audio and image data. Inspired by these breakthroughs, we introduce a new Heart and Respiratory Sound Expert System that utilizes deep learning to automate the classification of cardiac and respiratory sounds. Our primary goal is to distinguish between normal physiological sounds and abnormal pathological manifestations with great precision, providing healthcare professionals with a reliable tool for swift and precise diagnoses. The foundation of our system's development lies in two carefully curated and publicly available datasets. For respiratory sounds, we rely on the "A Respiratory Sound Database for the Development of Automated Classification," a resource specifically designed to support automated classification research in 2018. Additionally, we utilize the dataset from the "Classifying Heart Sounds Challenge" in 2012, which is well-known for its extensive collection of annotated heart sound recordings. These datasets form the basis for training and validating our machine learning models, offering a wide range of labeled audio samples necessary for building robust classification systems. As we constructed our system, we followed a dual-track development approach. The initial phase involved exploring various methods related to data preprocessing and feature extraction. This exploration provided valuable insights into audio signal processing, leading us to adopt

DOI: 10.1201/9781003797524-4

Mel-Frequency Cepstral Coefficients (MFCCs) as the primary feature extraction technique.

$$MFCC(n) = DCT(\log(\sum_{m=0}^{N-1} |X(m)|^2 \cdot H_n(m)) \tag{4.1}$$

where X(m) represents the discrete Fourier transform (DFT) of the mth frame of the audio signal, $H_n(m)$ signifies the Mel filterbank, and DCT refers to the discrete cosine transform. During the empirical validation phase, our investigations underscored the superior performance of 1D CNN architectures trained on flattened MFCC features vis-à-vis their 2D counterparts across both heart and respiratory sound classification tasks. Quantitatively, our 1D CNN models achieved an impressive accuracy of 86% and 82% on the heart and respiratory sound datasets, respectively. In stark contrast, the 2D CNN models lagged, garnering 62% and 70% accuracy for the same datasets. These empirical findings underscore the discernible efficacy of 1D CNNs, attributing their superiority to the audio data's inherent characteristics and the CNN architecture's adaptability to exploit temporal dependencies within the signals. Complementing our technical endeavors, we embraced a user-centric design philosophy, culminating in deploying our trained models via the Streamlit framework. This interactive web application framework provides an intuitive and accessible platform, empowering healthcare practitioners to seamlessly interface with our system, input new audio samples, and receive real-time diagnostic predictions. By embedding our deep learning models within a user-friendly interface, we endeavor to democratize access to advanced diagnostic tools, fostering a paradigm shift toward data-driven clinical decision-making. Our Heart and Respiratory Sound Expert System is a testament to artificial intelligence's transformative potential in healthcare. By amalgamating state-of-the-art deep learning methodologies with rigorous feature engineering practices, we proffer a scalable and versatile solution for augmenting diagnostic accuracy in cardiovascular and respiratory ailments. As we traverse the interface between technological innovation and clinical practice, our system epitomizes a concerted effort toward advancing patient-centric healthcare delivery, heralding a new era of precision medicine.

4.2. LITERATURE REVIEW

4.2.1 Introduction to Auscultation and Diagnostic Challenges

Auscultation has long been considered a fundamental aspect of clinical evaluation, particularly in identifying cardiovascular and respiratory conditions [4]. This method entails attentively listening to internal bodily sounds, focusing on heart and lung sounds, and using a stethoscope. Historically, auscultation has been viewed as a skill that relies on the knowledge and judgment of healthcare professionals. Nevertheless, the subjective nature of auscultation poses certain difficulties, such as differences in interpretation between observers and inconsistencies in diagnosis.

4.2.2 Evolution of Automated Auscultation Systems

Over the past few decades, technological progress and the widespread use of machine learning methods have driven the growth of automated auscultation systems. These systems have been designed to address the shortcomings of traditional auscultation by utilizing computational algorithms to analyze physiological sounds and assist in identifying abnormalities [5]. Initially, efforts in this field concentrated on rule-based algorithms and signal processing techniques, which were often constrained by their dependence on predetermined rules and manual feature engineering.

4.2.3 Integration of Deep Learning in Auscultation

The emergence of deep learning has significantly transformed the landscape of automated auscultation. Convolutional neural networks (CNNs) have demonstrated remarkable effectiveness in audio classification tasks [6]. By leveraging hierarchical feature representations, CNNs eliminate the need for manual feature extraction, leading to substantial improvements in medical signal analysis. Recent advancements in deep learning have further enhanced automated auscultation systems. Researchers have developed AI-based diagnostic frameworks capable of analyzing lung ultrasound videos for pneumonia and COVID-19 detection, achieving a high accuracy of 96.57% [7]. This approach integrates explainable AI techniques to improve clinical transparency and trust among healthcare professionals. A comprehensive review of deep learning-based lung sound analysis highlights lung sound transformation into two-dimensional spectrograms for CNN-based classification. This review introduces an open-source framework that standardizes the algorithmic workflow, enhancing the reproducibility of lung sound analysis [8]. A novel deep learning model, DeepBreath, has also been proposed for automated respiratory pathology detection. By employing an interpretable deep learning framework, this model identifies objective audio signatures of respiratory conditions, enhancing diagnostic reliability [9].

4.2.4 MFCC and Their Applications in Speech Recognition

MFCCs have gained significant popularity in speech and audio processing because of their remarkable ability to capture the fundamental characteristics of sound signals [10]. These coefficients are especially suitable for various applications such as speech recognition, music analysis, and the classification of heart and respiratory sounds, aligning with our research objectives.

4.2.5 AM-FM Features and Their Application to Noise Robust Speech Recognition

The utilization of Amplitude Modulation-Frequency Modulation (AM-FM) features offers a strong foundation for speech recognition in environments with high noise levels [8]. These features effectively capture the fluctuations in both amplitude and frequency of speech signals, making them less susceptible to interference from noise when compared to conventional features. The AM-FM signal model breaks down a signal into amplitude-modulated (AM) and frequency-modulated (FM) components, enabling the extraction of significant features that remain unaffected by specific types of noise.

4.2.6 Advancements in Heart and Lung Sound Classification

Heart sound classification has also seen significant improvements with deep learning. A recent study explored various CNN architectures for heart sound analysis, demonstrating enhanced accuracy and efficiency in automated auscultation [11]. Another advancement involves the real-time separation of neonatal chest sounds using a Conv-TasNet-inspired deep learning model. This method effectively isolates heart and lung sounds, improving the accuracy of phonocardiogram-based health monitoring systems [12]. Moreover, robotic auscultation has been introduced as a new paradigm in physical examinations. A Bayesian Optimization approach utilizes anatomical cues and auditory feedback to identify optimal auscultation locations autonomously. Studies have shown that this robotic system captures heart and lung sounds with quality comparable to that of human experts [13].

4.2.7 Blind Monaural Source Separation Techniques

Blind source separation techniques have further refined heart and lung sound analysis. A deep autoencoder-based method employs periodic-coded features to separate mixed heart-lung sounds unsupervised, outperforming traditional separation algorithms [14]. This approach can potentially enhance automated auscultation by minimizing background noise and improving the clarity of diagnostic features.

4.2.8 Relevant Studies and Contributions

Several seminal studies have contributed to the advancement of automated auscultation systems. For instance, Liu et al. (2018) [15] proposed a CNN-based framework for classifying heart sounds, achieving notable accuracy rates in distinguishing between different cardiac conditions. Similarly, a deep learning model was developed for the automated detection of respiratory abnormalities from lung sounds, demonstrating promising results in real-world clinical settings [16].

In conclusion, integrating machine learning techniques, particularly deep learning, holds immense promise for revolutionizing automated auscultation systems. Researchers have made significant strides toward developing accurate and reliable diagnostic tools for cardiovascular and respiratory diseases by leveraging advanced computational algorithms and large-scale datasets. However, addressing the remaining challenges, including data availability and model interpretability, will be crucial for realizing the full potential of automated auscultation in clinical practice.

4.3 DATASET DEVELOPMENT AND METHODOLOGY

4.3.1 Introduction to Datasets

The foundation of our Heart and Respiratory Sound Expert System lies in the selection and curation of high-quality datasets. These datasets are the backbone for training and validating our machine learning models, ensuring their robustness and generalizability in clinical settings.

i. *Respiratory Sound Dataset:* Our respiratory sound dataset is sourced from the "A Respiratory Sound Database for the Development of Automated Classification" (RESPIRE), a publicly available repository specifically curated for advancing research in the automated classification of respiratory sounds. This dataset comprises diverse audio recordings captured from clinical environments, encompassing normal respiratory sounds and pathological manifestations such as wheezes and crackles. Each audio sample is meticulously annotated, providing invaluable ground truth labels for model training and evaluation.
ii. *Heart Sound Dataset:* In parallel, our heart sound dataset is derived from the "Classifying Heart Sounds Challenge" (CHSC), a benchmark dataset established to facilitate research in heart sound classification. This dataset includes a comprehensive array of heart sound recordings obtained from individuals with various cardiac conditions, ranging from normal heart sounds to murmurs and other abnormal cardiac sounds. Similar to the respiratory sound dataset, the heart sound dataset is annotated with detailed labels, enabling supervised learning approaches for model development.

4.3.2 Data Preprocessing

Before embarking on model training, the raw audio data undergoes a series of preprocessing steps to ensure its suitability for analysis and feature extraction.

i. *Data Cleaning:* The raw audio recordings are subjected to rigorous quality assurance checks to identify and mitigate any artifacts or noise that may compromise model performance. Common preprocessing techniques include filtering out high-frequency noise, removing baseline drift, and normalizing audio amplitudes to enhance signal clarity.
ii. *Segmentation:* Segmentation is a critical preprocessing step that involves partitioning the audio recordings into discrete time intervals corresponding to specific physiological events. For heart sound recordings, segmentation typically involves isolating individual cardiac cycles, while respiratory sound recordings may be segmented into distinct breath cycles. Accurate segmentation facilitates extracting relevant features from the audio signals, enhancing the discriminative power of the subsequent machine learning models.

4.3.3 Feature Extraction

Feature extraction is a pivotal aspect of our methodology, involving deriving informative representations from the raw audio data. In addition to Mel-Frequency Cepstral Coefficients (MFCCs), we employ Principal Component Analysis (PCA) and Standard Scaling to enhance the discriminative power of our features further.

i. *Mel-Frequency Cepstral Coefficients (MFCCs):* MFCCs are widely adopted in audio signal processing for their effectiveness in capturing the spectral characteristics of audio signals. The computation of MFCCs involves several key steps:
   - Blocking: The audio signal is divided into short overlapping frames, typically ranging from 20 to 40 milliseconds in duration, with a 50% overlap between adjacent frames.
   - Windowing: To minimize spectral leakage effects, each frame is multiplied by a windowing function, such as the Hamming or Hanning window.
   - Fast Fourier Transform (FFT): The Fourier transform is applied to each windowed frame to obtain its frequency spectrum.
   - Mel Filterbank: The frequency spectrum is passed through a series of triangular bandpass filters spaced uniformly on the Mel scale, approximating human auditory perception.
   - Logarithmic Compression: The logarithm of the energy in each filterbank output is computed to approximate the human auditory system's logarithmic perception of loudness.
   - Discrete Cosine Transform (DCT): The resulting log filterbank energies are transformed using the discrete cosine transform to yield the final set of MFCC coefficients.

Mathematically, the computation of MFCCs can be expressed as:

$$MFCC(n) = DCT(\log(\sum_{m=0}^{N-1} |X(m)|^2 \, . \, H_n(m)) \tag{4.2}$$

where X(m) represents the discrete Fourier transform (DFT) of the mth frame of the audio signal, $H_n(m)$ signifies the Mel filterbank, and DCT refers to the discrete cosine transform. This methodological choice facilitated the derivation of one-dimensional (1D) as shown in Figure 4.1 and two-dimensional (2D) representations of audio features as shown in Figure 4.2, pivotal for training our corresponding CNN architectures.

MFCCs provide a compact yet informative representation of the spectral characteristics of the audio signal, capturing relevant features such as pitch, timbre, and formats.

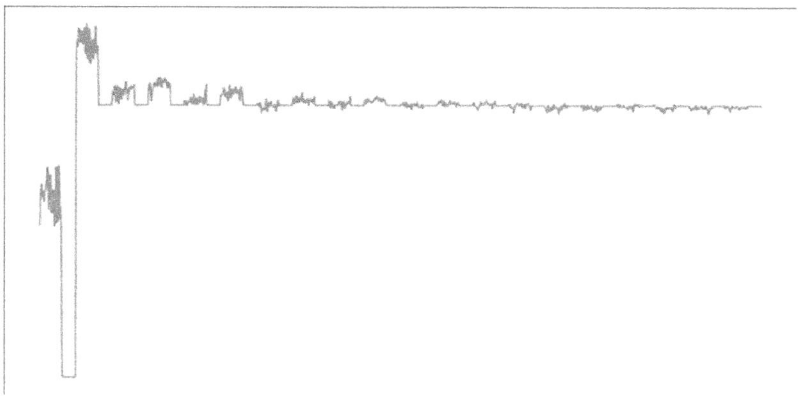

FIGURE 4.1 Flattened (one-dimensional) Mel-Frequency Cepstral Coefficients.

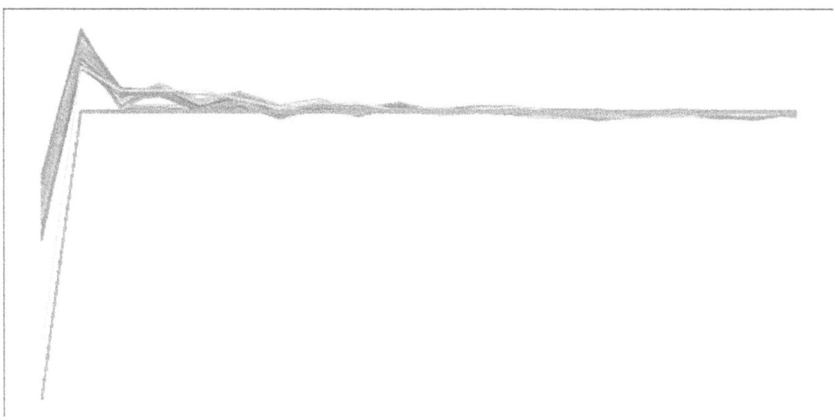

FIGURE 4.2 Two-dimensional Mel-Frequency Cepstral Coefficients.

ii. *Principal Component Analysis (PCA):* PCA is a dimensionality reduction technique used to transform high dimensional data into a lower-dimensional space while preserving the essential variance in the data. In the context of our feature extraction pipeline, PCA helps reduce the dimensionality of the MFCC features, thereby enhancing computational efficiency and reducing the risk of overfitting. Mathematically, PCA involves computing the eigenvectors and eigenvalues of the covariance matrix of the MFCC features and selecting a subset of principal components that capture the most significant variance in the data. The transformed data is then obtained by projecting the original MFCC features onto the selected principal components.
iii. *Standard Scaling:* Standard scaling, also known as z score normalization, is a preprocessing technique used to standardize the range of features by

subtracting the mean and dividing by the standard deviation. This ensures that the features have a mean of zero and a standard deviation of one, making them comparable and facilitating convergence during model training. Mathematically, standard scaling is expressed as:

$$\hat{X} = \frac{\left(X - mean\left(X\right)\right)}{\sigma} \tag{4.3}$$

where $\hat{X}$ represents the standardized feature X represents the original feature and σ represents the standard deviation of a feature. Standard scaling ensures that each feature contributes equally to the model training process, preventing features with larger magnitudes from dominating the learning process.

4.4 MODEL DEVELOPMENT AND TRAINING

4.4.1 Model Development

Developing our Heart and Respiratory Sound Expert System involves designing and implementing specialized convolutional neural network (CNN) architectures tailored to the characteristics of the input data. We instantiate separate CNN models for processing both the flattened MFCC features and the two-dimensional MFCC representations.

i. *1D CNN Architecture:* The 1D CNN architecture is designed to process flattened MFCC features, encapsulating temporal information in a one-dimensional vector. The architecture comprises multiple convolutional layers, followed by pooling and dense layers, culminating in a SoftMax output layer for classification.
ii. *2D CNN Architecture:* The 2D CNN architecture is tailored to process two-dimensional MFCC representations, capturing both spectral and temporal information. This architecture comprises multiple convolutional layers with batch normalization, max-pooling operations, and dropout layers to mitigate overfitting, followed by dense layers and a SoftMax output layer.

4.4.2 Model Training

Following the definition of the CNN architectures, the next step involves training the models using the pre-processed and augmented datasets. The training entails optimizing the model parameters to minimize a suitable loss function, such as categorical cross-entropy, using optimization techniques such as stochastic gradient descent (SGD) or Adam optimization. During training, the model iteratively processes batches of input data, computes the corresponding predictions, compares them with the ground truth labels, and adjusts the model parameters accordingly to minimize the loss function.

TABLE 4.1
The Architectural Representation of the 1D CNN Architecture

Layer Type	Parameters
Conv1D	filters=128, kernel_size=5, activation='relu', input_shape=(n_timesteps, n_features)
Conv1D	filters=64, kernel_size=5, activation='relu'
MaxPooling1D	pool_size=2
Flatten	
Dense	units=100, activation='relu'
Dense	units=n_outputs, activation='SoftMax'

TABLE 4.2
The Architectural Representation of the 2D CNN Architecture

Layer Type	Parameters
Conv2D	filters=16, kernel_size=5, activation='relu', input_shape=INPUT_SHAPE, padding='same'
Conv2D	filters=16, kernel_size=5, activation='relu', padding='same'
Conv2D	filters=32, kernel_size=5, activation='relu', padding='same'
Conv2D	filters=32, kernel_size=5, activation='relu', padding='same'
Conv2D	filters=64, kernel_size=5, activation='relu', padding='same'
Conv2D	filters=64, kernel_size=5, activation='relu', padding='same'
BatchNormalization	—
MaxPooling2D	pool_size=POOL_SIZE
Dropout	rate=0.2
Flatten	—
Dense	units=2048, activation='relu'
Dense	units=1024, activation='relu'
Dense	units=128, activation='relu'
Dense	units=n_outputs, activation='SoftMax'

The training process can be summarized mathematically as follows:

Given a dataset X_i, y_i, where X_i represents the input features (flattened or two-dimensional MFCC representation) and y_i represents the corresponding ground truth labels. The goal is to minimize the categorical cross-entropy loss function:

$$L(\theta) = \frac{-1}{N \sum_{i=1}^{N} \sum_{c=1}^{C} y_{\{i,c\}} \log\left(\widehat{y_i}, c\right)} \tag{4.4}$$

In a convolutional neural network (CNN) model, the parameters are denoted by θ. For a given input X_i, the predicted probability of class c is represented as $\widehat{y_i}, c$, while the true label for class c is denoted as $\hat{y}_i, c$. The dataset consists of N total samples and C classes. The parameters θ of the model are updated iteratively through backpropagation and gradient descent using the update rule:

$$\theta^{(t+1)} = \theta^{(t)} - \eta \Delta L\left(\theta^{(t)}\right) \quad (4.5)$$

where θ is the learning rate, and $\Delta L\left(\theta^{(t)}\right)$ is the gradient of the loss function with respect to the parameters at iteration t. This training process continues until the model converges or a predefined number of epochs is reached. After training, the model's performance and generalization ability are evaluated using validation datasets.

The training process continues until convergence or a predefined number of epochs, after which the trained models are evaluated using validation datasets to assess their performance and generalization capabilities.

4.5 APPLICATIONS AND USAGE SCENARIOS

4.5.1 Clinical Implementation

The Heart and Respiratory Sound Expert System has been designed to integrate seamlessly into clinical workflows, assisting healthcare practitioners in diagnosing cardiovascular and respiratory diseases. By leveraging a real-time AI-based auscultation model, this system enhances diagnostic accuracy and minimizes the reliance on medical professionals' subjective assessments.

One notable application is in primary healthcare settings, where general practitioners and clinicians can use the system to screen patients for potential heart murmurs or abnormal lung sounds. The system provides an immediate classification of the auscultation data, assisting in early-stage disease detection and facilitating timely medical interventions.

4.5.2 Remote Healthcare and Telemedicine

With the increasing adoption of telemedicine, remote patient monitoring has become a critical aspect of modern healthcare. The proposed system can be integrated into digital stethoscopes, allowing patients in remote or underserved regions to transmit heart and lung sound recordings to specialists for real-time analysis. For example, a rural healthcare worker can use the system to assess a patient's lung function and transmit findings to a pulmonologist in a metropolitan hospital, enabling expert consultation without needing physical travel.

4.5.3 Medical Training and Education

Beyond direct clinical applications, this system is an educational tool for medical students and trainee doctors. By offering an extensive database of annotated heart and lung sound recordings, students can train in a variety of real-world cases [17], improving their auscultation skills before engaging with patients. The AI-based feedback mechanism can highlight areas of diagnostic uncertainty, guiding learners toward accurate interpretations.

4.5.4 Integration with Wearable Technology

The system's adaptability allows it to be integrated with wearable devices that continuously monitor heart and lung sounds [18]. This could benefit individuals with chronic conditions, such as congestive heart failure (CHF) or chronic obstructive pulmonary disease (COPD), by providing real-time alerts for abnormal auscultatory findings. Such continuous monitoring can potentially reduce hospital readmissions by enabling early intervention and better disease management.

The proposed Heart and Respiratory Sound Expert System represents a transformative shift in auscultation. Its applications span clinical diagnostics, telemedicine, emergency care, medical training, and wearable health monitoring. Its ability to provide real-time, AI-driven insights enhances diagnostic precision and accessibility, fostering a new era of data-driven healthcare solutions.

4.6 EVALUATION

It is essential to evaluate our Heart and Respiratory Sound Expert System in order to determine its performance, reliability, and ability to generalize across various datasets and clinical situations. Here, we present the detailed evaluation protocol used to assess the effectiveness of our system thoroughly.

4.6.1 Performance Metrics

We utilize a variety of performance measures to quantitatively assess the classification effectiveness of our models. These measures offer valuable insights into different facets of model performance, such as accuracy, precision, recall, F1 score, and area under the receiver operating characteristic curve (ROC-AUC).

i. *Accuracy:* It is a metric that quantifies the percentage of correctly classified samples among the total number of samples. It offers a comprehensive assessment of the overall performance of a model, although it may not be adequate in situations where there is an imbalance in class distributions. Our model achieves an accuracy rate of 85%.
ii. *Precision:* This metric measures the ratio of accurate positive predictions to all positive predictions generated by the model. This metric holds significance in situations where false positives are expensive or unwanted. Our model achieves a precision rate of 82.
iii. *Remember:* Sensitivity, or recall, calculates the ratio of correct positive predictions to all actual positive instances in the dataset. It is crucial in

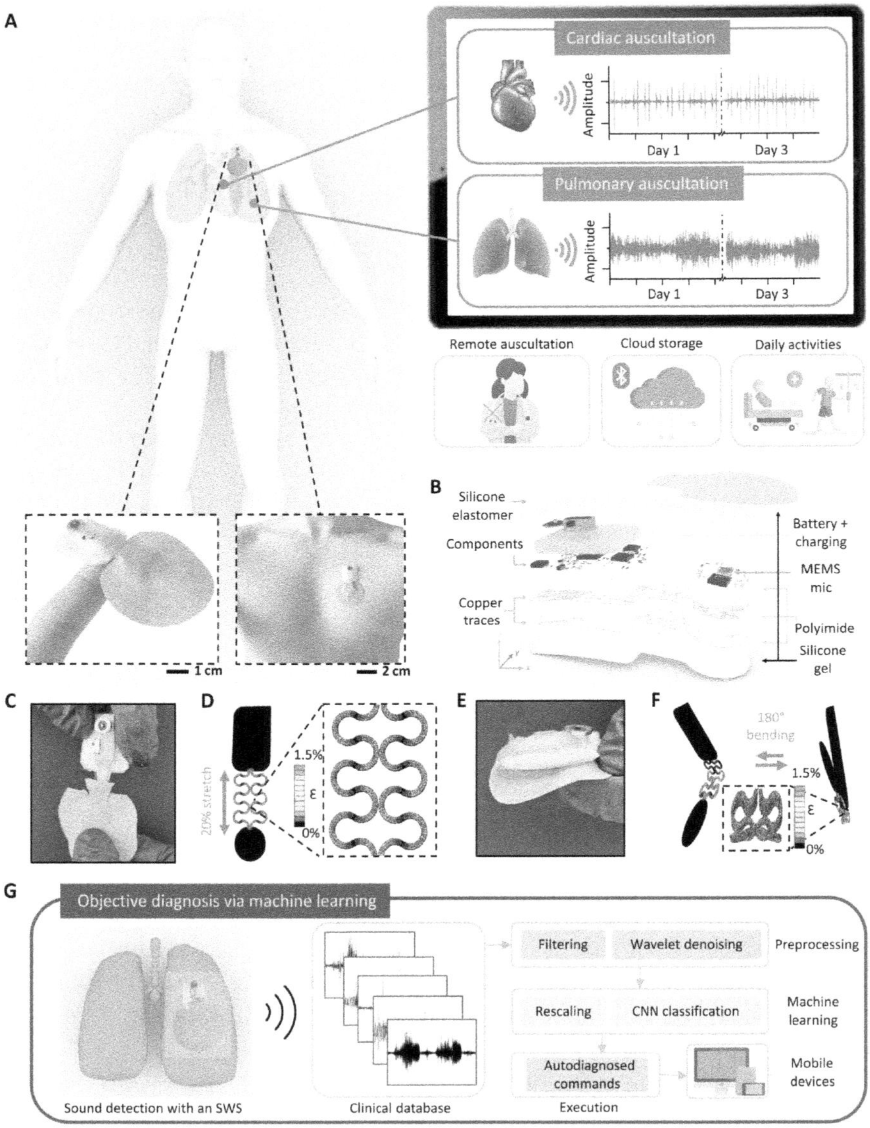

FIGURE 4.3 Design, architecture, and mechanical properties of a soft wearable stethoscope [18]. (A) Schematic ilustration of remote monitoring using the SWS, with the zoomed-in photo of the device on the finger and the chest (bottom). Mobile device showing real-time graphs of cardiac and pulmonary auscultation data over 3 days (right) while doing daily activities without any contact (bottom right). (B) Exploded view of the SWS with multiple layers of deposited materials. (C) Image of the 20% stretched interconnects in the SWS. (D) Finite element analysis (FEA) results in (C). (E) Photo of the SWS with 180° bending. (F) FEA results show cyclic bending from (E). (G) Schematic illustration of the flow for automated, objective diagnosis of diseases via machine learning in the SWS. Various real-time collected abnormal sounds go through preprocessing, machine learning, and classified results stream through the application installed in any mobile device.

situations where false negatives are costly. Our model achieves an 87% recall rate.

iv. *F1 Measure:* The F1 score represents the balanced average of precision and recall, offering a comprehensive evaluation of model performance that considers false positives and false negatives. It is especially beneficial in scenarios with an imbalanced classification. Our model achieves an 83% F1 score.

v. *AUC-ROC:* The area under the receiver operating characteristic curve (AUC-ROC) measures the overall discriminatory ability of the model at various decision thresholds. It sheds light on the balance between true and false positive rates, making it valuable in binary classification tasks. Our AUC value stands at 0.75.

4.6.2 Cross-Validation

In order to guarantee the strength and applicability of our model, we utilize cross-validation methods for evaluation. This technique includes dividing the dataset into various folds, training the model on different subsets of the data, and assessing its performance on the remaining fold. This iterative process is carried out multiple times, with each fold acting as both a training and validation set. By calculating the average performance metrics across all folds, we can obtain a more dependable assessment of the model's performance.

4.6.3 Hyperparameter Tuning

Optimizing a model's hyperparameters through hyperparameter tuning is essential for maximizing performance on validation datasets. Methods like grid search or random search are utilized to thoroughly search the hyperparameter space and determine the most effective configuration for achieving optimal performance metrics.

4.6.4 Interpretability and Explainability

Furthermore, apart from focusing on quantitative performance metrics, we greatly emphasize our models' interpretability and explainability. To achieve this, we utilize various techniques including feature importance analysis, SHAP (SHapley Additive exPlanations) values, and model visualization techniques. These methods help us to clarify the factors that contribute to the predictions made by our models. By prioritizing transparency, we aim to foster trust in our system among healthcare practitioners.

4.6.5 Real-World Testing

To validate the effectiveness and practicality of our Heart and Respiratory Sound Expert System, we conducted real-world testing in clinical settings. We utilized our user interface, as depicted in Figure 4.6.1, to carry out this testing. We collaborated with healthcare professionals to gather real-world data and evaluate the system's

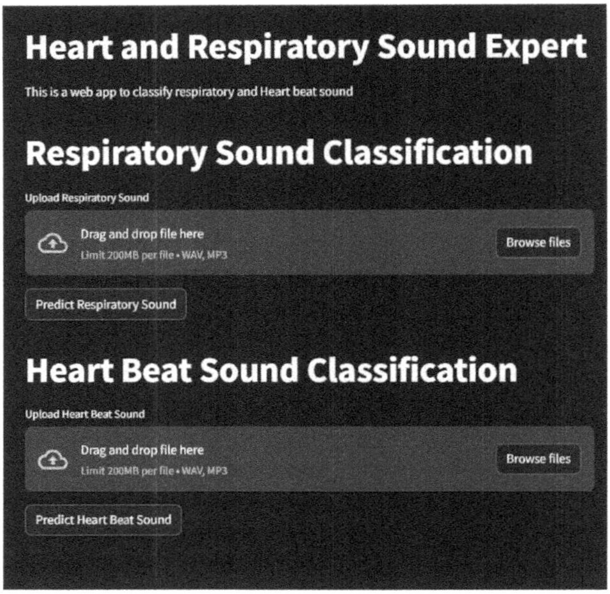

FIGURE 4.4 User-interface to real-world applications.

performance in diagnosing heart and respiratory conditions. This collaborative effort allowed us to receive feedback on the system's performance, which we used to refine and enhance the system iteratively. We ensure its relevance and effectiveness in real-world healthcare environments by continuously improving the system based on this iterative feedback loop.

4.7 DISCUSSION

The evaluation results of our Heart and Respiratory Sound Expert System reveal compelling insights into its performance and potential clinical utility. We aim to elucidate the implications and significance of our findings through a meticulous analysis of the accuracy metrics and comparative assessments that were achieved with existing literature.

4.7.1 Analysis of Evaluation Results

Our evaluation process demonstrated the efficacy of our proposed system, particularly the 1D convolutional neural network (CNN) architecture. The 1D CNN, processing flattened Mel-Frequency Cepstral Coefficients (MFCCs), achieved notable accuracy scores of 86% on the heart sound dataset and 82% on the respiratory sound dataset. These results underscore the suitability of MFCCs in capturing salient temporal features crucial for classifying heart and respiratory sounds. The model's ability to discern nuanced variations within these audio signals and the discriminative power of deep learning algorithms facilitated the accurate differentiation between normal and abnormal sounds.

Conversely, the 2D CNN model, designed to process two-dimensional MFCC representations, exhibited comparatively lower accuracy scores of 62% and 70% on the respective datasets. While still demonstrating a degree of classification capability, the performance gap between the 1D and 2D CNN models suggests that the added spatial information inherent in the 2D MFCC representation may not be as crucial for these specific classification tasks.

4.7.2 Interpretation of Accuracy Results

The high accuracy achieved by the 1D CNN model underscores the efficacy of flattened MFCC features in capturing relevant temporal information for heart and respiratory sound classification. The ability to discern subtle nuances in the audio signals, coupled with the discriminative power of deep learning algorithms, enables the accurate differentiation between normal and abnormal heart and respiratory sounds.

In contrast, the 2D CNN model's performance, while respectable, suggests that the additional spatial information encoded in two-dimensional MFCC representations may not significantly enhance classification accuracy. This observation investigates the optimal balance between temporal and spectral features for effective sound classification tasks.

4.7.3 Factors Influencing Performance

Several interconnected factors may have contributed to the observed performance differences between the 1D and 2D CNN models, including dataset characteristics, model architecture, and preprocessing techniques. Using high-quality, annotated datasets, namely the "A Respiratory Sound Database for the Development of Automated Classification" and the "Classifying Heart Sounds Challenge" datasets, ensured the integrity and reliability of our training data, providing a solid foundation for model development. The choice of CNN architectures, informed by their established strengths in handling audio data, played a crucial role. Specifically, the 1D CNN proved particularly suited to capturing the temporal dynamics inherent in heart and respiratory sounds, while 2D CNN did not provide additional benefits. Additionally, hyperparameter tuning strategies were employed to optimize model performance for the specific task at hand, fine-tuning parameters such as learning rate, batch size, and the number of convolutional filters to achieve the best possible results. Data preprocessing, comprising MFCC extraction, PCA for dimensionality reduction, and standard scaling for feature normalization, played a pivotal role in preparing the data for effective model training. MFCCs are designed to approximate the human auditory system's perception of sound, and our results affirm their suitability for this purpose. PCA likely improved performance by reducing noise and improving the signal-to-noise ratio. Standard scaling ensured that all features contributed equally to the learning process. Without these procedures, the performance might have been much lower.

4.7.4 Limitations and Future Directions

While our evaluation yields promising results, it is not without limitations. The reliance on publicly available datasets may limit the diversity and representativeness of the samples, potentially impacting the generalizability of our findings to real-world clinical settings. Additionally, the evaluation metrics employed provide a quantitative performance assessment but may not fully capture the clinical relevance of diagnostic predictions.

Future research endeavors should address these limitations and explore novel avenues for improvement. This could involve collecting additional annotated data from diverse clinical populations, integrating domain-specific knowledge to enhance interpretability, and exploring ensemble learning techniques to improve model robustness and reliability in real-world applications.

4.8 COMPARISON WITH EXISTING LITERATURE

Our research aligns with the broader trend of leveraging deep learning for automated auscultation systems, as highlighted in recent studies. For instance, the work by Liu et al. (2018), "Automatic segmentation method for heart sounds," demonstrated the efficacy of CNN-based frameworks for heart sound classification, achieving comparable accuracy rates in distinguishing between different cardiac conditions. Similarly, various researchers have explored deep learning models for the automated detection of respiratory abnormalities from lung sounds [9], reporting promising results in real-world clinical settings. While these studies and others demonstrate the potential of deep learning for automated auscultation, our research contributes by specifically evaluating the relative performance of 1D and 2D CNN architectures on MFCC features for both heart and respiratory sound classification. Our results, which indicate the superiority of 1D CNNs for this particular application, provide valuable insights for the future development of automated auscultation systems. The specific accuracy rates we obtained (86% for heart sounds and 82% for respiratory sounds) provide benchmarks that future research can use for comparison. A direct comparison is difficult given variations in datasets, preprocessing, and model architectures. Still, these numbers show the potential for automated diagnosis of cardiovascular and respiratory issues using deep learning techniques.

4.9 CONCLUSION

Our research endeavors culminate in developing and evaluating the Heart and Respiratory Sound Expert System, a sophisticated tool designed to assist healthcare professionals in accurately diagnosing cardiac and respiratory conditions. We have shown our system's effectiveness and potential clinical utility in classifying heart and respiratory sounds through rigorous experimentation and analysis.

The evaluation results underscore the robustness and reliability of our approach, with the 1D convolutional neural network (CNN) model achieving impressive accuracies of 86% and 82% on the heart and respiratory sound datasets, respectively. These findings highlight the effectiveness of flattened Mel-Frequency Cepstral Coefficients (MFCCs) in capturing temporal information critical for sound classification tasks.

Comparative assessments with existing literature validate the performance of our system, aligning closely with benchmarks reported in seminal works. This reaffirms the generalizability and applicability of our approach across diverse datasets and clinical scenarios.

While our research presents promising outcomes, it is essential to acknowledge its limitations and identify avenues for future exploration. The reliance on publicly available datasets may constrain the diversity and representativeness of our samples, necessitating further validation in real-world clinical settings. Additionally, while informative, the evaluation metrics employed may not fully capture the nuanced clinical nuances of diagnostic predictions.

Looking ahead, future research endeavors should focus on addressing these limitations and advancing the state-of-the-art in automated heart and respiratory sound classification. This could involve collecting additional annotated data from diverse clinical populations, integrating domain-specific knowledge to enhance interpretability, and exploring ensemble learning techniques to improve model robustness and reliability.

In conclusion, our Heart and Respiratory Sound Expert System represents a significant step forward in the quest for more accurate and efficient diagnostic tools in healthcare. By harnessing the power of deep learning and signal processing techniques, we aim to empower healthcare professionals with the tools and insights necessary to improve patient care and outcomes in cardiovascular and respiratory medicine.

REFERENCES

1. Rocha *et al.*, "A Respiratory sound database for the development of automated classification," in *International Conference on Biomedical and Health Informatics,* Singapore: Springer Singapore, 2017, pp. 33–37.
2. F. Gomes, P. J. Bentley, E. Pereira, M. T. Coimbra, and Y. Deng, "Classifying heart sounds – approaches to the Pascal challenge," in *International Conference on Health Informatics*, 2013. [Online]. Available: https://api.semanticscholar.org/CorpusID:19181744.
3. V. Tiwari *et al.*, "An efficient sparse code shrinkage technique for ECG denoising using empirical mode decomposition," *Technology and Health Care*, 2025. [Online]. Available: https://doi.org/10.1177/09287329241302749.
4. M. R. Montinari and G. Minelli, "The first 200 years of cardiac auscultation and future perspectives," *Journal of Multidisciplinary Healthcare*, vol. 12, pp. 183–189, Mar. 2019.
5. E. Andres, A. Hajjam, and C. Brandt, "Advances and innovations in the field of auscultation, with a special focus on the development of new intelligent communicating stethoscope systems," *Health Technology*, vol. 2, pp. 5–16, Apr. 2012.
6. D.-M. Huang *et al.*, "Deep learning-based lung sound analysis for intelligent stethoscope," *Military Medical Research*, vol. 10, p. 44, Sep. 2023.
7. "Researchers train AI to diagnose lung diseases," *Charles Darwin University*, [online]. Available: https://www.cdu.edu.au/news/researchers-train-ai-diagnose-lung-diseases. Accessed: Feb. 4, 2025.

8. V. T. Tiwari and S. Jyoti, "AM-FM features and their application to noise-robust speech recognition: A review," *The IUP Journal of Telecommunications,* vol. 2, no. 1, pp. 7–19, 2010.
9. J. Heitmann *et al.*, "DeepBreath—Automated detection of respiratory pathology from lung auscultation in 572 pediatric outpatients across 5 countries," *NPJ Digital Medicine*, vol. 6, no. 1, p. 104, 2023.
10. "V. Tiwari, "MFCC and its applications in speaker recognition," 2010. [online]. Available: https://api.semanticscholar.org/CorpusID:212584631.
11. Q. Zhao *et al.*, "Deep learning in heart sound analysis: From techniques to clinical applications," *Health Data Science*, vol. 4, p. 0182, 2024. [Online]. Available: https://spj.science.org/doi/abs/10.34133/hds.0182.
12. Y. Y. Poh *et al.*, "Real-time neonatal chest sound separation using deep learning," 2023. [Online]. Available: https://arxiv.org/abs/2310.17116.
13. Y. Zhu, A. Smith, and K. Hauser, "Automated heart and lung auscultation in robotic physical examinations," 2022. [Online]. Available: https://arxiv.org/abs/2201.09511.
14. K.-H. Tsai *et al.*, "Blind monaural source separation on heart and lung sounds based on periodic-coded deep autoencoder," *IEEE Journal of Biomedical and Health Informatics*, vol. 24, no. 11, pp. 3203–3214, Nov. 2020. [Online]. Available: http://dx.doi.org/10.1109/JBHI.2020.3016831.
15. Q. Liu, X. Wu, and X. Ma, "An automatic segmentation method for heart sounds," *BioMedical Engineering Online*, vol. 17, no. 1, p. 106, Aug. 2018.
16. C. Wall *et al.*, "A deep ensemble neural network with attention mechanisms for lung abnormality classification using audio inputs," *Sensors*, vol. 22, no. 15, 2022. [Online]. Available: https://www.mdpi.com/1424-8220/22/15/5566.
17. S. Rasouli, D. Alkurdi, and B. Jia, "The role of artificial intelligence in modern medical education and practice: A systematic literature review," *medRxiv*, 2024. [Online]. Available: https://www.medrxiv.org/content/early/2024/07/26/2024.07.25.24311022.
18. S. H. Lee *et al.*, "Fully portable continuous real-time auscultation with a soft wearable stethoscope designed for automated disease diagnosis," *Science Advances*, vol. 8, no. 21, p. eabo5867, 2022. [Online]. Available: https://www.science.org/doi/abs/10.1126/sciadv.abo5867.

5 Individual Discriminating Power Assessment of ECG Multi-Scale Entropies for Cardiovascular Disease Detection

Pedro Ribeiro, João Alexandre Marques Lobo, and Pedro Miguel Rodrigues

5.1 INTRODUCTION

In recent years, a notable surge in computational power has been driven by advanced hardware, parallel computing, cloud resources, and increased data accessibility. These developments have significantly enhanced machine learning (ML) applications to support CVDs' detection (Azmi et al. 2022). The rise of patients with cardiovascular diseases has been a major concern for the world population. According to the World Health Organization, 32% of global mortality is attributed to cardiovascular diseases (CVDs), which affect heart function and condition, with the most prevalent being arrhythmias, cardiac arrests, and heart failure (World Health Organization 2021), with an increase until 28% for cases like heart stroke over a 20-year period (Lim 2013). Heart disease is a term for health issues that affect the heart's function and condition. There are different types of heart disease, including:

- **Myocardial Infarction:** Also known as heart attack, it is often caused by a decrease or stoppage of the blood flow to a portion of the heart. Typically, this is the result of a blood clot in the epicardial artery that supplies that portion of the myocardium (Byrne et al. 2023; Saleh and Ambrose 2018).
- **ST/T Change:** As the name implies, ST/T is a group of cardiovascular diseases that affect the ST segment and the T wave portions of the ECG signal (Wohlfart 1987). Some of the changes present in the database used in this chapter were long QT-interval, ischemic ST/T changes, and physiological

DOI: 10.1201/9781003797524-5

nature changes compatible with abnormalities in the electrolytes (Wagner et al. 2020; Wagner et al. 2022).

- **Conduction Disturbance:** These are a group of diseases that affect the electrical conduction of the heart. Some of the diseases present in the database are Left Anterior Fascicular Block, Incomplete Bundle Branch Block, and first-degree AV Block (Chiu et al. 2008).
- **Hypertrophy:** it is defined as the increase in mass, which is associated with changes in the heart structure. These changes come with altered ECG patterns. Some examples of these kinds of diseases are Left Ventricular Hypertrophy, Left Atrial Overload/Enlargement, and Right Ventricular Hypertrophy (Bacharova and Estes 2017; Baghdadi et al. 2023).

The early and correct diagnosis can make a difference in the outcomes of the disease. In some cases, the early diagnosis can make the difference between life and death for a patient (Baghdadi et al. 2023). Electrocardiogram (ECG), more specifically the 12-lead ECG, is a key diagnostic test for CVDs, assessing risk, and identifying CVDs (Ribeiro et al. 2024). However, to counter the recent significant increase, strategies such as early diagnosis or prognosis can reduce the impact caused by CVDs on the patient (Karunathilake, Ganegoda, and others 2018). This study aims to:

- Introduce 18 multi-scale Entropies (*ApEn*, *SampEn*, *FuzzEn*, *K2En*, *PermEn*, *CondEn*, *DistEn*, *DispEn*, *SpecEn*, *SyDyEn*, *IncrEn*, *CoSiEn*, *PhasEn*, *SlopEn*, *BubbEn*, *GridEn*, *EnofEn*, and *AttnEn*) extracted from ECG signals under 1s 50% overlapping analyses using rectangular windows.
- Improve the discrimination between healthy control and CVDs using the extracted features' power.
- Evaluate the performance of multi-scale features by inputting them into a comprehensive number of ML classifiers.
- Provide a model that uses a simple tool based on very accessible ECG parameters to discriminate and generate a prediction to determine whether the patients have a CVD.

Table 5.1 presents state-of-the-art studies on distinguishing between healthy controls and CVD patients using the same dataset.

5.2 METHODOLOGY

5.2.1 Experimental Setup

The study was accomplished by using MATLAB, version R2022a for the features extraction, and Python (version 3.10.4) was used to develop and implement various ML models and generate a discrimination report based on the obtained results. The computer used for this study was a MacBook Pro 14 with an M1 Pro (8-core CPU, 14-core GPU) and 16 GB RAM.

TABLE 5.1
Report of State-of-the-Art Literature on the Same Database

Ref	Year	Comparison Group (Number of participants)	Features Extracted	Classifier	Validation	Accuracy	F1-Score
(Karthik et al. 2022)	2022	All vs. All (2965)	Features extracted from DLECG-CVD	DLECG-CVD	Hold-on	88.44%	90.82%
(Chumachenko et al. 2022)	2022	Norm (674) vs. MI (2022)	BPM, IBI, SDNN, RMSSD	Random Forest	Hold-on	99.63%	99.26%
(Pałczyński et al. 2022)	2022	Norm (758) vs. Abnormal (539)	Features extracted from FSL	FSL + SVM	Cross-validation	91.30%	90.50%
(Śmigiel, Pałczyński, and Ledziński 2021)	2021	Norm (1465) vs. Abnormal (1095)	Shannon entropy, Approximate entropy, Sample entropy, Permutation entropy, Spectral entropy, SVD entropy, Rényi entropy, Tsallis entropy and Extropy	CNN	Hold-on	89.20%	89.10%
(Śmigiel 2022)	2022	Norm (1469) vs. Abnormal (1083)	Orthogonal Matching Pursuit features similar to the median R-peak or the QRS extraction	XGBoost	Cross-validation	90.60%	90.40%
Present Study	2025	Healthy Control(100) vs. CVD(100)	18 Multi-scale Entropies	RF or KNN or SVC	Hold-on	95%	94.74%

5.2.2 The Database

The present study used 200 participants from the PTB-XL [7,8] randomly selected from a set of 21799 ECG records. Reducing the instances has been done so as not to overuse the statistical analysis method. Healthy control and CVD group (Myocardial Infarction, ST/T Change, Conduction Disturbance, and Hypertrophy) were formed with 100 instances each for the next stages. Each 10-second ECG sample includes 12 leads (I, II, III, αVr, αVl, αVf, V1, V2, V3, V4, V5, and V6), recorded at a 500 Hz sampling frequency.

5.2.3 ECG Filtering

This process comprehends the application of an elliptical band-pass filter with order 32 plus frequency cut-offs 1 Hz and 40 Hz, a *Steepness* of 0.85, and a *StopBandAttenuation* of 60 db to each ECG signal lead of every included patient. Figure 5.1 illustrates the filter application on a raw ECG signal.

5.2.4 Signal Normalization

The ECG signals, $x(n)$, were normalized according to the following equation (Rodrigues et al. 2021).

$$x(n) = \frac{x(n)}{\sum_{n=0}^{N-1} x^2(n)} \tag{5.1}$$

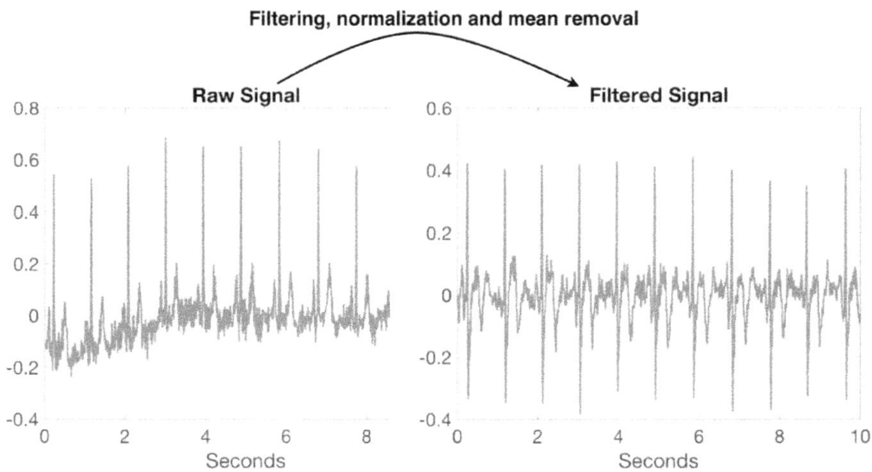

FIGURE 5.1 Filter application.

5.2.5 Windowing Process and Multi-Scale Entropy Extraction

A windowing process for multi-scale Entropy extraction was applied; it comprises a sliding rectangular window analysis of 1-second length with an overlap of 50%. Figure 5.2 illustrates the process used for this work.

Evaluating signals using different entropy metrics is crucial because each metric captures unique aspects of the complexity and irregularity of the signal. Therefore, extracting different entropy metrics is vital for comprehensive signal analysis as: (1) Entropy metrics like Sample Entropy and Distribution Entropy have different sensitivities to patterns and noise (e.g., sample entropy is more robust to noise and can better handle short data lengths, while Distribution Entropy is more sensitive to the overall distribution of values (Borowska 2015; C. Liu et al. 2018)); (2) different entropy measures can capture various aspects of a signal's complexity an dynamics. For example, Permutation Entropy is particularly good at detecting changes in the temporal order of values, which can be crucial to understanding the underlying dynamics of a system (Borowska 2015; Kay et al. 2024); (3) different fields may require different entropy measures. For example, in biomedical signal processing, certain entropy measures might be better suited for detecting specific physiological states or conditions (Borowska 2015; Araújo, Teixeira, and Rodrigues 2022; Silva, Batista, and Rodrigues 2022; Silva et al. 2023; Richman and Moorman 2000). Based on the previously mentioned reasons, we applied a comprehensive set of entropy metrics in this study to ensure we extract the most relevant information from the data, thereby maximizing the final discrimination results. Thus, for all study participants per each signal's leads and window of analysis, 18 Multi-scale-based Entropies were extracted. The 18 Entropies are described below:

- **Approximate Entropy** (*ApEn*) has the equation defined as

$$ApEn(m,r) = \lim_{N \to \infty} \left[\phi m(r) - \phi m + 1(r) \right], \tag{5.2}$$

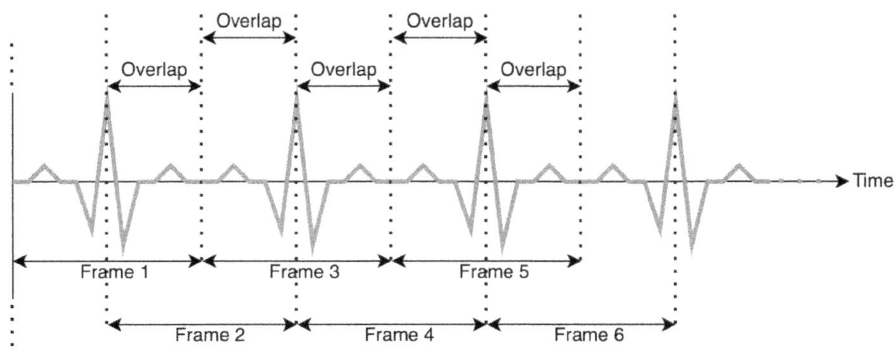

FIGURE 5.2 Windowing process illustration.

where ϕ is the Heaviside step dimension, and m is the dimension (Caesarendra et al. 2013).

- **Sample Entropy** (*SampEn*) is defined as

$$SampEn(m,r,N) = -\ln\left(\frac{n^{m+1}}{n^{m}}\right), \tag{5.3}$$

where m is the length of the vector, r is the tolerance, N is the total size of the vector, and n is the vector portion that is being analyzed (Richman, Lake, and Moorman 2004).

- **Fuzzy Entropy** (*FuzzEn*) is defined as

$$FuzzEn(x,m,r,n_e,d) = -\ln\left(\frac{\psi^{m+1,d}(n_e,r)}{\psi^{m,d}(n_e,r)}\right), \tag{5.4}$$

where $\psi^{m,d}(n_e,r)$ is defined as

$$\psi^{m,d}(n_e,r) = \frac{\sum_{\Lambda=1}^{N-md}\sum_{\lambda=1,\lambda\neq\Lambda}^{N-md}\exp\left(-\frac{\Delta_{\Lambda,\lambda}^{n_e}}{r}\right)}{(N-md)(N-md-1)}, \tag{5.5}$$

in which r is the resolution and m is the dimension (Azami et al. 2019).

- **Kolmogorov Entropy** (*K2En*) – in this study, the *K2En* refers to the second-order Kolmogorov entropy and the equation is defined as

$$K2En = \lim_{\varepsilon\to 0}\lim_{d\to\infty}\frac{\ln\left[\frac{C_d(\varepsilon)}{C_{d+1}(\varepsilon)}\right]}{\tau}, \tag{5.6}$$

where $C_d(\varepsilon)$ is the correlation integral (Gao, Wang, and Chen 2013).

- **Permutation Entropy** (*PermEn*) is defined as

$$PermEn(m) = -\sum_{v=1}^{k} P_v \ln P_v, \tag{5.7}$$

where P is the probability distribution for each symbol (Bian et al. 2012).

- **Conditional Entropy** (*CondEn*) has the equation defined as

$$CondEn(L/L-1) = E(L) - E(L-1), \tag{5.8}$$

where E is the Shannon Entropy, and L is the dimension (Porta et al. 1998).

- **Distribution Entropy** (*DistEn*) is defined as

$$DistEn = -\sum_{t=1}^{M} p_t \log_2(p_t), \tag{5.9}$$

where p is the probability of each bin (Li et al. 2015).

- **Dispersion Entropy** (*DispEn*) is defined as

$$DispEn = -\sum_{\pi=1}^{c^m} p(\pi_{v_0v_1\ldots v_{m-1}}) \ln(p(\pi_{v_0v_1\ldots v_{m-1}})), \tag{5.10}$$

where $\pi_{v_0v_1\ldots v_{m-1}}$ is the dispersion pattern and c^m is the potential dispersion patterns (Rostaghi and Azami 2016).

- **Spectral Entropy** (*SpecEn*) has a formula defined as

$$SpecEn = -\sum_{f=0}^{f_n} S(f) \log S(f), \tag{5.11}$$

where $S(f)$ is the power spectrum and f_n is the upper limit frequency (Inouye et al. 1991).

- **Symbolic Dynamic Entropy** (*SyDyEn*) is defined as

$$SyDyEn = -\sum_{l=1}^{4^m} p(l) \log p(l), \tag{5.12}$$

where $p(l)$ is the probability of occurrence (Wang et al. 2015).

- **Increment Entropy** (*IncrEn*) is defined as

$$IncrEn = -\frac{\sum_{n=1}^{(2q+1)^m} p(w_n)\log p(w_n)}{m-1}, \tag{5.13}$$

where $p(w_n)$ is the frequency of each unique word, q is the quantifying precision, and m is the dimension (X. Liu et al. 2018).

- **Cosine Similarity Entropy** (*CoSiEn*) has a formula defined as

$$CoSiEn = -B_{(\varepsilon)}^{(m)}(r_{CSE})\log_2 B_{(\varepsilon)}^{(m)}(r_{CSE}) + \left(1 - B_{(\varepsilon)}^{(m)}(r_{CSE})\right)\log_2\left(1 - B_{(\varepsilon)}^{(m)}(r_{CSE})\right), \tag{5.14}$$

where $B_{(\varepsilon)}^{(m)}(r_{CSE})$ is the global probability of occurrences of similar patterns and r_{CSE} is the tolerance (Chanwimalueang and Mandic 2017).

- **Phase Entropy** (*PhasEn*) is defined as

$$PhasEn = -\frac{\sum_{i=1}^{k} p(i)\log p(i)}{\log k}, \tag{5.15}$$

where the $p(i)$ is the probability distribution and k is the maximum sector of i (Rohila and Sharma 2019).

- **Slope Entropy** (*SlopEn*) is defined as the computation of a subsequence

of symbols. Those symbols are defined by

$$\begin{cases} d > \gamma \rightarrow 2 \\ d \leq \gamma \;\&\; d > \delta \rightarrow 1 \\ |d| \leq \delta \rightarrow 0 \\ d\langle -\delta \;\; d\rangle - \gamma \rightarrow -1 \\ d < -\gamma \rightarrow -2 \end{cases} \tag{5.16}$$

where d is the difference between two consecutive samples and γ and δ are thresholds (Cuesta-Frau et al. 2020).

- **Bubble Entropy** (*BubbEn*) is defined as

$$BubbEn = \frac{H_{swaps}^{m+1} - H_{swaps}^{m}}{\log\left(\frac{m+1}{m-1}\right)}, \tag{5.17}$$

where H_{swaps}^{m} is the conditional Rényi entropy (Manis, Aktaruzzaman, and Sassi 2017).

- **Gridded Distribution Entropy** (*GridEn*) is defined as

$$GridEn = -\sum_{j=1}^{n^2} p_j \log p_j, \tag{5.18}$$

where j is the jth grid and the p_j is the probability of each grid (Yan et al. 2019).

- **Entropy of Entropy** (*EnofEn*) can be defined as

$$EnofEn = -\sum_{l=1}^{s_2} p_l \ln p_l, \tag{5.19}$$

where l is the level index (Hsu et al. 2017).

- **Attention Entropy** (*AttnEn*) is defined as

$$AttnEn = -\sum_{j=0}^{d_2} a_{i,j} \log a_{i,j}, \tag{5.20}$$

where $a_{i,j}$ are the attention weights between the positions i and j (Attanasio et al. 2022).

Each Multi-scale Entropy has been extracted from scales 1 to 3 (scale 1: 0 – 250 Hz, scale 2: 0 – 125 Hz, and scale 3: 0 – 93.3 Hz), where each scale includes downsampled versions of the original signal, adjusted by the respective scale factor. Figure 5.3 illustrates the way the Multi-scale part of the Entropy process operates.

5.2.6 Data Compressor

Taking into consideration that the 18 Entropies were extracted from (x) 3 scales under sliding window analyses over time, 6 distinct statistical functions acted like

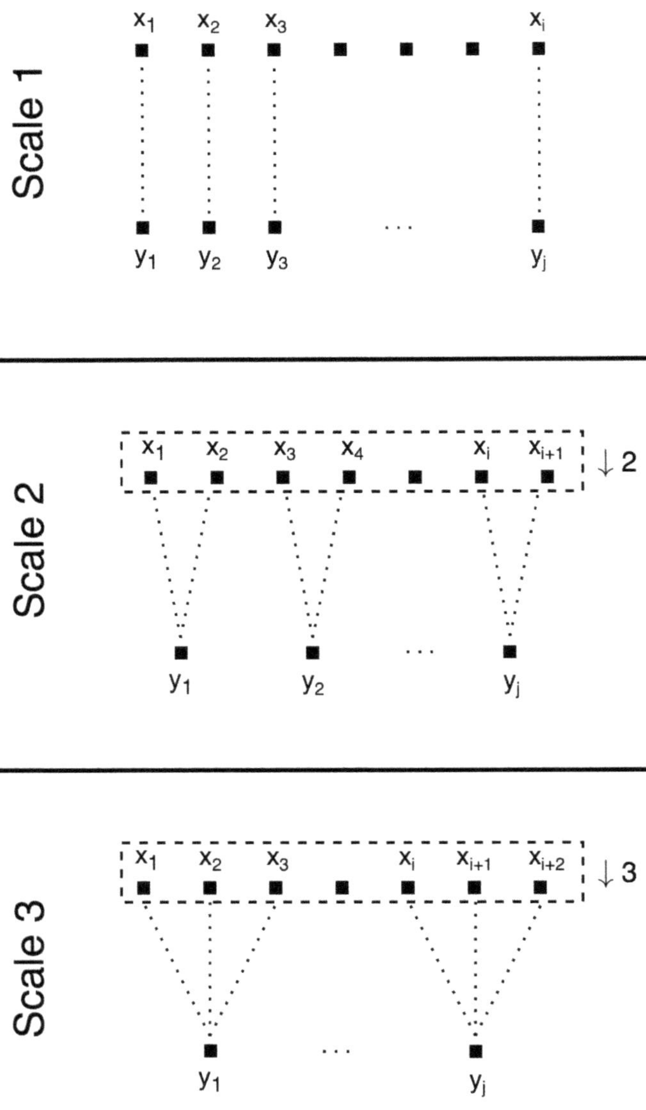

FIGURE 5.3 Multi-scale diagram decomposition.

time-data compressors (Ribeiro et al. 2023) per scale, reducing the dimensional problem for ML and statistical analyses. The six statistical used functions were:

- **Average** (Avg) is calculated by the sum of values in the vector and then divided by the length of the vector (Peck, Olsen, and Devore 2008). The equation is defined as

$$Avg = \frac{\sum_{n=1}^{N} x(n)}{N}, \tag{5.21}$$

where N is the length of the vector, and x is the vector.

- Standard Deviation (Std) is a measure of how dispersed the data is relative to the mean (Peck, Olsen, and Devore 2008) and can be defined as

$$Std = \sqrt{\frac{\sum_{n=1}^{N} |x(n) - Avg|^2}{N-1}} \tag{5.22}$$

- **95th Percentile** ($P95$) is the number that is equal to or greater than 95% of the values present in a vector (Rosner 2010). *P95* is obtained by ordering the values in increasing order and using the formula

$$n_{P95} = 0.95 * K, \tag{5.23}$$

where n_{P95} is the $P95$ position in a vector and K is the number of samples.

- **Variance** (Var) is the spread of numbers in a vector (Rosner 2010) and is defined as

$$Var = \frac{\sum_{n=1}^{N} |x(n) - Avg|^2}{N-1} \tag{5.24}$$

- **Median** (Med) is the value separating the highest values in half from the lowest values. Med is obtained by arranging the values in ascending order and using the equation

$$n_{Med} = 0.5 * K, \tag{5.25}$$

where n_{Med} is the Med position in an array and K is the number of samples (Rosner 2010).

- **Kurtosis** (Kur) measures how a distribution differs from a normal distribution. The equation is defined as

$$Kur = \frac{\sum_{n=1}^{N} |x(n) - Avg|^4}{Std^4} \tag{5.26}$$

5.2.7 Feature Selection by Statistical Analysis

T-test statistical tool has been used to evaluate the individual discriminating power of features to differentiate between binary classes per scale and lead. This stage was used to perform a feature pre-triage for the ML stage, where only the distributions of features that proved to be statistically relevant with the p-value < 0.05 were selected to be present to the ML entries for discrimination.

5.2.8 Machine Learning Approaches

A total of 19 Scikit-learn-classifiers (Pordeus et al. 2023; Ribeiro et al. 2024) have been selected for discrimination between the two classes by evaluating each selected feature's discrimination power in an 80/20 training/testing split evaluation. The classifiers used in this study are listed and explained in Table 5.2.

Fig. 5.4 summarizes all the methodological approaches applied in the present work.

5.3 RESULTS

Figure 5.5 shows a bar graph with the total number of statistical analyses that presented significant differences per scale and lead.

Figure 5.6 shows a heat-map that indicates the best classification results per lead. To build the heat-map per lead, the best Entropy feature has been selected based on its *Accuracy* to discriminate between the Healthy control and the CVD group.

Figure 5.7 illustrates the total number of statistical analyses that presented significant differences per scale and per feature in the form of a bar graph.

Figure 5.8 presents a heat-map showing the best classification results per lead.

5.4 DISCUSSION

A total of 3498 statistical analyses were done; after that, only the analysis with significant differences ($p<0.05$) was used for the Machine learning discrimination. The percentage of statistical analyses with significant differences was 16.58% (580 out of 3498).

Figure 5.5 shows the number of statistical analyses that present significant differences per lead; in this graph, we can see that Lead *III* obtained the highest number of statistical differences with 60 out of 580 (10.34%). *Scale 3* was the scale with the highest number of distributions with statistical differences, with 210 distributions out of 580 (36.21%). Figure 5.7 allows us to get a similar conclusion as the previous table regarding *Scale 3*. This table, however, details the number of significant

TABLE 5.2
Description of the 19 Scikit-Learn Classifiers Used in This Study

Classifier	Hyperparameter	Definition
Support-vector Machines (SVC)	Default parameters + Gamma set to "auto"	SVC is a powerful classification method that finds the optimal hyperplane to separate different classes in the feature space. It works well for both linear and non-linear data by using kernel functions to transform the data into higher dimensions (Chang and Lin 2011).
Gaussian Process Classifier (GauPro)	Default parameters + 1.0*RBF(1.0)	This classifier uses a Gaussian process to define a distribution over possible functions that fit the data. It provides probabilistic predictions and is particularly useful for small datasets with complex relationships. The RBF kernel defines the covariance function, which helps in capturing the smoothness of the data (Rasmussen 2006).
Linear SVC (LinSVC)	Default parameters	LinSVC is a linear classifier that uses the same principles as SVC but is optimized for large datasets. It is efficient and scales well with the number of samples and features. It uses a linear kernel and is implemented in terms of liblinear, which allows for more flexibility in the choice of penalties and loss functions (Fan et al. 2008).
SGD Classifier (SGD)	Default parameters (e.g., max iter was 100, and tol was 0.001)	This classifier uses stochastic gradient descent to optimize linear models. It is suitable for large-scale learning and can handle various loss functions, making it versatile for different types of classification problems (Newton, Yousefian, and Pasupathy 2018).
KNearest Neighbors Classifier (KNN)	Default parameters (e.g., 5 neighbors and uniform weights)	KNN is a simple, instance-based learning algorithm that classifies a sample based on the majority vote of its k-nearest neighbors. It is intuitive and effective for small datasets with clear class boundaries (Cunningham and Delany 2021).
Logistic Regression (LogReg)	Default parameters + solver set to "lbfgs"	LogReg is a linear model used for binary classification. It estimates the probability that a given input belongs to a particular class using the logistic function. The solver "lbfgs" is used for optimization, which is efficient for small to medium-sized datasets (LaValley 2008).
Logistic RegressionCV (LogRegCV)	Default parameters + cv set to 3	This is an extension of Logistic Regression that includes cross-validation to automatically select the best regularization parameter, improving the model's generalization performance. The cv parameter is set to 3, meaning it uses 3-fold cross-validation (LaValley 2008).
Bagging Classifier (BaggC)	Default parameters (e.g., Decision Tree Classifier as the base estimator)	BaggC is an ensemble method that combines multiple base classifiers trained on random subsets of the data. It reduces variance and improves the stability and accuracy of the model (Breiman 1996).

(Continued)

TABLE 5.2 CONTINUED
Description of the 19 Scikit-Learn Classifiers Used in This Study

Classifier	Hyperparameter	Definition
ExtraTrees Classifier (ExTreeC)	Default parameters + n estimators set to 300	This ensemble method builds multiple randomized decision trees and averages their predictions. It is similar to Random Forest but introduces more randomness to reduce overfitting (Geurts, Ernst, and Wehenkel 2006).
Random Forest Classifier (RF)	Default parameters + the max depth, n estimators, and max features set to 5, 300, and 1, respectively	RF is an ensemble method that constructs multiple decision trees and merges their predictions. It is robust to overfitting and provides high accuracy for various classification tasks (Breiman 2001).
Gaussian Naive Bayes (GauNB)	Default parameters	GauNBis a probabilistic classifier based on Bayes' theorem. It assumes that features follow a Gaussian distribution and is particularly effective for high-dimensional data (Anand et al. 2022).
Decision Tree Classifier (DeTreeC)	Default parameters + max depth set to 5	DeTreeC splits the data into subsets based on feature values, creating a tree-like model of decisions. It is easy to interpret and can handle both numerical and categorical data (Breiman et al. 2017).
MLP Classifier (MLP)	Default parameters + alpha set to 1, and max iter equal to 1000	MLP is a neural network model with an input layer, one hidden layer, and an output layer. It uses forward propagation to pass input data through the network, applying a weighted sum and an activation function at each neuron to introduce non-linearity. The model calculates the loss by comparing the output to the target values and adjusts the weights through backward propagation to minimize this loss. Key parameters include alpha, which helps prevent overfitting by penalizing large weights, and max iter, which sets the maximum number of iterations for convergence. MLPs are versatile and can handle both classification and regression tasks, but they can be computationally intensive and require careful tuning of hyperparameters (Haykin 2008).
AdaBoost Classifier (AdaBoost)	Default parameters	AdaBoost is an ensemble method that combines multiple weak classifiers to form a strong classifier. It adjusts the weights of incorrectly classified samples to focus on difficult cases (Chengsheng, Huacheng, and Bing 2017).
Linear Discriminant Analysis (LinDis)	Default parameters	LinDis is a linear classifier that projects the data onto a lower-dimensional space to maximize class separability. It is effective for datasets with well-separated classes (Tharwat 2016).

(Continued)

TABLE 5.2 CONTINUED
Description of the 19 Scikit-Learn Classifiers Used in This Study

Classifier	Hyperparameter	Definition
Quadratic Discriminant Analysis (QuadDis)	Default parameters	QuadDis is similar to LinDis but allows for quadratic decision boundaries. It is useful when the class distributions have different covariances (Tharwat 2016).
OneVsRest Classifier (OvsR)	Default parameters + random state equal to 0	This strategy is used for multiclass classification by fitting one classifier per class. Each classifier predicts whether a sample belongs to its class or not (Vogiatzis et al. 2021).
Gradient Boosting Classifier (GradBoost)	Default parameters	GradBoost is an ensemble method that builds trees sequentially to minimize the loss function. It is highly effective for both classification and regression tasks (Natekin and Knoll 2013).
SGD Classifier (SGDC)	Default parameters	It uses stochastic gradient descent for optimization. It is efficient for large-scale learning and supports various loss functions (Newton, Yousefian, and Pasupathy 2018).

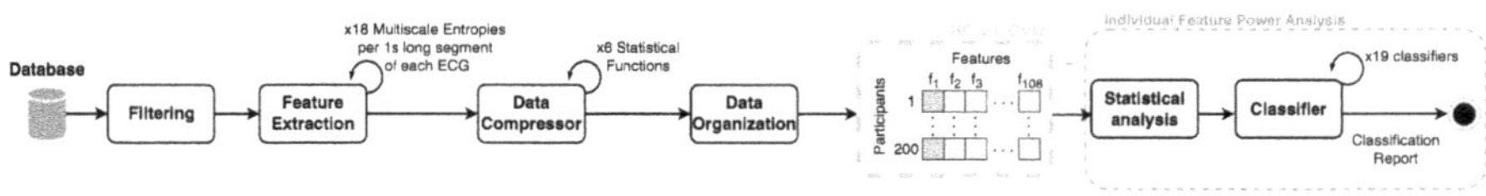

FIGURE 5.4 Workflow diagram.

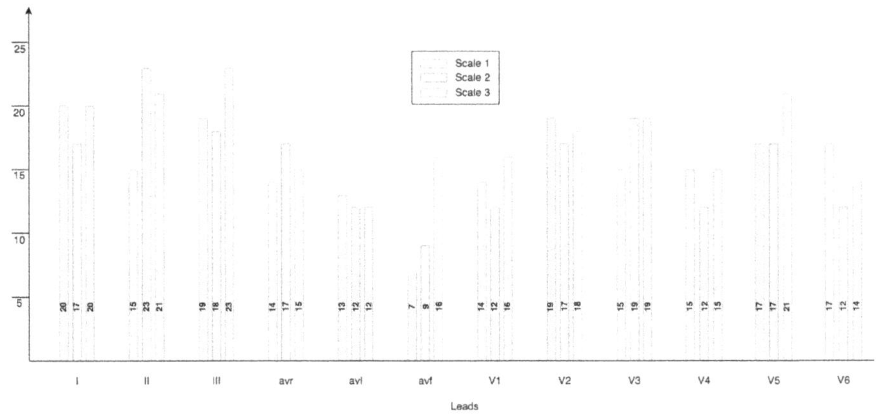

FIGURE 5.5 Total number of statistical analyses with significant differences per scale per lead.

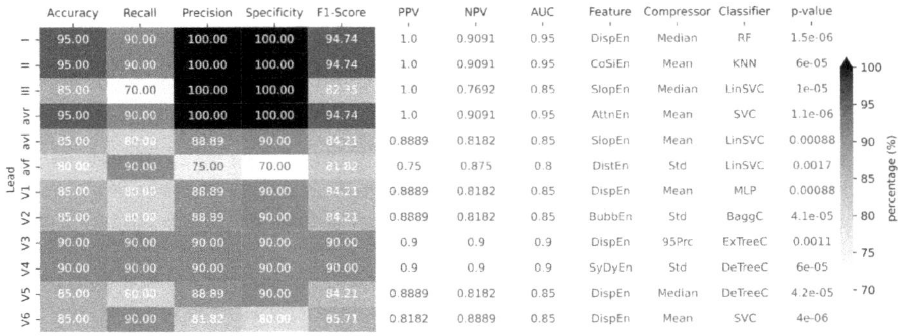

FIGURE 5.6 Best classification results per lead.

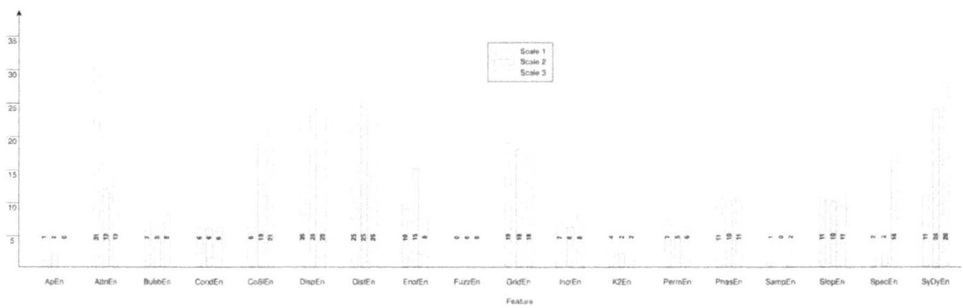

FIGURE 5.7 Total number of statistical analyses with significant differences per scale per feature.

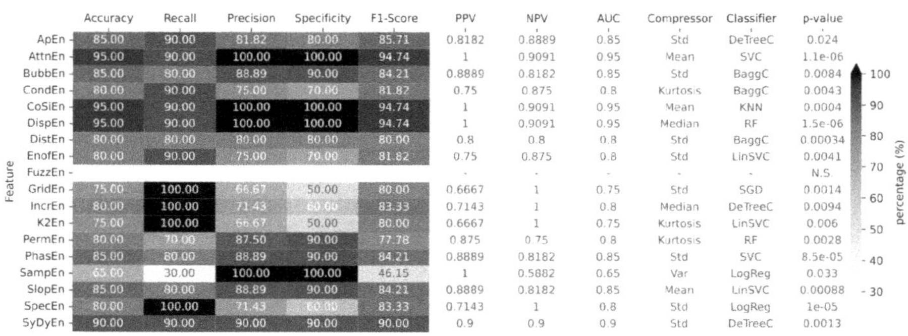

FIGURE 5.8 Best classification results per feature.

statistical distributions per feature. Notably, the features with the highest number of significant distributions were *DispEn* and *DistEn*, each with 75 distributions out of 580, accounting for 12.93%.

Figure 5.6 shows the best classification results per lead. The best overall results were found in the leads *I*, *II*, and *avr* with the *Accuracy*, *Recall*, *Precision*, *Specificity*,

F1Score, *PPV*, *NPV*, and *AUC* reaching 95%, 90%, 100%, 100%, 94.74%, 1, 0.9091, and 0.95, respectively. The feature that showed better adaptation to the CVD's activity along the leads was *DispEn*, appearing in 50% (6 out of 12) as the best one for discrimination between classes along leads. The *Mean* was the compressor that showed the best ability to emphasize the capability of the extracted features to discriminate along the lead, representing 41.67% (5 out of 12).

Figure 5.8 shows the best classification results per feature for all analyses. The best overall results were found by using the features *AttnEn* and *DispEn* with the discrimination *Accuracy*, *Recall*, *Precision*, *Specificity*, *F1Score*, *PPV*, *NPV*, and *AUC* reaching 95%, 90%, 100%, 100%, 94.74%, 1, 0.9091, and 0.95, respectively. The feature *FuzzEn* did not show statistically significant differences across all its distributions, and as a result, it was excluded from the input set for the ML classifiers.

In Table 5.1, we can see that our approach proved to have a better performance than 80% (4 out of 5) of the state-of-the-art studies, with an accuracy improvement ranging between 3.7 percentage points and 5.8 percentage points.

We can also see that, as far as we know, this is the first time that Multi-scale Entropy analyses have been applied to ECG signals for CVD's detection. However, our study used only 200 samples, which is a small sample size compared to the state-of-the-art works in Table 1.

5.5 CONCLUSION

For this research, 18 Multi-scale Entropies (ApEn, SampEn, FuzzEn, K2En, PermEn, CondEn, DistEn, DispEn, SpecEn, SyDyEn, IncrEn, CoSiEn, PhasEn, SlopEn, BubbEn, GridEn, Enof En and AttnEn) were extracted from 200 records in a well-known ECG database (PTB-XL dataset). From the recorded 12 leads per patient, each signal lead underwent a 1-second length with a 50% overlapped rectangular windowing process over time for extracting a total of 18 features per window. At the end of the process, each feature time series was compacted by six statistics. The individual power was accessed to discriminate between the Normal class (Healthy controls) and the abnormal class (CVD patients).

The *Accuracy* discrimination results ranged between 65% and 95%. The results demonstrate that the applied method is a robust tool for effectively distinguishing between Healthy patients and patients with CVDs through the analysis of ECG signals. The level of detail and discrimination achieved surpasses what is typically observed in state-of-the-art studies using the same dataset and classes.

Although our results indicate strong performance in differentiating between healthy controls and CVD patients, this study utilized only a small portion of the available database. Future studies should apply the algorithm to the entire dataset to verify and generalize its performance on a larger scale.

ACKNOWLEDGMENTS

This work was supported by National Funds from FCT – Fundação para a Ciência e a Tecnologia through project UIDB/50016/2020.

REFERENCES

Anand, M. Vijay, B. KiranBala, S. R. Srividhya, Kavitha C., Mohammed Younus, and Md Habibur Rahman. 2022. 'Gaussian Naïve Bayes Algorithm: A Reliable Technique Involved in the Assortment of the Segregation in Cancer'. Edited by Praveen Kumar ReddyM . *Mobile Information Systems* 2022 (June). Hindawi Limited: 1–7. doi:10.1155/2022/2436946.

Araújo, Teresa, João Paulo Teixeira, and Pedro Miguel Rodrigues. 2022. 'Smart-Data-Driven System for Alzheimer Disease Detection through Electroencephalographic Signals'. *Bioengineering* 9 (4). MDPI AG: 141. doi:10.3390/bioengineering9040141.

Attanasio, Giuseppe, Debora Nozza, Dirk Hovy, and Elena Baralis. 2022. 'Entropy-Based Attention Regularization Frees Unintended Bias Mitigation from Lists'. *ArXiv Preprint.*

Azami, Hamed, Peng Li, Steven E. Arnold, Javier Escudero, and Anne Humeau-Heurtier. 2019. 'Fuzzy Entropy Metrics for the Analysis of Biomedical Signals: Assessment and Comparison'. *IEEE Access* 7. IEEE: 104833–104847.

Azmi, Javed, Muhammad Arif, Md Tabrez Nafis, M. Afshar Alam, Safdar Tanweer, and Guojun Wang. 2022. 'A Systematic Review on Machine Learning Approaches for Cardiovascular Disease Prediction Using Medical Big Data'. *Medical Engineering & Physics* 105. Elsevier: 103825.

Bacharova, Ljuba, and E. Harvey Estes. 2017. 'Left Ventricular Hypertrophy by the Surface ECG'. *Journal of Electrocardiology* 50 (6). Elsevier: 906–908.

Baghdadi, Nadiah A., Sally Mohammed Farghaly Abdelaliem, Amer Malki, Ibrahim Gad, Ashraf Ewis, and Elsayed Atlam. 2023. 'Advanced Machine Learning Techniques for Cardiovascular Disease Early Detection and Diagnosis'. *Journal of Big Data* 10 (1). Springer: 144.

Bian, Chunhua, Chang Qin, Qianli D. Y. Ma, and Qinghong Shen. 2012. 'Modified Permutation-Entropy Analysis of Heartbeat Dynamics'. *Physical Review E—Statistical, Nonlinear, and Soft Matter Physics* 85 (2). APS: 21906.

Borowska, Marta. 2015. 'Entropy-Based Algorithms in the Analysis of Biomedical Signals'. *Studies in Logic, Grammar and Rhetoric* 43 (1). Walter de Gruyter GmbH: 21–32.

Breiman, Leo. 1996. 'Bagging Predictors'. *Machine Learning* 24 (2). Springer Science and Business Media LLC: 123–140. doi:10.1007/bf00058655.

Breiman, Leo. 2001. 'Random Forests'. *Machine Learning* 45 (1). Springer Science and Business Media LLC: 5–32. doi:10.1023/a:1010933404324.

Breiman, Leo, Jerome H. Friedman, Richard A. Olshen, and Charles J. Stone. 2017. *Classification and Regression Trees.* Routledge. doi:10.1201/9781315139470.

Byrne, Robert, Xavier Rossello, J. Coughlan, Emanuele Barbato, Colin Berry, Alaide Chieffo, Marc Claeys, et al. 2023. '2023 ESC Guidelines for the Management of Acute Coronary Syndromes'. *European Heart Journal* 13 (1). Oxford University Press (OUP): 55–161.

Caesarendra, Wahyu, Buyung Kosasih, Kiet Tieu, and Craig A. S. Moodie. 2013. 'An Application of Nonlinear Feature Extraction – A Case Study for Low Speed Slewing Bearing Condition Monitoring and Prognosis'. In *2013 IEEE/ASME International Conference on Advanced Intelligent Mechatronics.* Wollongong: IEEE.

Chang, Chih-Chung, and Chih-Jen Lin. 2011. 'LIBSVM: A Library for Support Vector Machines'. *ACM Transactions on Intelligent Systems and Technology* 2 (3). Association for Computing Machinery (ACM): 1–27. doi:10.1145/1961189.1961199.

Chanwimalueang, Theerasak, and Danilo P. Mandic. 2017. 'Cosine Similarity Entropy: Self-Correlation-Based Complexity Analysis of Dynamical Systems'. *Entropy* 19 (12). MDPI: 652.

Chengsheng, Tu, Liu Huacheng, and Xu Bing. 2017. 'AdaBoost Typical Algorithm and Its Application Research'. Edited by Bing Xu and Yinong Chen. *MATEC Web of Conferences* 139. EDP Sciences: 222. doi:10.1051/matecconf/201713900222.

Chiu, Shuenn-Nan, Jou-Kou Wang, Mei-Hwan Wu, Chi-Wei Chang, Chun-An Chen, Ming-Tai Lin, En-Ting Wu, et al. 2008. 'Cardiac Conduction Disturbance Detected in a Pediatric Population'. *The Journal of Pediatrics* 152 (1). Elsevier: 85–89.

Chumachenko, Dmytro, Mykola Butkevych, Daniel Lode, Marcus Frohme, SchmailzlKurt J. G. , and Alina Nechyporenko. 2022. 'Machine Learning Methods in Predicting Patients with Suspected Myocardial Infarction Based on Short-Time HRV Data'. *Sensors* 22 (18). MDPI: 7033.

Cuesta-Frau, David, Jakub Schneider, Eduard Bakštein, Pavel Vostatek, Filip Spaniel, and Daniel Novák. 2020. 'Classification of Actigraphy Records from Bipolar Disorder Patients Using Slope Entropy: A Feasibility Study'. *Entropy* 22 (11). MDPI: 1243.

Cunningham, Pádraig, and Sarah Jane Delany. 2021. 'K-Nearest Neighbour Classifiers – A Tutorial'. *ACM Computing Surveys* 54 (6). Association for Computing Machinery (ACM): 1–25. doi:10.1145/3459665.

Fan, Rong-En, Kai-Wei Chang, Cho-Jui Hsieh, Xiang-Rui Wang, and Chih-Jen Lin. 2008. 'LIBLINEAR: A Library for Large Linear Classification'. *The Journal of Machine Learning Research* 9. JMLR. org: 1871–1874.

Gao, Lin, Jue Wang, and Longwei Chen. 2013. 'Event-Related Desynchronization and Synchronization Quantification in Motor-Related EEG by Kolmogorov Entropy'. *Journal of Neural Engineering* 10 (3). IOP Publishing: 36023.

Geurts, Pierre, Damien Ernst, and Louis Wehenkel. 2006. 'Extremely Randomized Trees'. *Machine Learning* 63 (1). Springer Science and Business Media LLC: 3–42. doi:10.1007/s10994-006-6226-1.

Haykin, Simon O. 2008. *Neural Networks and Learning Machines.* 3rd ed. Upper Saddle River, NJ: Pearson.

Hsu, Chang Francis, Sung-Yang Wei, Han-Ping Huang, Long Hsu, Sien Chi, and Chung-Kang Peng. 2017. 'Entropy of Entropy: Measurement of Dynamical Complexity for Biological Systems'. *Entropy* 19 (10). MDPI: 550.

Inouye, Tsuyoshi, Kazuhiro Shinosaki, H. Sakamoto, Seigo Toi, Satoshi Ukai, Akinori Iyama, Y. Katsuda, and M. Hirano. 1991. 'Quantification of EEG Irregularity by Use of the Entropy of the Power Spectrum'. *Electroencephalography and Clinical Neurophysiology* 79 (3). Elsevier: 204–210.

Karthik, S., M. Santhosh, M. S. Kavitha, and A. Christopher Paul. 2022. 'Automated Deep Learning Based Cardiovascular Disease Diagnosis Using ECG Signals'. *Computer Systems Science and Engineering* 42 (1). Computers, Materials and Continua (Tech Science Press): 183–199.

Karunathilake, Sachith Paramie, Gamage Upeksha Ganegoda, and others. 2018. 'Secondary Prevention of Cardiovascular Diseases and Application of Technology for Early Diagnosis'. *BioMed Research International* 2018. Hindawi: 9, Article ID: 5767864. doi:10.1155/2018/5767864.

Kay, Bill, Audun Myers, Thad Boydston, Emily Ellwein, Cameron Mackenzie, Iliana Alvarez, and Erik Lentz. 2024. 'Permutation Entropy for Signal Analysis'. *Discrete Mathematics & Theoretical Computer Science* 26 (1), Permutation... (Special issues). Centre pour la Communication Scientifique Directe (CCSD). doi:10.46298/dmtcs.12644.

LaValley, Michael P. 2008. 'Logistic Regression'. *Circulation* 117 (18). Ovid Technologies (Wolters Kluwer Health): 2395–2399. doi:10.1161/circulationaha.106.682658.

Li, Peng, Chengyu Liu, Ke Li, Dingchang Zheng, Changchun Liu, and Yinglong Hou. 2015. 'Assessing the Complexity of Short-Term Heartbeat Interval Series by Distribution Entropy'. *Medical & Biological Engineering & Computing* 53. Springer: 77–87.

Lim, Gregory B. 2013. 'Global Burden of Cardiovascular Disease'. *Nature Reviews Cardiology* 10 (2). Nature Publishing Group UK London: 59.

Liu, Chengyu, Julien Oster, Erik Reinertsen, Qiao Li, Lina Zhao, Shamim Nemati, and Gari D. Clifford. 2018. 'A Comparison of Entropy Approaches for AF Discrimination'. *Physiological Measurement* 39 (7). IOP Publishing: 74002. doi:10.1088/1361-6579/aacc48.

Liu, Xiaofeng, Xue Wang, Xu Zhou, and Aimin Jiang. 2018. 'Appropriate Use of the Increment Entropy for Electrophysiological Time Series'. *Computers in Biology and Medicine* 95. Elsevier: 13–23.

Manis, George, M. D. Aktaruzzaman, and Roberto Sassi. 2017. 'Bubble Entropy: An Entropy Almost Free of Parameters'. *IEEE Transactions on Biomedical Engineering* 64 (11). IEEE: 2711–2718.

Natekin, Alexey, and Alois Knoll. 2013. 'Gradient Boosting Machines, a Tutorial'. *Frontiers in Neurorobotics* 7. Frontiers Media SA. doi:10.3389/fnbot.2013.00021.

Newton, David, Farzad Yousefian, and Raghu Pasupathy. 2018. 'Stochastic Gradient Descent: Recent Trends'. In *Recent Advances in Optimization and Modeling of Contemporary Problems*, 193–220. INFORMS. doi:10.1287/educ.2018.0191.

Pałczyński, Krzysztof, Sandra Śmigiel, Damian Ledziński, and Sławomir Bujnowski. 2022. 'Study of the Few-Shot Learning for ECG Classification Based on the PTB-XL Dataset'. *Sensors* 22 (3). MDPI: 904.

Peck, Roxy, Chris Olsen, and Jay L Devore. 2008. *Introduction to Statistics and Data Analysis.* Belmont: Cengage Learning.

Pordeus, Daniel, Pedro Ribeiro, Laíla Zacarias, João Paulo Madeiro, Joao Alexandre Lobo Marques, Pedro Miguel Rodrigues, Camila Leite, Manoel Alves Neto, Arnaldo Aires Peixoto Jr, and Adriel de Oliveira. 2023. 'Classification of Severity of COVID-19 Patients Based on the Heart Rate Variability'. In *Computerized Systems for Diagnosis and Treatment of COVID-19*, edited by Joao Alexandre Lobo Marques, and Simon James Fong, 155–177. Springer International Publishing.

Porta, Alberto, Giuseppe Baselli, Diego Liberati, Nicola Montano, Chiara Cogliati, Tomaso Gnecchi-Ruscone, Alberto Malliani, and Sergio Cerutti. 1998. 'Measuring Regularity by Means of a Corrected Conditional Entropy in Sympathetic Outflow'. *Biological Cybernetics* 78. Springer: 71–78.

Rasmussen, Carl Edward. 2006. *Gaussian Processes for Machine Learning.* Cambridge, MA: MIT Press.

Ribeiro, Pedro, João Alexandre Lobo Marques, Daniel Pordeus, Laíla Zacarias, Camila Ferreira Leite, Manoel Alves Sobreira-Neto, Arnaldo Aires Peixoto, Adriel de Oliveira, João Paulo do Vale Madeiro, and Pedro Miguel Rodrigues. 2024. 'Machine Learning-Based Cardiac Activity Non-Linear Analysis for Discriminating COVID-19 Patients with Different Degrees of Severity'. *Biomedical Signal Processing and Control* 87 (January). Elsevier BV: 105558. doi:10.1016/j.bspc.2023.105558.

Ribeiro, Pedro, Daniel Pordeus, Laíla Zacarias, Camila Leite, Manoel Alves Neto, Arnaldo Aires Peixoto Jr, Adriel de Oliveira, João Paulo Madeiro, João Alexandre Lobo Marques, and Pedro Miguel Rodrigues. 2023. 'Evaluation of ECG Non-Linear Features in Time-Frequency Domain for the Discrimination of COVID-19 Severity Stages'. In *Computerized Systems for Diagnosis and Treatment of COVID-19*, edited by Joao Alexandre Lobo Marques, and Simon James Fong, 137–154. Springer International Publishing.

Richman, Joshua S., Douglas E. Lake, and J. Randall Moorman. 2004. 'Sample Entropy'. *Methods in Enzymology* 384: 172–184. Elsevier.

Richman, Joshua S., and J. Randall Moorman. 2000. 'Physiological Time-Series Analysis Using Approximate Entropy and Sample Entropy'. *American Journal of Physiology-Heart and Circulatory Physiology* 278 (6). American Physiological Society: H2039–H2049. doi:10.1152/ajpheart.2000.278.6.h2039.

Rodrigues, Pedro, Bruno Bispo, Carolina Garrett, Dilio Alves, Joao Teixeira, and Diamantino Freitas. 2021. 'Lacsogram: A New EEG Tool to Diagnose Alzheimers Disease'. *IEEE Journal of Biomedical and Health Informatics* 25 (9). Institute of Electrical and Electronics Engineers (IEEE): 3384–3395.

Rohila, Ashish, and Ambalika Sharma. 2019. 'Phase Entropy: A New Complexity Measure for Heart Rate Variability'. *Physiological Measurement* 40 (10). IOP Publishing: 105006.

Rosner, Bernard. 2010. *Fundamentals of Biostatistics*. Boston: Duxbury Press.

Rostaghi, Mostafa, and Hamed Azami. 2016. 'Dispersion Entropy: A Measure for Time-Series Analysis'. *IEEE Signal Processing Letters* 23 (5). IEEE: 610–614.

Saleh, Moussa, and John A. Ambrose. 2018. 'Understanding Myocardial Infarction'. *F1000Research* 7. Faculty of 1000 Ltd.

Silva, Gabriel, Patrícia Batista, and Pedro Miguel Rodrigues. 2022. 'COVID-19 Activity Screening by a Smart-Data-Driven Multi-Band Voice Analysis'. *Journal of Voice*, November. Elsevier BV. doi:10.1016/j.jvoice.2022.11.008.

Silva, Martim, Pedro Ribeiro, Bruno C. Bispo, and Pedro Miguel Rodrigues. 2023. 'Detecção Da Doença de Alzheimer Através de Parâmetros Não-Lineares de Sinais de Fala'. In *Anais Do XLI Simpósio Brasileiro de Telecomunicações e Processamento de Sinais*. Sociedade Brasileira de Telecomunicações.

Śmigiel, Sandra. 2022. 'ECG Classification Using Orthogonal Matching Pursuit and Machine Learning'. *Sensors* 22 (13). MDPI: 4960.

Śmigiel, Sandra, Krzysztof Pałczyński, and Damian Ledziński. 2021. 'ECG Signal Classification Using Deep Learning Techniques Based on the PTB-XL Dataset'. *Entropy* 23 (9). MDPI: 1121.

Tharwat, Alaa. 2016. 'Linear vs. Quadratic Discriminant Analysis Classifier: A Tutorial'. *International Journal of Applied Pattern Recognition* 3 (2). Inderscience Publishers: 145. doi:10.1504/ijapr.2016.079050.

Vogiatzis, Antonios, Georgios Chalkiadakis, Konstantia Moirogiorgou, and Michalis Zervakis. 2021. 'A Novel One-vs-Rest Classification Framework for Mutually Decisions by Independent Parallel Classifiers'. In *2021 IEEE International Conference on Imaging Systems and Techniques (IST)*. IEEE.

Wagner, Patrick, Nils Strodthoff, Ralf-Dieter Bousseljot, Dieter Kreiseler, Fatima I. Lunze, Wojciech Samek, and Tobias Schaeffter. 2020. 'PTB-XL, a Large Publicly Available Electrocardiography Dataset'. *Scientific Data* 7 (1). Springer Science and Business Media LLC.

Wagner, Patrick, Nils Strodthoff, Ralf-Dieter Bousseljot, Wojciech Samek, and Tobias Schaeffter. 2022. 'PTB-XL, a Large Publicly Available Electrocardiography Dataset (version 1.0.3)'. PhysioNet. RRID:SCR_007345. https://doi.org/10.13026/kfzx-aw45.

Wang, Jian, Ting Li, Rong Xie, Xin-min Wang, and Yu-yan Cao. 2015. 'Fault Feature Extraction for Multiple Electrical Faults of Aviation Electro-Mechanical Actuator Based on Symbolic Dynamics Entropy'. In *2015 IEEE International Conference on Signal Processing, Communications and Computing (ICSPCC)*, 1–6. Ningbo, Zhejiang: IEEE.

Wohlfart, B. 1987. 'A Simple Model for Demonstration of STT-Changes in ECG'. *European Heart Journal* 8 (4). Oxford University Press: 409–416.

World Health Organization. 2021. 'Cardiovascular Diseases (CVDs)'. https://www.who.int/news-room/fact-sheets/detail/cardiovascular-diseases-(cvds). (accessed October 5, 2023).

Yan, Chang, Peng Li, Changchun Liu, Xinpei Wang, Chunyan Yin, and Lianke Yao. 2019. 'Novel Gridded Descriptors of Poincaré Plot for Analyzing Heartbeat Interval Time-Series'. *Computers in Biology and Medicine* 109. Elsevier: 280–289.

6 Development of a Far Infrared Thermal Sensor-Based Contactless Breath Rate Measuring System with a Constraint on Resources

Sukesh Rao, Roopa B Hegde, and Sanith Bangera

6.1 INTRODUCTION

Breathing or respiration is considered one of the important physiological activities in every living organism. The process of inhaling and exhaling the air is considered respiration or breathing, and the number of such events in unit time is regarded as breath rate (BR) or respiratory frequency (Smith et al. 2011; A-Khalidi et al. 2011; Parkes 2011; Cretikos et al. 2008). In humans, BR varies with different age groups. The standard BR is found to be 12 to 20 beats per minute (BPM) in resting adults (Chourpiliadis and Bharadwaj 2022), 21 to 34 BPM in children, and 40 to 60 BPM in infants (Hermansen and Mahajan 2015). Every individual will have different breathing patterns and breath rates depending on the environment and activities performed. BR can be considered an essential marker of illness in certain clinical events such as cardiac arrest, respiratory alkalosis, hyperventilation, stress, anxiety, and nervousness (Basu et al. 2017; Roelofs 1985). This can provide information on the physiological changes that occur in the human body, such as physical and emotional stress. A study (Fieselmann et al. 1993) reported that BR higher than 27 BPM represented cardiac arrest, a cardiovascular disease event (CVD event), and BR in the range of 25–29 BPM was found to be critical. Abnormal BR per minute may differ from person to person. However, recent evidence suggests that BR greater than 20 BPM may require medical assistance. Hence, BR can be a vital parameter in providing suitable pre-hospital care.

DOI: 10.1201/9781003797524-6

Several methods are used to monitor the BR in humans. The technique can be classified as contact-based, non-contact, or contactless (Jin et al. 2005, Massaroni et al. 2019; Maurya et al. 2021). Contact-based respiration rate monitoring instruments include acoustic methods, airflow sensors, chest abdominal movement detection, Transcutaneous CO_2 Monitoring, Oximetry probes, and ECG-derived devices used in clinical practices (Jin et al. 2005; Folke et al. 2003; Helfenbein et al. 2014; Pereira et al. 2015; Nam et al 2016; Tipparaju et al. 2020). In an acoustic method, a microphone is placed close to the respiratory airways or over the throat to detect sound variations (Massaroni et al. 2019). Different types of time and frequency domain analyses are performed to estimate the parameters related to the respiratory system (Fei et al. 2005). A major drawback with acoustic-based respiratory monitoring is that speaking, snorting, coughing, etc., makes it difficult to predict accurate values. The airflow-based method uses different sensors on the airflow path near the nasal end to detect the BR (Jiang et al. 2020; Rosengarten et al. 2003). The airflow-based method includes pressure sensors (Fan et al. 2018), temperature sensors (Basra et al. 2017), and CO_2 sensors (Massaroni et al. 2019) for measuring the BR. Inhaling and exhaling air pressure can be used as an indicator for BR using a pressure sensor. The inhaling air temperature is lower than the exhaling air temperature as the exhaling air contains more CO_2 concentration (Angelova et al. 2021; Anghel and Iacobescu 2013). Temperature and CO_2 sensors are used to detect this variation in respiratory monitoring systems. During the inhaling and exhaling, the chest and abdominal wall provide movement. The displacement in the chest wall can be measured using the non-invasive type of strain gauge pressure or force sensors (Al-Halhouli et al. 2021).

There is also evidence of monitoring BR using blood oxygen saturation levels obtained using photoplethysmography (Charlton et al. 2018). ECG can also be used to record BR (Charlton et al. 2018). These methods pose limitations on accuracy, mainly due to motion artifacts. Placing the sensor, especially on infants, is a most difficult issue as they do not feel comfortable, making it challenging to get an accurate reading. According to the literature, non-contact or contactless sensors are ideal for breath rate estimation (Massaroni et al. 2018). Radar-based (Lauteslager et al. 2021) optical and thermal image sensor-based (Yang et al. 2022; Takahashi et al. 2021) respiratory estimation systems are also commonly used. Thermal and optical sensor-based BR monitoring systems are found to be inexpensive, off-the-shelf, and contactless measuring systems for respiration signals. Image sensors for BR estimation have been tested with different spectral bands such as visible light (Bartula et al. 2013), long-wave infrared (Pereira et al. 2015; Abbas et al. 2011), and mid-wave infrared (Jin and Pavlidis 2010; Lewis et al. 2011). Infrared thermography (IRT) is a new technology used to capture an image based on the thermal waves emitted by different objects (Pereira et al. 2014). IRT technology has been used to capture thermal images around the nostrils, and different algorithms have been used to get the best possible BR (Abbas et al. 2011; Jin and Pavlidis 2010; Lewis et al. 2011; Fei and Pavlidis 2007).

At present, the commonly used BR estimation method requires the attachment of sensors to the human body. This not only causes discomfort but also causes errors due to the body's movement. Such systems fail to estimate BR without contacting, which was essential during the pandemic. Also, the current systems are expensive and burdened with computational expenses. Researchers have developed contactless methods for BR estimation to address the challenges in recent years. This study introduces a cost-effective and robust contactless BR estimation method. The primary objective of this paper is to design a non-invasive system that measures BR by analyzing facial temperature variations around the nostril region. The proposed system utilizes a far infrared thermal sensor to capture temperature changes in the nostril area. Subsequently, the collected sensor data undergo processing and analysis in the frequency domain to derive the BR. The key contributions of this work are as follows.

- Development of a setup to acquire and process the breath data through far infrared sensor.
- Two novel pre-processing methods are proposed to provide better insight into far infrared sensors' data acquisition methods.
- A computationally efficient algorithm to compute BR using frequency domain information.

The subsequent sections are organized as follows: Section 6.2 outlines the setup details of the breath rate estimation. Section 6.3 provides the details of the breath rate detection algorithm followed by Section 6.4 presenting the results and discussions while Section 6.5 concludes the experimental-based study.

6.2 SETUP FOR CONTACTLESS DATA ACQUISITION SYSTEM

BR is estimated through a far infrared thermal sensor, which detects temperature changes associated with inhalation and exhalation during every breath. For this exploration, an MLX90640 far infrared thermal sensor array with a resolution of 32 x 24 pixels is employed to capture real-time thermal image frames and subsequently save them in CSV file format. Figure 6.1(a) shows the functional block diagram of the proposed BR system and the experimental setup employed for data acquisition (Figure 6.1(b)).

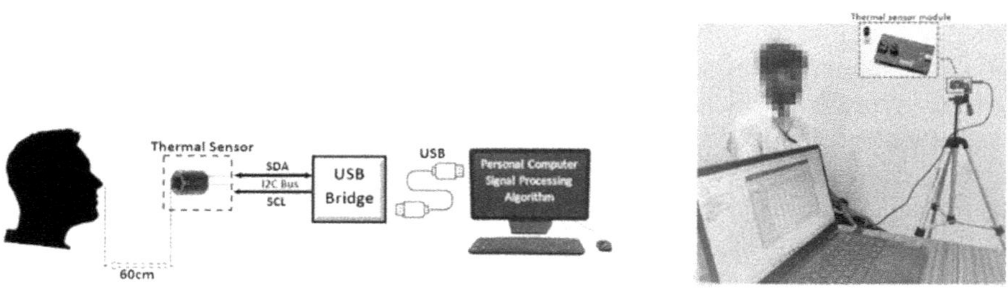

(a) (b)

FIGURE 6.1 (a) System block diagram of BR estimation, (b) experimental setup.

The MLX90640 is a far infrared thermal sensor that can detect temperature changes from objects in its field of view. It works by detecting the infrared radiation emitted by objects in the far infrared spectrum, typically between 7 and 14 microns. The sensor uses 32x24 infrared thermopile sensors, each of which measures the temperature of a small area of the sensor's field of view. These thermopile sensors are designed to absorb infrared radiation and convert it into an electrical signal, which is then processed by the sensor's on-board processing unit. It is necessary to interface it with a microcontroller or computer using a serial interface to use the MLX90640. The sensor can be programmed to output temperature data in various formats, including raw temperature data, temperature maps, and digital temperature readings. In the proposed work, raw temperature data are acquired to estimate the BR.

Breath patterns are acquired from 10 participants (with their consent) in a sitting position. The sensor is placed approximately 60 cm from the nostril region, as shown in Figure 6.1. The distance between the sensor and the participant is decided empirically. The sensor data is recorded for one minute, and it is stored in the CSV file for further processing. The participants were also informed to count the number of breaths they exhaled during the data collection for one minute. The counted exhaling rate is noted as the actual BPM, and the experimental results are compared with these values to validate the predicted BR by the proposed system.

The MLX90640 is programmed with initial parameters to decide on the quality of the image frames. The parameters include emissivity, a measure of IR energy emission; frame rate, which is the number of frames captured per second; and resolution, and filter gain. The sensor parameter values used during data acquisition are listed in Table 6.1. Emissivity is a measure of thermal emission, and its value provides the efficiency with which a surface emits IR energy compared to an ideal black body. Human skin shows an emissivity close to 0.98 (Charlton et al. 2020), and hence, an emissivity of 0.98 is set to ensure accurate temperature readings near the nostril region. The sensor has thermal image resolution of 32 x 24 sensing elements, and this is sufficient for measuring thermal changes. This enables to estimate breathing frequency over the nostril region. Additionally, a high frame rate is required for detecting a periodic rise and fall in temperature due to breathing. Hence, a frame rate of 64 per second is considered in the proposed method. Further, breathing is a slow

TABLE 6.1
Sensor (MLX90640) Parameters

Parameter	Value
Emissivity	0.98
Resolution	32x24 pixels
Frame Rate	64 Hz
Filter Gain	10

periodic change in temperature affected by sensor noise and thermal fluctuations. Therefore, a filter is used to suppress the noise with a gain of 10.

Data visualization is achieved per the format prescribed in the MLX90640 technical datasheet. This allows the user to visualize data as thermal image of size 32x24. To limit the processing region and complexity, a small area around the nostril region is considered for further processing. As per the sensor settings, around 3840 frames are obtained per person. These are stored as 1D vectors in CSV format. To confirm the nostril region, these 1D values are read and converted to thermal images of size 32x24 for visualization of the required region. The thermal images highlight the temperature variations when mapped to suitable colors. The regions with high temperature values appear dark red, and the regions with less temperature appear blue. However, visualization is not mandatory, as each pixel is already in degrees Celsius and can be directly analyzed by considering maximum temperature regions. In the proposed method, the data acquired from the sensor are converted to images to select the region around the nostril accurately.

6.2.1 BR Detection Method

The flow diagram of the BR estimation system is depicted in Figure 6.2. To begin the estimation process, the data stored in the CSV file is read and subjected to processing using MATLAB 2022. This software facilitates the computations and analysis required to estimate the BR accurately.

In the proposed work, two methods namely maximum temperature (MT) and fixed position (FP) are employed to estimate BR and validate the correctness of the experimentations.

6.2.1.1 Pre-processing of Sensor Data

In the proposed approach, processing is limited to the region around the nostril. This is achieved by selecting the region around the nostril using the visualization method. A 1D vector array is converted to a thermal image to select an appropriate region. The maximum temperature region in the thermal image appears dark red after color

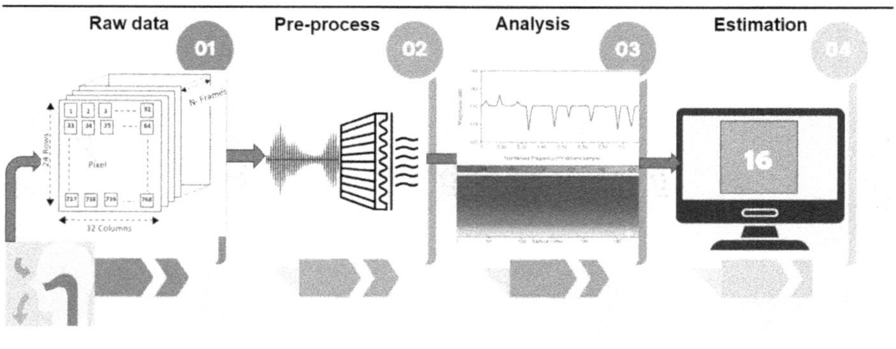

FIGURE 6.2 Functional flow diagram of the BR detection.

mapping. This confirms the region around the nostril for further processing. Based on this, the thermal images are cropped to obtain a small subset image of size 11x13 by determining the coordinates of the pixel having the maximum temperature. A bounding box is inserted on the original thermal image to test the chosen region's correctness. Both the MT and FP methods are applied to the cropped images.

6.2.1.2 Maximum Temperature Method

In the MT method, the maximum pixel value from the cropped image is determined as indicated in Figure 6.3(a) and stored in the variable named 'max_value'. This is repeated for each frame; therefore, the length of 'max_value' is the same as the number of frames per minute. Random fluctuations in the sensor readings have interfered with the 'max_value'.

6.2.1.3 Fixed Position Method

In the FP method, the location in the cropped region is fixed, as shown in Figure 6.3(b), and the corresponding pixel value is stored in a variable named 'fixed_value' and repeated for all the frames, resulting in a vector length equal to the number of frames per minute. The region is fixed empirically. Both 'max_value' and 'fixed_value' vectors are tested for the possible estimation of the BR. In real-time data acquisition, the presence of noise is unavoidable. The acquired breathing data has noise components at higher frequencies than the breathing frequency. Hence, a low-pass filter is used to eliminate the noise components present in the data. In the present approach, a low-pass finite impulse response (FIR) filter is used to eliminate high-frequency components from the stored vectors (above 100 BPM or 1.6 Hz) as described in Equation (6.1). Output is characterized by delayed versions of the input signal.

$$y[n] = \sum_{n=0}^{k} b_n x[n] \tag{6.1}$$

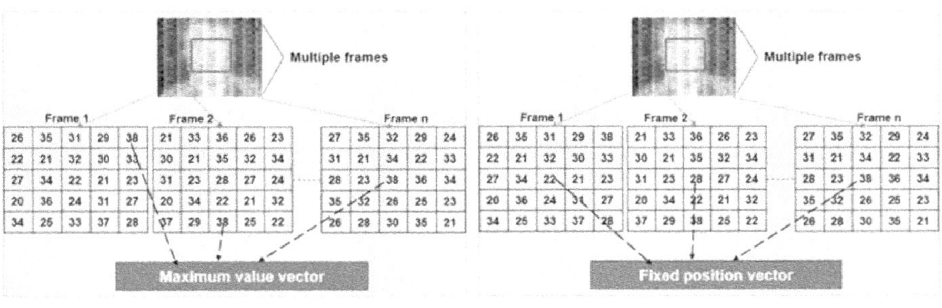

(a) (b)

FIGURE 6.3 (a) Selection of maximum value from the cropped section of frame. (b) Selection of fixed position value from the cropped section of frame.

where x[n] is 'max_value' or 'fixed_value' based on the approach, y[n] is the filtered output signal, and b is the scale factor of the delayed version of the input corresponding to filter coefficients. In the present study, 100 filter coefficients are considered with a frequency of 1.6 Hz. The filtered signal is interfered with low-frequency noise as well. Such interference cannot be eliminated using the linear filter. The time domain variations in the signal do not reveal the BR due to the presence of fluctuations. The filtered data is subjected to Fourier transform (FT) using the Fast Fourier transform (FFT) method as described in Equation (6.2). The nearest frequency information corresponding to the BR is predicted in the proposed method.

$$Y[k] = \sum_{n=0}^{N-1} y[n] e^{\frac{j2\pi kn}{N}} \tag{6.2}$$

where Y[k] is the frequency domain representation of the filtered time domain representation of y[n].

In the FFT approach, an N value of 3000 is used to compute FFT, and frequency resolution is computed. To count the BR accurately, the analysis is limited between 0.2 and 0.5 Hz. The lower and upper bounds are selected based on the possible lower and upper count of BR among the acquired data. In the dataset, 12 BPM is the lower value, and 28 BPM is the upper value of the count. To limit the frequency range, we considered the lower breath rate value of 8 and the upper BR value of 30 per second. Further, the lower and upper values are divided by the frequency resolution value, and the same is plotted in the frequency domain. The location of the maximum peak gives the BR count when mapped in the time domain. Implementation steps for the same are given in Algorithm 6.1.

Algorithm 6.1: Breath rate count

1) Read sensor data in .csv format
2) Convert each row into image of size 24X32
3) Crop the images to select region around the nostril
4) Get the maximum pixel/fixed position pixel value from each cropped image
5) Save the maximum values as row vector
6) Apply FIR filter
7) Apply FFT on filtered data
8) Map the frequency domain data for the duration of 60 seconds
9) Determine the BR count from the location of maximum peak of the mapped data

6.3 RESULTS AND DISCUSSIONS

In this section, results obtained from the different stages of the BR estimation system are presented. The stages of the proposed system include data acquisition, pre-processing of raw data, DFT, and the actual BR estimation process. The acquired data is initially in the form of a 1D vector, which is converted into images to facilitate better visualization. The resulting images are represented in grayscale, as depicted in Figure 6.4(a). The images are mapped using the 'jet' color map to determine the necessary region effectively, as shown in Figure 6.4(b). The color mapping helps to confirm the region with the maximum temperature, which typically appears around the nostril region. To further refine the selection process, the image's centroid is calculated, and the region around the centroid is chosen, as demonstrated in Figure 6.4(c). The size of this selected region is determined empirically to ensure coverage of the area around the nose.

In the MT method, the maximum pixel value from the cropped image is determined and stored in the variable named 'max_value'. In the FP approach, the pixel value from a fixed position is determined and stored in the variable named 'fixed_value'. The data is acquired for one minute, as shown in Figure 6.5. It can be observed from Figure 6.5(a) that the raw data is noisy, and it is hard to analyze in the existing form. From the plot, it can be concluded that the required signal of interest is in the lower frequency band (less than 1 Hz). The typical BR is 10 to 40 bpm or 0.167 Hz to 0.67 Hz. It is essential to filter the 'max_value' and 'fixed_value' vectors using an LPF. In this experiment, the LPF cut-off frequency is selected as 1.6 Hz. Figure 6.6 represents the time and frequency domain changes in the filtered signals of the MT and FP methods.

Since the maximum temperature around the nostril is considered, the peaks in the plot represent a number of exhales. However, it is challenging to decide the threshold value to count the number of peaks as the variations of peaks are wide. Also, it is well-known that time domain data is hard to analyze. Hence, the filtered data is converted to the frequency domain to determine the BR. The frequency domain analysis is band-limited to 0.2 to 0.5 Hz. However, to perform uniform computation, the frames for the calculation of DFT resolution are fixed to 3000. Hence, the frequency resolution in DFT becomes 0.02 Hz. This resolution will provide around 15 frequency point to determine the BR within the ROI of 0.2 to 0.5 Hz.

The peak magnitude corresponding to the frequency on the x-axis is chosen as the BR estimate. Figure 6.7 shows the estimated BR using the MP and FP methods and the values are 20.8 BPM and 26.6 BPM, respectively. During the experimentation, the actual BR recorded was 20 BPM. The BR estimation algorithm was evaluated on 10 healthy participants aged between 25 and 40 years. The BR obtained from the algorithm is labeled as the estimated BR, while each participant's count of exhale

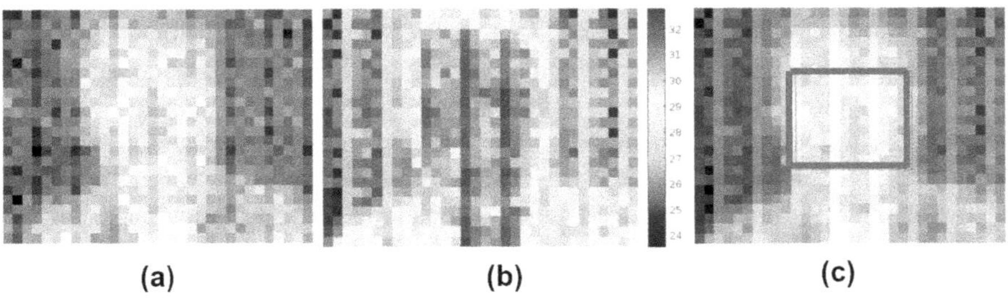

FIGURE 6.4 Region selection for processing: (a) image representation of sensor data, (b) color-mapped image, and (c) cropped region.

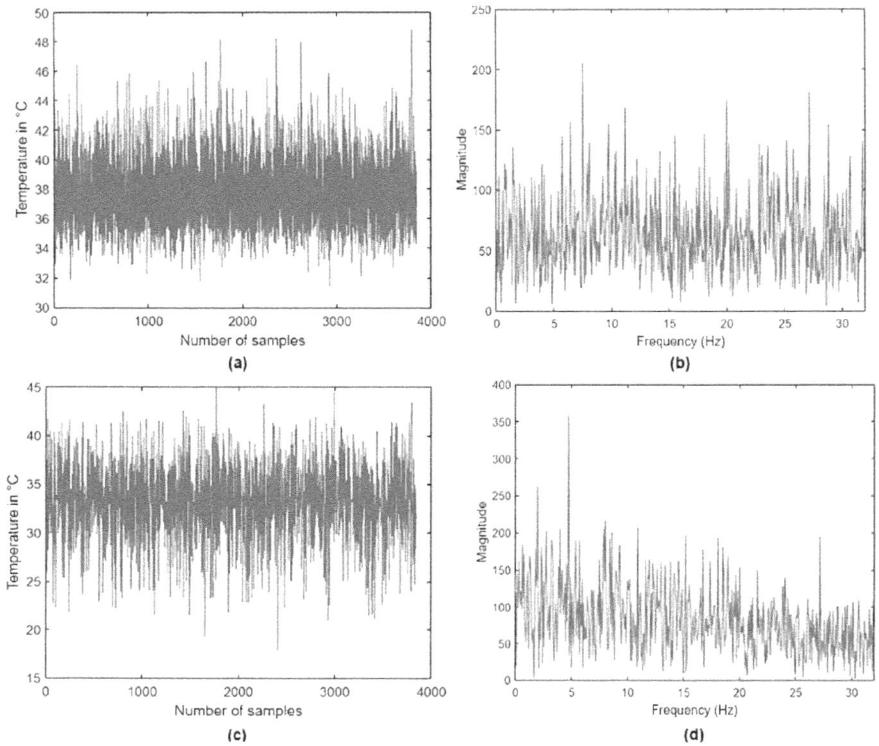

FIGURE 6.5 Time domain representation, top row: (a) Time domain data from MP method, (b) 100-point DFT of MP data, (c) time domain data from FP method, and (d) 100-point DFT of FP data.

events is labeled as the actual BR. The actual BR, estimated BR, and absolute error are tabulated in Table 6.2 for both the MP and FP methods. Mean absolute error (MAE) is calculated using the equation as given in Equation (6.3).

$$MAE = \frac{1}{N}\sum_{i=1}^{N}\left|X_i - X\right| \tag{6.3}$$

where N is the number of tests, X is the actual BR, and Xi is the estimated BR.

Figure 6.8 shows the mean and standard deviation (SD) values for the actual and estimated methods with error bars representing SD. The accrual BR shows a mean value of 20.8, while the MP method and FP method show mean value of 21.16 and 22.26, respectively. Additionally, the SD value for MP method is closer to the SD of the actual BR, and hence the MP method is more suitable compared to the FP method.

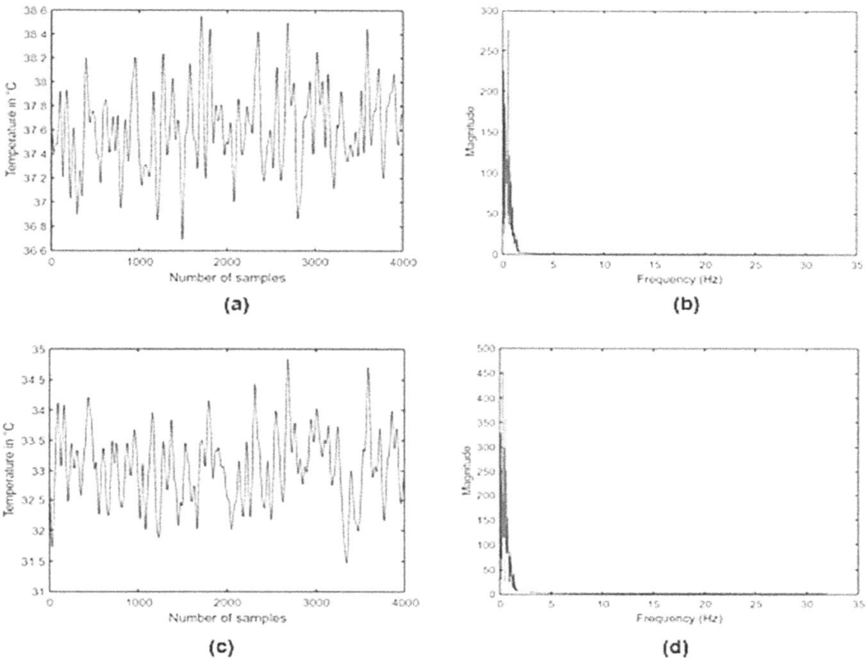

FIGURE 6.6 MP and FP method data after LPF: (a) time domain data from MP method (filtered), (b) 100-point DFT, (c) time domain data from FP method (filtered), and (d) 100-point DFT.

6.4 PERFORMANCE EVALUATION

To determine the correlation between the actual BR and estimated BR, we computed the Pearson's correlation coefficient (PCC) using the formula in Equation (6.4).

$$PCC = \sum \frac{(AR - M_{ER})(ER - M_{AR})}{\sqrt{(DS_{AR})(DS_{ER})}} \tag{6.4}$$

where AR is actual BR, ER is estimated BR, MAR and MER are mean values, DSAR and DSER are deviation squared values of the actual and estimated BR. PCC of 0.9545 and −0.2635 are obtained for actual BR and estimated BR, respectively. Further, to measure the strength of association between the actual BR and estimated BR, Spearman's rho is calculated using the formula given in Equation (6.5).

$$SR = 1 - \frac{6 \sum D^2}{N(N^2 - 1)} \tag{6.5}$$

where SR is Spearman's rho, D is the difference between actual BR and estimated BR, and N is the number of tests.

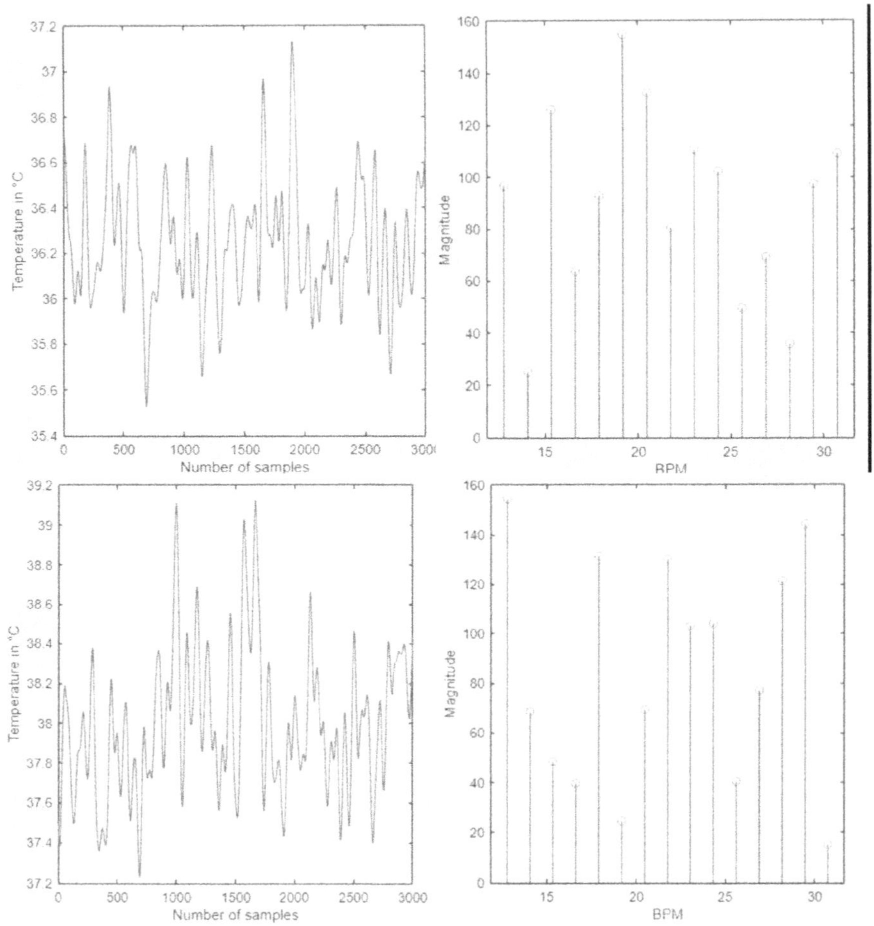

FIGURE 6.7 Possible BR on frequency domain: (a) 3000 point samples of MP data, (b) DFT of MP data, (c) 3000 point samples of FP data, and (d) DFT of FP data.

The performances of MT and FP methods are listed in Table 6.3, and it is evident that the error rate is lower in the case of MT method. The PCC value of 0.9545 indicated a strong positive correlation between the actual and estimated BR. Also, the SR value of 0.964 discloses that the association between actual BR and estimated BR is considerably significant. It is evident from Figure 6.9 that there is a strong correlation between actual BR and estimated BR in the case of MT method compared to that of FP method. The error in the BR estimate is mainly due to the noise interference in far infrared activities. The sampling rate can be reduced to overcome the low-frequency distortion. However, the interested signal is already in the very low-frequency range; it may still deteriorate the quality of the data.

Automated estimation of BR is addressed by several research groups, as mentioned in the introduction. However, in the proposed approach, a far infrared thermal

TABLE 6.2
Comparison of Actual BR and Estimated BR

Sl. No	Actual BR	Estimated BR in BPM (MP method)	Absolute Error	Estimated BR in BPM (FP method)	Absolute Error
1	23	21	2	23.04	0.04
2	21	23	2	20.63	0.37
3	12	13.8	1.8	23.92	11.92
4	17	16	1	22.68	5.68
5	19	20.9	1.9	21.94	2.94
6	20	20.8	0.8	26.6	6.6
7	28	26.6	1.4	19.25	8.75
8	25	26.2	1.2	15.84	9.16
9	27	28.2	1.2	28.20	1.2
10	16	15.1	0.9	25.14	10.04

sensor is used to estimate BR in real time. The use of far infrared sensor with 32x 24-pixel resolution for BR estimation is a novel approach, and the sensor used in our approach is a low-cost device; hence, it can be used in low-resource settings. The method used for estimating BR in the proposed approach is simple and does not require computationally efficient processors. Also, the BR estimation is independent of a person's slight movement. A comparison of the proposed method with the state-of-the-art approaches is provided in Table 6.4. A few researchers (Pereira et al. 2015;

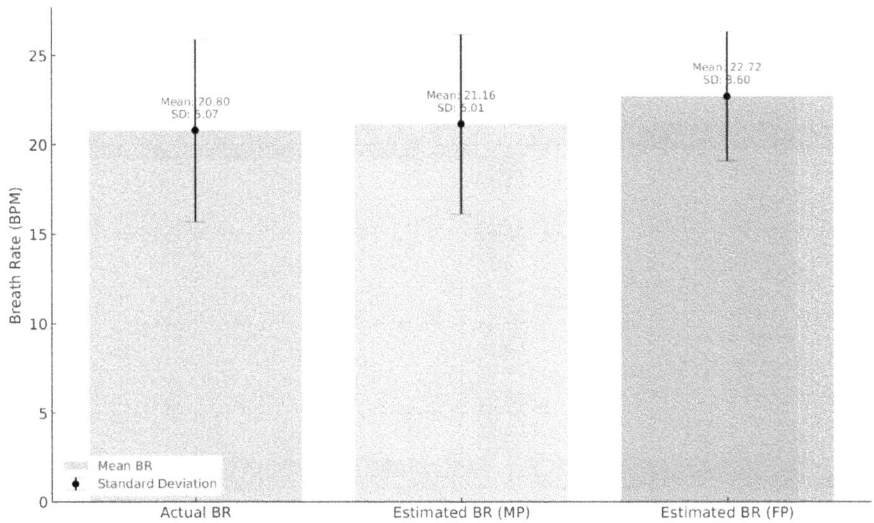

FIGURE 6.8 Mean and standard deviation of the actual and estimated BR.

TABLE 6.3
Performance Metrics

	MAE	PCC	SR
MT method	1.42	0.9545	0.964
FP method	5.66	0.2635	0.384

Nam et al. 2016; Yang et al. 2022; Takahashi et al. 2021) found that the movement of participants may affect BR estimation with a camera-based system. Moreover, the high-resolution capturing system used in the state-of-the-art literature results in the requirement for high-end resources. Also, the cost of such devices is higher than that of far infrared thermal sensors. It can be observed from the table that the error rate of the proposed method using a low-cost far IR sensor is comparable with that of the state-of-the-art techniques. Also, the proposed BR estimation method is independent of the movement of the participants. Hence, the proposed contactless approach provides a sustainable solution for monitoring BR in low-resource settings. The far IR sensor can be used for temperature measurement and BR estimation by holding

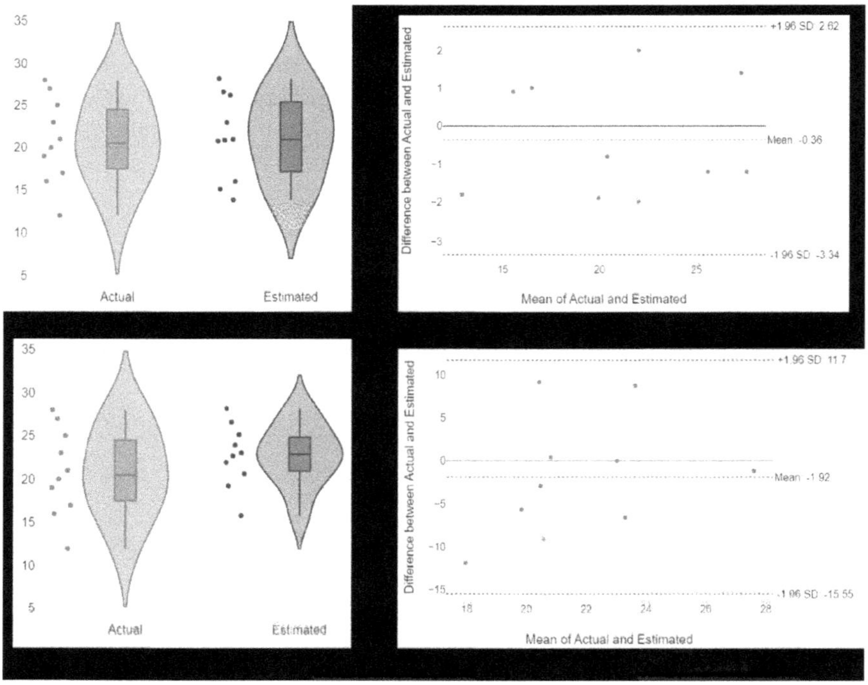

FIGURE 6.9 Violine (left) and Bland-Altman (right) plot: (a, b) MT method and (c, d) FP method.

TABLE 6.4
Comparison of the Proposed Approach with State-of-the-Art Literature

Paper	Approach	Result	Sensor Specifications
Pereira et al. 2015	Infrared thermal imaging (video recording), beat-to-beat intervals method	Error rate: 0.71–1.51	Thermal video recorder with 1280 × 1024 pixels
Nam et al. 2016	Cell-phone camera (invasive method). PSD of frequency domain signal	Average median error: 1.62	HTC One (M8) camera with 1080x1920 pixels
Yang et al. 2022	Thermal and RGB camera, CNN for ROI detection, time domain analysis	Absolute error: 1.47±1.33	Thermal camera resolution: 256 × 192, RGB camera resolution: 640 × 480
Takahashi et al. 2021	Thermal imaging camera, frequency domain analysis	MAE: 0.66 (−1.9 to 2.3)	Thermal sensor images with resolution 320 × 320
Bartula et al. 2013	Camera-based system (video stream)	Accuracy 85%	monochrome Near IR camera with 752 × 480 pixels
Abbas et al. 2011	Infrared thermography	MAE: 1.45	VarioCAM® hr head IR camera with 2,048 × 1,536 pixels
The proposed method	Far infrared thermal sensor, FFT	MAE: 1.42	MLX90640 with 32 × 24 pixels

the sensor at about 60 cm. The proposed system could be used in hospital care units, especially for neonatal applications. Infants and children are not allowed to undergo any testing. Hence, the proposed setup can be used for both temperature and BR estimation by mounting the sensor or by holding the sensor at a specified distance. We have acquired the data in a sitting position. However, it is not a mandatory posture. Data can be acquired even when a person is lying down. Hence, the setup can be used in intensive care units.

6.5 CONCLUSION

This paper presents a novel contactless and automated method for breath rate estimation utilizing a 32x24 pixel far infrared thermal sensor. The far infrared sensor is well-known for estimating the temperature of distant objects, a technique that gained popularity during the COVID-19 pandemic. Therefore, this study proposes an experimental investigation of BR estimation using the far-infrared sensor. The developed system analyzes the frame-by-frame pixels of the sensor data to estimate the BR through two distinct methods, namely the 'MT method' and the 'FP method'.

In the 'MT method', maximum temperature values around the nostril regions are processed, while in the 'FP method', a fixed position around the nostrils is selected, and temperature values in the chosen region are processed. Subsequently, the analysis and estimation of BR are conducted in the frequency domain. The obtained results reveal a mean absolute error of 1.42 BPM and 5.66 BPM for the 'MT' and 'FP' methods, respectively. The 'MT method' demonstrates better performance, indicated by a Pearson correlation coefficient (PCC) of 0.9545 and a sensitivity rate (SR) of 0.964. Thus, processing the maximum temperature around the nostril region offers promising results for monitoring BR using thermal sensors. Moreover, further research could be undertaken to minimize the error and to conduct clinical evaluations, thereby extending the potential applicability of the proposed method. Thus, using a far-infrared thermal sensor for non-invasive breath rate monitoring proves to be a promising solution, especially in real-time applications with low resource settings. The obtained results, exhibiting high accuracy and performance comparable to state-of-the-art methods, highlight the potential of this method for simultaneous monitoring of breath rate and body temperature. This approach holds significant implications for improving pre-hospital care and emergency response systems, enhancing healthcare outcomes in various scenarios.

STATEMENTS AND DECLARATIONS

Funding: No funds, grants, or other support were received during the preparation of this manuscript.

Competing Interests: The authors have no relevant financial or non-financial interests to disclose.

Consent to participate: The participants voluntarily involved in the study. It was conducted in the institution, and our colleagues voluntarily participated in the experimentation.

Data Availability: The data (.csv file) will be made available upon reasonable request to the corresponding author.

REFERENCES

A. Al-Halhouli, L. Al-Ghussain, S. El Bouri, H. Liu, and D. Zheng, "Clinical evaluation of stretchable and wearable inkjet-printed strain gauge sensor for respiratory rate monitoring at different measurements locations," *J. Clin. Monit. Comput.*, vol. 35, no. 3, pp. 453–462, 2021, doi: 10.1007/s10877-020-00481-3.

A. Basra, B. Mukhopadhayay, and S. Kar, "Temperature sensor based ultra-low cost respiration monitoring system," *2017 9th International Conference on Communication Systems and Networks (COMSNETS),* Bengaluru, India, 2017, pp. 530–535, doi: 10.1109/COMSNETS.2017.7945448.

A. Basu, A. Dasgupta, and A. Routray, "A thermographic method for detecting Respiratory Alkalosis by monitoring breath patterns," 2016 *Int. Conf. Syst. Med. Biol. ICSMB 2016*, pp. 26–30, Apr. 2017, doi: 10.1109/ICSMB.2016.7915080.

C. Chourpiliadis and A. Bhardwaj, "Physiology, respiratory rate," In: StatPearls [Internet]. Treasure Island (FL): StatPearls Publishing, 2025 Jan–. PMID: 30725991, 2022.

C. Massaroni, A. Nicolò, D. Lo Presti, M. Sacchetti, S. Silvestri, and E. Schena, "Contact-based methods for measuring respiratory rate," *Sensors (Switzerland)*, vol. 19, no. 4, pp. 1–47, 2019, doi: 10.3390/s19040908.

C. Massaroni, D. S. Lopes, D. Lo Presti, E. Schena, and S. Silvestri, "Contactless monitoring of breathing patterns and respiratory rate at the pit of the neck: A single camera approach," *J. Sensors*, vol. 2018, 2018, doi: 10.1155/2018/4567213.

C. B. Pereira, M. Czaplik, N. Blanik, R. Rossaint, V. Blazek, and S. Leonhardt, "Contact-free monitoring of circulation and perfusion dynamics based on the analysis of thermal imagery," *Biomed. Opt. Express*, vol. 5, no. 4, p. 1075, Apr. 2014, doi: 10.1364/BOE.5.001075.

C. B. Pereira, X. Yu, M. Czaplik, R. Rossaint, V. Blazek, and S. Leonhardt, "Remote monitoring of breathing dynamics using infrared thermography," *Biomed. Opt. Express*, vol. 6, no. 11, p. 4378, Nov. 2015, doi: 10.1364/BOE.6.004378.

C. B. Pereira, X. Yu, V. Blazek, and S. Leonhardt, "Robust remote monitoring of breathing function by using infrared thermography," in *Proc. Annu. Int. Conf. IEEE Eng. Med. Biol. Soc. EMBS*, vol. 2015-Novem, pp. 4250–4253, Nov. 2015, doi: 10.1109/EMBC.2015.7319333.

C. L. Hermansen and A. Mahajan, "Newborn respiratory distress," *Am. Fam. Physician*, vol. 92, no. 11, pp. 994–1002, 2015, doi: 10.1007/978-3-030-26044-6_157.

D. Fan, J. Yang, J. Zhang, Z. Lv, H. Huang, J. Qi, and P. Yang, "Effectively measuring respiratory flow with portable pressure data using back propagation neural network," *IEEE J. Transl. Eng. Heal. Med.*, vol. 6, no. December 2016, 2018, doi: 10.1109/JTEHM.2017.2688458.

E. Helfenbein, R. Firoozabadi, S. Chien, CarlsonE., and S. Babaeizadeh, "Development of three methods for extracting respiration from the surface ECG: A review," *J. Electrocardiol.*, vol. 47, no. 6, pp. 819–825, Nov. 2014, doi: 10.1016/J.JELECTROCARD.2014.07.020.

F. Yang, S. He, S. Sadanand, A. Yusuf, and M. Bolic, "Contactless measurement of vital signs using thermal and RGB cameras: A study of COVID 19-related health monitoring," *Sensors*, vol. 22, no. 2. 2022, doi: 10.3390/s22020627.

F. Q. Al-Khalidi, R. Saatchi, D. Burke, H. Elphick, and S. Tan, "Respiration rate monitoring methods: A review," *Pediatr. Pulmonol.*, vol. 46, no. 6, pp. 523–529, Jun. 2011, doi: 10.1002/PPUL.21416.

G. Rosengarten, B. Ahmed, and C. Marselli, "A novel method to measure respiratory airflow rate based on nasal pressure," *IFAC Proc. Vol.*, vol. 36, no. 15, pp. 415–419, 2003, doi: 10.1016/s1474-6670(17)33539-5.

G. F. Lewis, R. G. Gatto, and S. W. Porges, "A novel method for extracting respiration rate and relative tidal volume from infrared thermography," *Psychophysiology*, vol. 48, no. 7, pp. 877–887, Jul. 2011, doi: 10.1111/j.1469-8986.2010.01167.x.

J. Fei and I. Pavlidis, "Analysis of breathing air flow patterns in thermal imaging," *Conf Proc IEEE Eng Med Biol Soc*, vol. 2006, pp. 946–952, 2006, doi: 10.1109/IEMBS.2006.260117.

J. Fei and I. Pavlidis, "Virtual thermistor," in *Proc. 29th Annual International Conference of the IEEE Engineering in Medicine and Biology Society*, Aug. 2007, pp. 250–253, doi: 10.1109/IEMBS.2007.4352271.

Jin Fei and I. Pavlidis, "Thermistor at a distance: Unobtrusive measurement of breathing," *IEEE Trans. Biomed. Eng.*, vol. 57, no. 4, pp. 988–998, Apr. 2010, doi: 10.1109/TBME.2009.2032415.

Jin Fei, Zhen Zhu, and I. Pavlidis, "Imaging breathing rate in the CO2 absorption band," 2005 *IEEE Engineering in Medicine and Biology 27th Annual Conference*, Shanghai, 2005, pp. 700–705, doi: 10.1109/IEMBS.2005.1616510.

J. F. Fieselmann, M. S. Hendryx, C. M. Helms, and D. S. Wakefield, "Respiratory rate predicts cardiopulmonary arrest for internal medicine inpatients," *J. Gen. Intern. Med.*, vol. 7, pp.354–360, 1993, doi: 10.1007/BF02600071. PMID: 8410395.

K. Abbas, K. Heimann, K. Jergus, T. Orlikowsky, and S. Leonhardt, "Neonatal non-contact respiratory monitoring based on real-time infrared thermography," *Biomed. Eng. Online*, vol. 10, Oct. 2011, doi: 10.1038/415035A.

L. Maurya, P. Kaur, D. Chawla, and P. Mahapatra, "Non-contact breathing rate monitoring in newborns: A review," *Comput. Biol. Med.*, vol. 132, May 2021, doi: 10.1016/j.compbiomed.2021.104321.

M. Bartula, T. Tigges, and J. Muehlsteff, "Camera-based system for contactless monitoring of respiration," in *Proc. 35th Annual International Conference of the IEEE Engineering in Medicine and Biology Society (EMBC)*, Jul. 2013, pp. 2672–2675, doi: 10.1109/EMBC.2013.6610090.

M. Charlton, S. A. Stanley, Z. Whitman, V. Wenn, T. J. Coats, M. Sims, and J. P. Thompson, "The effect of constitutive pigmentation on the measured emissivity of human skin," *PLoS One*, vol. 15, no. 11, p. e0241843, Nov. 2020, doi: 10.1371/journal.pone.0241843.

M. Folke, L. Cernerud, M. Ekström, and B. Hök, "Critical review of non-invasive respiratory monitoring in medical care," *Med. Biol. Eng. Comput.*, vol. 41, no. 4, pp. 377–383, 2003, doi: 10.1007/BF02348078.

M.-A. Anghel and F. Iacobescu, "The influence of temperature and CO2 in exhaled breath," *16th International Congress of Metrology*, vol. 10012, p. 10012, 2013, doi: 10.1051/metrology/201310012.

M. A. Cretikos, R. Bellomo, K. Hillman, J. Chen, S. Finfer, and A. Flabouris, "Respiratory rate: The neglected vital sign," *Med. J. Aust.*, vol. 188, no. 11, pp. 657–659, Jun. 2008, doi: 10.5694/J.1326-5377.2008.TB01825.X.

P. H. Charlton, D. A. Birrenkott, T. Bonnici, M. A. F. Pimentel, A. E. W. Johnson, J. Alastruey, L. Tarassenko, P. J. Watkinson, R. Beale, and D. A. Clifton, "Breathing rate estimation from the electrocardiogram and photoplethysmogram: A review," *IEEE Rev. Biomed. Eng.*, vol. 11, pp. 2–20, Oct. 2018, doi: 10.1109/RBME.2017.2763681.

R. A. Angelova, D. Markov, R. Velichkova, P. Stankov, and I. Simova, "Exhaled carbon dioxide as a physiological source of deterioration of indoor air quality in non-industrial environments: Influence of air temperature," *Energies*, vol. 14, no. 23, 2021, doi: 10.3390/en14238127.

R. Parkes, "Rate of respiration: The forgotten vital sign," *Emerg. Nurse*, vol. 19, no. 2, pp. 12–17, May 2011, doi: 10.7748/EN2011.05.19.2.12.C8504.

S. M. Roelofs, "Hyperventilation, anxiety, craving for alcohol: A subacute alcohol withdrawal syndrome," *Alcohol*, vol. 2, no. 3, pp. 501–505, 1985, doi: 10.1016/0741-8329(85)90123-5.

Smith Ian E., John Mackay, Nahla Fahrid, and Don Krucheck, "Respiratory rate measurement: A comparison of methods," *Brit Journal of Healthcare Assistants*, vol. 5, no. 1, pp. 18–23, 2011, doi: 10.12968/BJHA.2011.5.1.18.

T. Jiang, Lirong Deng, Wenying Qiu, Jiaming Liang, Yichuan Wu, Zhichun Shao, Dongkai Wang, Min Zhang, Xiang Qian, Junwen Zhong, Xiaohao Wang, and Liwei Lin, "Wearable breath monitoring via a hot-film/calorimetric airflow sensing system," *Biosens. Bioelectron.*, vol. 163, Sep. 2020, doi: 10.1016/J.BIOS.2020.112288.

T. Lauteslager, M. Maslik, F. Siddiqui, S. Marfani, G. D. Leschziner, and A. J. Williams, "Validation of a new contactless and continuous respiratory rate monitoring device based on ultra-wideband radar technology," *Sensors*, vol. 21, no. 12, 2021, doi: 10.3390/s21124027.

V. V. Tipparaju, D. Wang, J. Yu, F. Chen, F. Tsow, E. Forzani, N. Tao, and X. Xian, "Respiration pattern recognition by wearable mask device," *Biosens. Bioelectron.*, vol. 169, Dec. 2020, doi: 10.1016/J.BIOS.2020.112590.

Y. Takahashi, Yi Gu, Takaaki Nakada, Ryuzo Abe, and Toshiya Nakaguchi, "Estimation of respiratory rate from thermography using respiratory likelihood index," *Sensors*, vol. 21, no. 13, pp. 4406, 2021, doi: 10.3390/s21134406. PMID: 34199084; PMCID: PMC8271612.

Y. Nam, Y. Kong, B. Reyes, N. Reljin, and K. H. Chon, "Monitoring of heart and breathing rates using dual cameras on a smartphone," *PLoS One*, vol. 11, no. 3, Mar. 2016, doi: 10.1371/JOURNAL.PONE.0151013.

7 Electrocardiographic Signature Assessment of Post-COVID-19 Syndrome via Machine Learning Algorithms in Patients with Comorbid Cardiovascular Conditions

Pedro Ribeiro, João Alexandre Marques Lobo, Maria Inês Barbosa, Clarice Cristina Cunha de Souza, Cristine Mayara Cavalcante Camerino, Daniel Pordeus, Camila Ferreira Leite, João Paulo Madeiro, and Pedro Miguel Rodrigues

7.1 INTRODUCTION

Coronavirus Disease 2019 (COVID-19) is a viral disease caused by the clinical manifestation of infection with Severe Acute Respiratory Syndrome Coronavirus-2 (SARS-CoV-2) (Agrawal et al. 2022; Angeli et al. 2022). This is a contagious infection that spreads rapidly through respiratory droplets expelled into the air when an infected person coughs or sneezes (Agrawal et al., 2022; Ribeiro et al. 2023), and it has significantly impacted global health, contributing to unprecedented morbidity and mortality worldwide (Shah et al., 2022; Pordeus, Ribeiro, Zacarias, de Oliveira, et al. 2023). According to the World Health Organization, by September 2025, more than 778 million COVID-19 cases had been reported, and over 7 million people had

DOI: 10.1201/9781003797524-7

died from the disease (World Health Organization 2024). Additionally, a significant proportion of patients continue to experience functional limitations and a decline in quality of life after recovery (Shah et al., 2022).

The clinical spectrum of COVID-19 ranges from asymptomatic infection, which occurs in a substantial proportion of individuals, to mild presentations such as fever, headache, myalgia, sore throat, cough, and anosmia, which may progress to severe viral pneumonia with potential development of acute respiratory distress syndrome and multi-organ failure (Asarcikli et al. 2022; Pordeus et al. 2023). In addition, COVID-19 has also been associated with a broad range of cardiovascular complications, including myocardial injury, myocarditis, acute myocardial infarction, stress cardiomyopathy, heart failure, arrhythmias, and thromboembolic events (Angeli et al. 2022; Chevrot et al. 2022; Agrawal et al. 2022). Even after recovery from acute COVID-19, some individuals experience persistent or newly emerging symptoms, a condition often described as long COVID or post-acute COVID-19 syndrome (PACS). Risk factors for developing PACS may include advanced age, female sex, hospitalization during acute COVID-19, symptom burden, and pre-existing comorbidities such as cardiovascular disease (Sha'ari et al. 2024). These manifestations can lead to functional impairment and reduced quality of life. However, current evidence regarding their duration and long-term outcomes remains limited (Shah et al. 2022; Soeiro and Pêgo-Fernandes 2021; Asarcikli et al. 2022). Moreover, there is still no clear definition of PACS cardiac changes, and cardiac abnormalities associated with it remain poorly characterized (Roca-Fernandez et al. 2023). This is especially true for patients with pre-existing cardiovascular conditions (Sha'ari et al. 2024). The electrocardiogram (ECG) is a simple, widely available, and rapidly performed examination used to identify cardiac abnormalities, including COVID-19–related cardiac changes, by recording the heart's electrophysiological activity (Agrawal et al. 2022; Hrebenyk et al. 2024; Moreno-Sánchez et al. 2024). While effective, the interpretation of ECG recordings is often time-consuming for cardiologists. Therefore, there is a growing need to develop artificial intelligence–based methods capable of analyzing and interpreting variability in ECG signals (Ribeiro, Marques, and Rodrigues 2023), particularly in patients with long COVID-19 and previously cardiac comorbidities (Agrawal et al. 2022; Moreno-Sánchez et al. 2024). ECG abnormalities during acute COVID-19 usually include medication-induced QTc prolongation, ST-T changes indicative of myocarditis, and various arrhythmias (Mehraeen et al. 2020). However, to date, only a limited number of studies have investigated ECG alterations specifically associated with long COVID-19 (Chevrot et al. 2022).

Recent research has applied machine learning (ML) to analyze and characterize PACS conditions. Studies have employed ML models to differentiate post-COVID-19 patients from healthy controls using ECG features (Agrawal et al. 2022; Stasenko et al. 2023) and metabolic profiles (Oropeza-Valdez et al. 2024), as well as to identify structural and functional alterations through imaging (Li et al. 2022; Fujimoto et al. 2025). Another approach reported in the literature involves the use of wearable-derived physiological data to model heart rate variability (HRV) across

COVID-19 and post-COVID-19 states (Sanches et al. 2025), or the use of Electronic Health Record data to predict the probability of developing PACS and/or to identify patient subphenotypes based on comorbidities and clinical patterns (Pfaff et al. 2022; Zhang et al. 2022; Antony et al. 2023; Bergquist et al. 2024; Jayavelu et al. 2025). Furthermore, immunological and hormonal biomarker analyses using ML models have been developed to diagnose Long COVID (Klein et al. 2023) automatically. However, to the authors' knowledge, no study has specifically compared individuals with pre-existing cardiovascular disease who had Long COVID-19 with those who did not.

Therefore, the primary objectives of this study are twofold: (1) assess Electrocardiographic Signatures by identifying and characterize specific ECG patterns associated with PACS in patients with comorbid cardiovascular conditions; (2) conduct a comparative discriminant analysis of ECG data between two groups of patients with pre-existing cardiac diseases using an end-to-end ML complexity framework—Group 1, Patients with cardiac pathologies but no history of COVID-19 infection (CVD + No COVID); Group 2, Patients with cardiac pathologies who have developed PACS (CVD + Had COVID).

7.2 METHODOLOGY

7.2.1 Experimental Setup

Feature extraction was performed in MATLAB R2022a, while Python 3.10.4 (scikit-learn) was used to develop and evaluate ML models and to generate discrimination reports. All experiments were run on a 14-inch MacBook Pro with an M1 Pro (8-core CPU, 14-core GPU) and 16 GB of RAM.

7.2.2 The Database

This quantitative, cross-sectional descriptive study was conducted at Hospital Universitário Walter Cantídio (HUWC), Fortaleza, Ceará, Brasil, from December 2023 to May 2024. The study received ethical approval from the Committee for Research on Humans (CAAE: 75377123.4.0000.5045).

The recruitment process began with an initial screening of 30 individuals. To be included, participants had to be over 18 years old, diagnosed with heart disease, and provide informed consent. Two participants from this group were excluded because they used mechanical ventilation. The remaining 28 participants had their vital signs and ECG data recorded.

Following data collection, an additional 10 participants were excluded: six due to significant interference with their HRV measurements and four due to incomplete data labels. This process resulted in a final dataset of 18 participants (44% female), with all data sampled at 256 Hz. For a detailed overview of the recruitment and selection process, please refer to the flowchart in Figure 7.1.

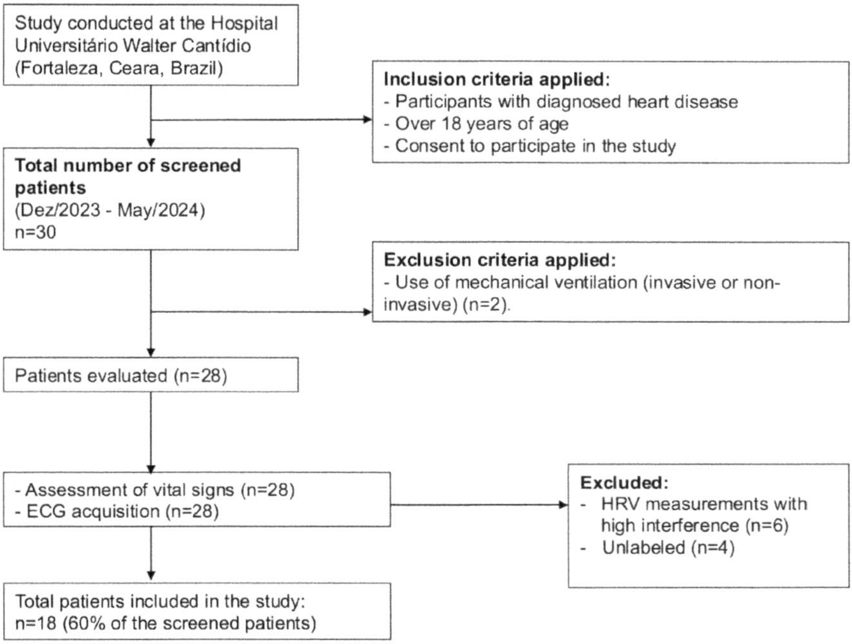

FIGURE 7.1 Flowchart of the participant flow diagram showing the recruitment, inclusion criteria, and exclusions of the cross-sectional study.

7.2.3 ECG Filtering

Each ECG signal lead from every participant was processed using an elliptical band-pass filter. This filter was configured with an order of 32, frequency cut-offs at 1 Hz and 40 Hz, a steepness of 0.85, and a stop-band attenuation of 60 dB.

7.2.4 Signal Normalization

The ECG signals, denoted as $x(n)$, were normalized to have unit energy. This was achieved by dividing each sample by the square root of the mean of the squared signal values, as described in the following equation (Rodrigues et al., 2021).

$$x(n) = \frac{x(n)}{\sqrt{\frac{\sum_{n=0}^{N-1} x^2(n)}{N}}} \tag{7.1}$$

Figure 7.2 illustrates 5 seconds of the ECG signal after filtering and normalization, for each class.

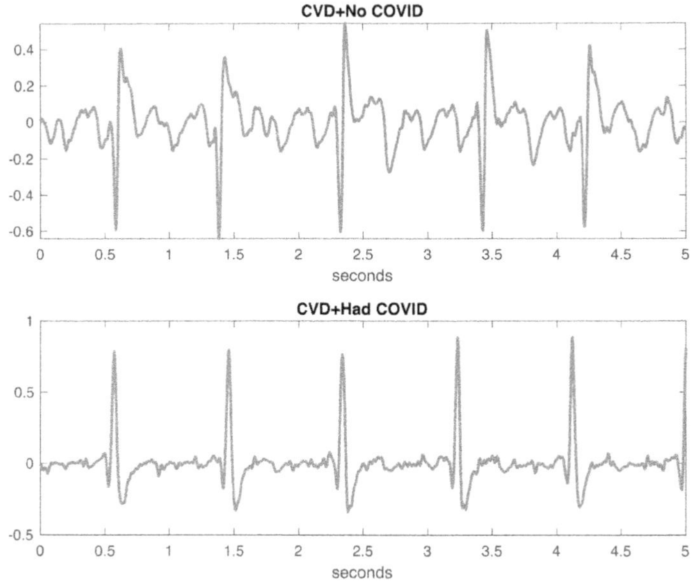

FIGURE 7.2 5-second ECG signal example of each class after normalization and filtering.

7.2.5 ECG Multi-band Decomposition via Wavelet Transform and Feature Extraction

The Discrete Wavelet Transform (DWT) is a powerful technique for analyzing non-stationary signals, such as ECGs. It decomposes a signal into various frequency bands (sub-bands) at different resolutions, providing a detailed time-frequency representation that is ideal for feature extraction (Guido 2022; Rioul and Vetterli 1991). The decomposition process is performed using a filter bank, which consists of a low-pass filter and a high-pass filter (Malvar 1992; Martin Vetterli and Jelena Kovačević 1995). At each level of decomposition, the signal is passed through both filters according to the following steps:

1. The DWT uses an analysis scale function, $\left(\tilde{\phi}_1(n)\right)$, and an analysis wavelet function, $\left(\tilde{\Psi}_1(n)\right)$, which are defined by the impulse responses of the low-pass $\left(h\_LP(n)\right)$ and high-pass $\left(h\_HP(n)\right)$ filters, respectively:

$$\tilde{\phi}_1(n) = h\_LP(n) \tag{7.2}$$

$$\tilde{\Psi}_1(n) = h\_HP(n) \tag{7.3}$$

2. Recursive Decomposition: The signal is decomposed recursively. The scaling and wavelet functions at a level i+1 are derived from the scaling function at the previous level i:

$$\tilde{\phi}_{i+1}(n) = \tilde{\phi}_i(n/2) * \tilde{\phi}_1(n) \tag{7.4}$$

$$\tilde{\Psi}_{i+1}(n) = \tilde{\phi}_i(n) * \tilde{\Psi}_1(n/2^i) \tag{7.5}$$

where $*$ denotes the convolution operation.

3. Sub-band Signal Computation: The signal in the m-th sub-band, $x_m(n)$, is computed by convolving the original signal $x(k)$ with the appropriate analysis filter, $h_m(n)$, and then downsampling:
   a. For the approximation sub-band ($m = 0$): $x_0(n) = \Sigma\left[x(k) * h_0(2^s n - k)\right]$
   b. For the detail sub-bands ($m = 1, 2, \ldots, S$): $x_m(n) = \Sigma\left[x(k) * h_m(2^{s-m+1} n - k)\right]$

Figure 7.3 shows the equivalent filter bank and the subband decomposition; ω denotes the angular frequency. For this study, each ECG signal was decomposed into sub-bands up to level three (S = 3), using the Symlet7 wavelet, which has demonstrated strong performance in ECG analysis (Chen et al. 2020; Ribeiro et al. 2024). The resulting sub-band signals, $x_m(n)$, were resampled to the original sampling rate using a wavelet interpolation method to ensure consistency.

7.2.6 Feature Extraction

After that, 10 nonlinear features were collected from the signal's full-band and sub-bands every 1s within a sliding rectangular non-overlapped windowing analysis.

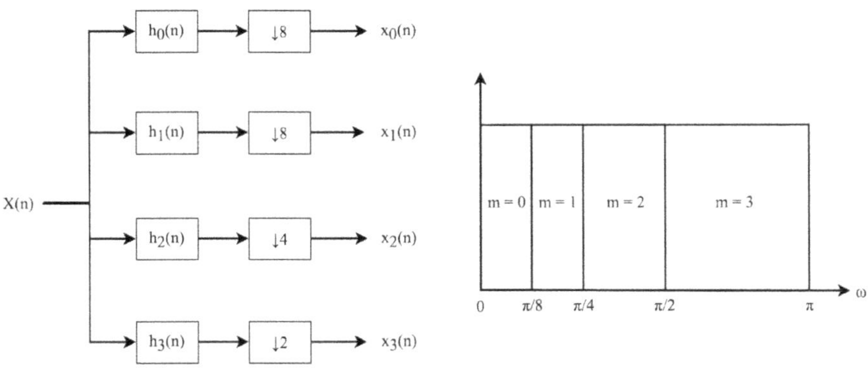

(a) Equivalent filter bank (b) Nonuniform sub-band division

FIGURE 7.3 Equivalent filter bank and sub-band division (ω: angular frequency).

Below are the details of the 10 nonlinear features extracted from the ECG signals, including their definitions and corresponding equations.

1. **Approximate Entropy (AE)**: AE assesses the likelihood that similar patterns within a time series remain consistent when new data points are included. A lower AE value suggests more regular or predictable data, while a higher value indicates greater complexity or irregularity.

$$AE(m,r) = \lim_{N\to\infty} \Theta^m(r) - \Theta^{m+1}(r), \tag{7.6}$$

Θ is the Heaviside step function and can be defined as

$$\Theta^m(r) = \frac{\sum_i \ln\left[C_i^m(r)\right]}{N-m+1}, \tag{7.7}$$

where r denotes a predetermined tolerance, N is the number of data points in the time series, and m is the dimension (Caesarendra et al. 2013).

2. **Correlation Dimension (CD)**: CD measures the self-similarity of a signal. Higher values indicate greater complexity and less internal similarity.

$$CD = \lim_{M\to\infty} \frac{2\sum_{i=1}^{M-k}\sum_{j=i+k}^{M} \Theta(l\,|\,X_i - X_j\,|)}{M^2}, \tag{7.8}$$

where Θ(x) is the Heaviside step function, X_i and X_j are position vectors on the attractor, l is the distance under consideration, k is the summation offset, and M is the number of reconstructed vectors from x (Caesarendra et al. 2013).

3. **Detrended Fluctuation Analysis (DFA)**: DFA measures the statistical self-affinity of a signal, quantifying long-range correlations in a time series.

$$DFA(n) = \sqrt{\frac{\sum_{k=1}^{N}\left[y(k) - y_n(k)\right]^2}{N}}, \tag{7.9}$$

where N is the length, $y_n(k)$ is the local trend, and $y(k)$ is defined as

$$y(k) = \sum_{i=1}^{k}\left[x(i) - \bar{x}\right], \tag{7.10}$$

with $x(i)$ as the inter-beat interval and $\bar{x}$ as its average (Hardstone et al. 2012).

4. **Energy (En)**: In the context of signal processing, energy represents the capacity of the system to perform work and is calculated as the sum of the squared amplitudes of the signal (Sundararajan 2015).

$$En = \sum_{n=0}^{N-1} | x(n) |^2 \tag{7.11}$$

5. **Higuchi Fractal Dimension (H)**: This feature estimates the fractal dimension of a time series, providing a measure of its complexity.

$$H = \frac{\ln\left(L(k)\right)}{\ln\left(\frac{1}{k}\right)}, \tag{7.12}$$

where k is the number of composed sub-series, and $L(k)$ is the averaged curve size (Silva et al. 2023).

6. **Hurst Exponent (EH)**: The Hurst Exponent quantifies how chaotic or unpredictable a time series is by measuring its long-term memory.

$$K_q(\tau) \sim \left(\frac{\tau}{\nu}\right)^{qEH(q)}, \tag{7.13}$$

with

$$K_q(\tau) = \frac{\left(| X(t+\tau) - X(t) |^q\right)}{\left(| X(t) |^q\right)}, \tag{7.14}$$

where q is the order moments of the distribution increments, ν is the time resolution, τ is the incorporation time delay of the attractor, and t is the period of a given time series signal $X(t)$ (Garcia et al., 2022).

7. **Katz Fractal Dimension (K)**: This feature estimates the fractal dimension through a waveform analysis of a time series (Garcia et al. 2022).

$$K = \frac{\log(n)}{\log(n) + \log\left(\frac{max_n\left(\sqrt{(n-1)^2 + \left(x(n) - x(1)\right)^2}\right)}{\sum_{n=2}^{N}\sqrt{1 + \left(x(n-1) - x(n)\right)^2}}\right)}, \tag{7.15}$$

8. **Lyapunov Exponent (ELy)**: The Lyapunov Exponent evaluates a system's predictability and its sensitivity to initial conditions by measuring the rate of separation of infinitesimally close trajectories in phase space.

$$Ly(x_0) = \lim_{n \to \infty} \frac{\sum_{k=1}^{n} \ln |f'(x_k - 1)|}{n}, \tag{7.16}$$

where f' is the derivative of f (Silva, Batista, and Rodrigues 2022).

9. **Logarithmic Entropy (LE)**: LE quantifies the average amount of information (in bits) needed to represent each event in a probability distribution. Higher values indicate greater unpredictability or randomness (Sundararajan 2015).

$$LE = \sum_{n=1}^{N} \log_2 \left[|x(n)|^2 \right] \tag{7.17}$$

10. **Shannon Entropy (SE)** SE measures the uncertainty or randomness in a probability distribution. Higher entropy values indicate greater uncertainty, while lower values suggest more order or certainty (Sundararajan 2015).

$$SE = -\sum_{n=1}^{N} |x(n)|^2 \log_2 \left[|x(n)|^2 \right] \tag{7.18}$$

7.2.7 Data Compressor

To reduce the dimensionality of the feature space for ML analysis, six statistical functions were applied to the 10 nonlinear features extracted from the four signal bands (3 detail sub-bands + 1 approximation sub-band). This process, acting as a time-data compressor, resulted in a total of 480 features (10 features × 4 bands × 6 statistical functions).

The statistical functions used were Average (Avg), Standard Deviation (Std), 95th Percentile (P95), Variance (Var), Median (Med), and Kurtosis (Kur) (Peck, Olsen, and Devore 2008; Rosner 2010).

7.2.8 Machine Learning Approaches

A total of 19 classifiers from the Scikit-learn library were used to discriminate between the two classes ("Had COVID" vs. "No COVID"); check Table 7.1 for more details. A leave-one-out cross-validation (LOOCV) strategy was employed to evaluate the discriminative power of the selected features.

TABLE 7.1
Description of the 19 Scikit-Learn Classifiers Used in This Study

Classifier	Hyperparameters	Basic Definition
Support-Vector Machines (SVC)	γ='auto', kernel='rbf', C=1.0, probability=false + Default	A powerful classification method that finds an optimal hyperplane to separate classes in feature space. It uses kernel functions to handle nonlinear data by transforming it into higher dimensions.
Gaussian Process Classifier (GauPro)	1.0 * RBF(1.0), optimizer='fmin_l_bfgs_b', max_iter_predict=100, copy_X_train=true + Default	A probabilistic classifier that uses a Gaussian process to model a distribution over functions. It provides probabilistic predictions, making it useful for capturing uncertainty in small or complex datasets.
Linear SVC (LinSVC)	penalty='l2', loss='squared_hinge', dual=True + Default	A linear classifier optimized for large datasets, based on the liblinear library. It is highly efficient and scales well with the number of samples and features, using a linear kernel.
SGD Classifier (SGD)	max_iter=100, tol=0.001, penalty='l2', loss='hinge', alpha=0.0001 + Default	A versatile classifier that optimizes linear models using stochastic gradient descent. It is suitable for large-scale learning and can handle various loss functions for different classification problems.
K-Nearest Neighbors Classifier (KNN)	n_neighbors=5, weights='uniform', algorithm='auto' + Default	A simple, instance-based learning algorithm that classifies a sample based on the majority vote of its k-nearest neighbors. It is intuitive and effective for datasets with clear class boundaries.
Logistic Regression (LogReg)	solver='lbfgs', penalty='l2', C=1.0, max_iter=100 + Default	A linear model used for binary or multiclass classification. It estimates the probability that a given input belongs to a particular class by using the logistic (sigmoid) function.
Logistic RegressionCV (LogRegCV)	cv=3, penalty='l2', solver='lbfgs', max_iter=100 + Default	An extension of Logistic Regression that includes built-in cross-validation to automatically select the best regularization parameter, improving the model's generalization performance.
Bagging Classifier (BaggC)	n_estimators=10, max_samples=1.0, bootstrap=true + Default	An ensemble method that combines multiple base classifiers trained on random subsets of the data (with replacement). It reduces variance and improves the model's stability and accuracy.
Extra Trees Classifier (ExTreeC)	n_estimators=300, criterion='gini', max_features='auto', bootstrap=false + Default	An ensemble method that builds multiple randomized decision trees and averages their predictions. It introduces more randomness than Random Forest to further reduce overfitting.
Random Forest Classifier (RF)	max_depth=5, n_estimators=300, criterion='gini', bootstrap=true, min_samples_split=2 + Default	An ensemble method that constructs multiple decision trees during training and merges their predictions. It is robust against overfitting and provides high accuracy for various classification tasks.

(Continued)

TABLE 7.1 CONTINUED
Description of the 19 Scikit-Learn Classifiers Used in This Study

Classifier	Hyperparameters	Basic Definition
Gaussian Naive Bayes (GauNB)	priors=none, var_smoothing=1e-9, store_covariance=false + Default	A probabilistic classifier based on Bayes' theorem with a "naive" assumption of feature independence. It assumes that features follow a Gaussian distribution and is effective for high-dimensional data.
Decision Tree Classifier (DeTreeC)	max_depth=5, criterion='gini', splitter='best', min_samples_split=2 + Default	A model that splits data into subsets based on feature values, creating a tree-like structure of decisions. It is easy to interpret and can handle both numerical and categorical data.
MLP Classifier (MLP)	α=1, max_iter=1000, hidden_layer_sizes=100, activation='relu', solver='adam' + Default	A neural network model with an input layer, one or more hidden layers, and an output layer. It learns nonlinear relationships in data by adjusting weights through backpropagation.
AdaBoost Classifier (AdaBoost)	n_estimators=50, learning_rate=1.0, algorithm='SAMME.R' + Default	An ensemble method that sequentially combines multiple weak classifiers to form a strong classifier. It adjusts the weights of incorrectly classified samples to focus on difficult cases.
Linear Discriminant Analysis (LinDis)	solver='svd', shrinkage=none, priors=none + Default	A linear classifier that projects data onto a lower-dimensional space to maximize class separability. It is effective for datasets with well-separated classes.
Quadratic Discriminant Analysis (QuadDis)	reg_param=0.0, priors=none, store_covariance=false + Default	Similar to Linear Discriminant Analysis but allows for quadratic decision boundaries. It is useful when the class distributions have different covariances.
One-vs-Rest Classifier (OvsR)	estimator=LinearSVC(random_state=0), n_jobs=none, verbose=false + Default	A strategy used for multiclass classification by fitting one classifier per class. Each classifier is trained to distinguish its class from all other classes combined.
Gradient Boosting Classifier (GradBoost)	loss='log_loss', learning_rate=0.1, n_estimators=100 + Default	An ensemble method that builds trees sequentially, with each new tree trained to correct the errors of the previous ones. It is highly effective for both classification and regression.
SGD Classifier (SGDC)	penalty='l2', loss='hinge', alpha=0.0001 + Default	A versatile classifier that optimizes linear models using stochastic gradient descent. It is suitable for large-scale learning and can handle a variety of loss functions for different classification problems.

7.2.9 Classification Evaluation Metrics

To rigorously assess and compare the performance of the machine learning models, we utilized a comprehensive set of standard classification metrics. These metrics are derived from the four possible outcomes of a binary classification task, which are typically presented in a confusion matrix:

- **True Positives (TP):** The number of positive instances (e.g., "CVD + Had COVID") correctly classified as positive.
- **True Negatives (TN):** The number of negative instances (e.g., "CVD + No COVID") correctly classified as negative.
- **False Positives (FP):** The number of negative instances incorrectly classified as positive (a "Type I error").
- **False Negatives (FN):** The number of positive instances incorrectly classified as negative (a "Type II error").

The primary metric for ML performance evaluation:

- **Area Under the Receiver Operating Characteristic Curve (AUC)**: The AUC represents a model's ability to distinguish between the positive and negative classes across all possible classification thresholds. It is the area under the ROC curve, which plots the True Positive Rate (Recall) against the False Positive Rate. An AUC of 1.0 signifies a perfect classifier, while an AUC of 0.5 indicates performance no better than random chance. The AUC is particularly valuable as it provides a single, aggregate measure of performance that is robust to class imbalance (Nahm 2022).

While our primary metric for model comparison was the AUC, we also calculated several other metrics to gain a more granular understanding of model performance.

- **Accuracy (Acc)** measures the proportion of all instances that were correctly classified. While intuitive, it can be misleading in datasets with a significant class imbalance (Doğan 2019).

$$Acc = \frac{TP + TN}{TP + TN + FP + FN} \tag{7.19}$$

- **Recall (or Sensitivity)** measures the proportion of actual positive instances that were correctly identified by the model. High recall is crucial when the cost of false negatives is high (Doğan 2019).

$$Recall = \frac{TP}{TP + FN} \tag{7.20}$$

- **Specificity (Spec)** measures the proportion of actual negative instances that were correctly identified. It is the counterpart to recall (Hicks et al. 2022).

$$Spec = \frac{TN}{TN + FP} \tag{7.21}$$

- **Precision (or Positive Predictive Value, PPV)** measures the proportion of positive predictions that were actually correct. High precision is important when the cost of false positives is high (Doğan 2019).

$$Precision = \frac{TP}{TP + FP} \tag{7.22}$$

- **Negative Predictive Value (NPV)** measures the proportion of negative predictions that were actually correct (Safari et al. 2018).

$$NPV = \frac{TN}{TN + FN} \tag{7.23}$$

- **F1-Score** is the harmonic mean of Precision and Recall. It provides a single score that balances both metrics, making it particularly useful for evaluating models on imbalanced datasets where both precision and recall are important (Goutte and Gaussier 2005).

$$F1 - Score = 2 \cdot \frac{(Precision\ x\ Recall)}{(Precision + Recall)} \tag{7.24}$$

7.3 RESULTS

Figure 7.4 presents a detailed overview of the AUC distributions for all classifiers.
Table 7.2 indicates the best performance achieved results.

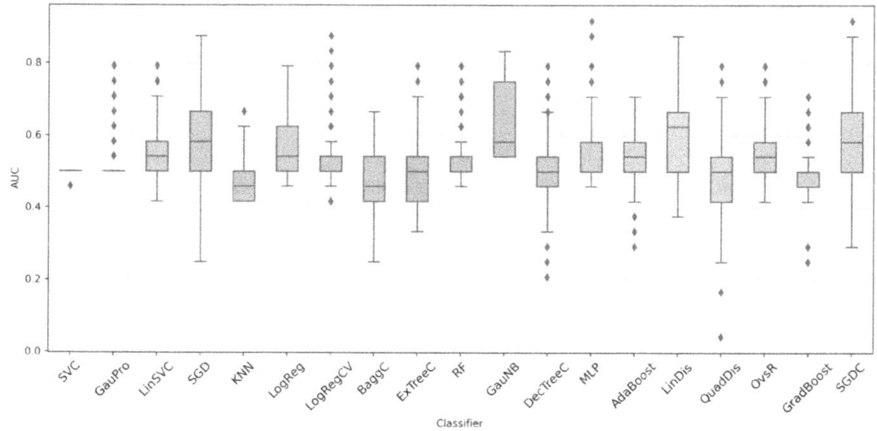

FIGURE 7.4 AUC Boxplots of every classifier's performance.

TABLE 7.2
Best Classification Results

Comparison Group	Algorithm	# of Features	Acc	Rec	Prec	Spec	NPV	F1-Score	AUC
CVD + Had COVID vs. CVD + No COVID	SGDC	5	94.44%	100%	92.30%	83.33%	100%	96.00%	0.9167

Figure 7.5 presents the confusion matrix for the best classification results located in Table 7.2.

Figure 7.6 shows the ROC curves for the best overall results.

7.4 DISCUSSION

The results depicted in Figure 7.4 demonstrate that, for the "CVD + Had COVID vs. CVD + No COVID" classification task, the MLP and SGDC classifiers exhibited the highest levels of performance. Notably, the SGDC model achieved a higher median AUC than the MLP, indicating superior discriminative capability. The boxplots provide additional insights, showing that: (1) differences in performance among most classifiers are relatively minor; (2) results are consistent across multiple models, suggesting an absence of selective reporting; (3) the choice of classifier exerts only a limited influence on overall model performance.

Collectively, these observations underscore the robustness and reliability of the findings. Among all classifiers evaluated, the SGDC model achieved the strongest overall results, with an *Acc* of 94.44%, *Rec* of 100%, *Prec* of 92.30%, *Spec* of 83.33%, *NPV* of 100%, *F1-score* of 96.00%, and an AUC of 0.9167. Figure 7.5 presents the confusion matrix corresponding to the best-performing model reported in Table 7.2. The results indicate that the "CVD + No COVID" class was classified correctly in 100% of cases (12 out of 12), whereas the "CVD + Had COVID" class was correctly classified in 83.33% of cases (5 out of 6), as demonstrated by checking the ROC curve presented in Figure 7.6.

One plausible explanation for these observations is the persistence of ECG alterations induced by COVID, which may continue to manifest during the post-acute

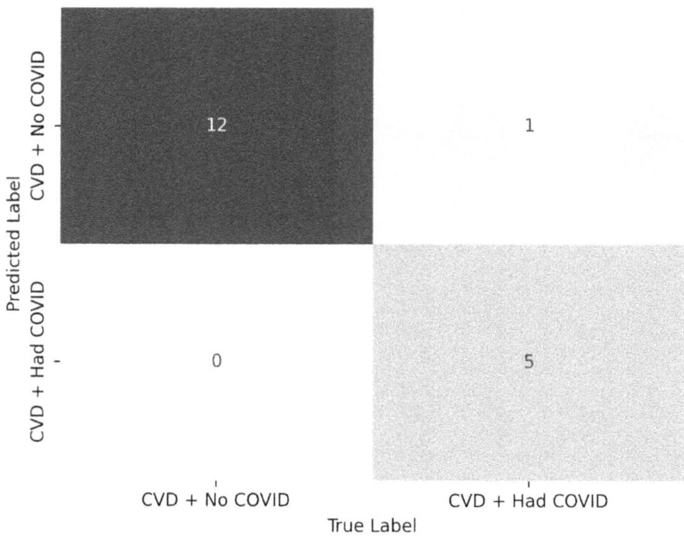

FIGURE 7.5 Confusion Matrix for the best classification results.

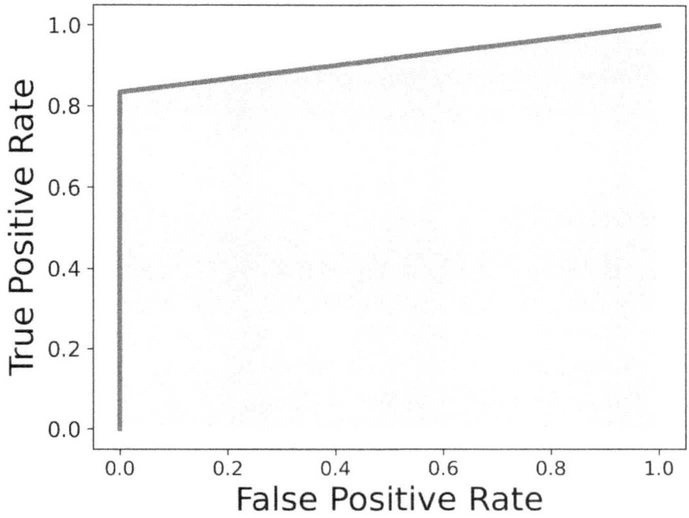

FIGURE 7.6 Best prediction results: ROC curves.

phase, as reflected in the present study. This interpretation is supported by evidence from a longitudinal investigation conducted by Xie et al. (2022), which examined the long-term cardiovascular outcomes associated with COVID-19. Their findings revealed a marked difference in the incidence of cardiovascular diseases before and after SARS-CoV-2 infection, with significantly higher rates observed during the post-infection period. Furthermore, the study reported a graded increase in cardiovascular risk proportional to the severity of the acute phase of the disease.

7.5 LIMITATIONS

Although the study demonstrates promising results, it is important to acknowledge certain limitations. First, the relatively small size of the dataset means that even a few misclassifications can lead to substantial fluctuations in performance metrics. Second, the dataset is unbalanced, which may introduce biases and increase the risk of overfitting the results.

7.6 CONCLUSION

This study assessed ECG signatures to identify patterns associated with PACS in patients with pre-existing cardiovascular conditions. By extracting ten nonlinear ECG features and summarizing them through statistical measures, we characterized distinctive signal behaviors potentially linked to prior COVID-19 infection.

A comparative discriminant analysis using an end-to-end machine learning framework successfully differentiated two patient groups: those with cardiac pathologies and no history of COVID-19, and those with cardiac pathologies who had recovered from COVID-19. The proposed approach achieved an accuracy of 94.44% and an AUC of 0.9167, demonstrating strong potential for clinical application. Nevertheless, the small and unbalanced dataset limits generalizability, highlighting the need for future studies with larger, more balanced cohorts to validate and strengthen these findings.

ACKNOWLEDGMENTS

This work was supported by National Funds from FCT - Fundação para a Ciência e a Tecnologia through project UIDB/50016/2020, Coordenação de Aperfeiçoamento de Pessoal de Nível Superior (CAPES) - Postgraduate Scholarship (cod 001), and Fundação Cearense de Apoio ao Desenvolvimento Científico e Tecnológico (FUNCAP) - Postgraduate Scholarship (cod 001).

REFERENCES

Agrawal, Amulya, Aniket Chauhan, Manu Kumar Shetty, Girish M P, Mohit D Gupta, and Anubha Gupta. 2022. “ECG-ICOVIDNet: Interpretable AI Model to Identify Changes in the ECG Signals of Post-COVID Subjects.” *Computers in Biology and Medicine* 146 (July): 105540. https://doi.org/10.1016/j.compbiomed.2022.105540.

Angeli, Fabio, Gianpaolo Reboldi, Antonio Spanevello, Roberto De Ponti, Dina Visca, Jacopo Marazzato, Martina Zappa, et al. 2022. “Electrocardiographic Features of Patients with COVID-19: One Year of Unexpected Manifestations.” *European Journal of Internal Medicine* 95 (January): 7–12. https://doi.org/10.1016/j.ejim.2021.10.006.

Antony, Blessy, Hannah Blau, Elena Casiraghi, Johanna J Loomba, Tiffany J Callahan, Bryan J Laraway, Kenneth J Wilkins, et al. 2023. “Predictive Models of Long COVID.” *EBioMedicine* 96 (October): 104777. https://doi.org/10.1016/j.ebiom.2023.104777.

Asarcikli, Lale Dinc, Mert İlker Hayiroglu, Altug Osken, Kivanc Keskin, Zeynep Kolak, and Tolga Aksu. 2022. “Heart Rate Variability and Cardiac Autonomic Functions in Post-COVID Period.” *Journal of Interventional Cardiac Electrophysiology* 63 (3): 715–721. https://doi.org/10.1007/s10840-022-01138-8.

Bergquist, Timothy, Johanna Loomba, Emily Pfaff, Fangfang Xia, Zixuan Zhao, Yitan Zhu, Elliot Mitchell, et al. 2024. “Crowd-Sourced Machine Learning Prediction of Long COVID Using Data from the National COVID Cohort Collaborative.” *EBioMedicine* 108 (October): 105333. https://doi.org/10.1016/j.ebiom.2024.105333.

Caesarendra, Wahyu, Buyung Kosasih, Kiet Tieu, and Craig A S Moodie. 2013. “An Application of Nonlinear Feature Extraction – A Case Study for Low Speed Slewing Bearing Condition Monitoring and Prognosis.” *2013 IEEE/ASME International Conference on Advanced Intelligent Mechatronics* (Wollongong), July 2013, 1613–1618. https://doi.org/10.1109/aim.2013.6584344.

Chen, You-Shyang, Ching-Hsue Cheng, Su-Fen Chen, and Jhe-You Jhuang. 2020. “Identification of the Framingham Risk Score by an Entropy-Based Rule Model for Cardiovascular Disease.” *Entropy* 22 (12): 1406. https://doi.org/10.3390/e22121406.

Chevrot, Gabriel, Marie Hauguel-Moreau, Marion Pépin, Antoine Vieillard-Baron, Anne-Sophie Lot, Mounir Ouadahi, Hélène Hergault, et al. 2022. “Electrocardiogram Abnormalities and Prognosis in COVID-19.” *Frontiers in Cardiovascular Medicine* 9 (October). https://doi.org/10.3389/fcvm.2022.993479.

Doğan, Onur. 2019. "Data Linkage Methods for Big Data Management in Industry 4.0." In *Optimizing Big Data Management and Industrial Systems With Intelligent Techniques*, 108–127. Hershey: IGI Global. https://doi.org/10.4018/978-1-5225-5137-9.ch005.

Fujimoto, Yu, Hiroki Abe, Tsuyoshi Eiro, Sakiko Tsugawa, Meiro Tanaka, Mai Hatano, Waki Nakajima, et al. 2025. "Systemic Increase of AMPA Receptors Associated with Cognitive Impairment of Long COVID." *Brain Communications* 7 (5). https://doi.org/10.1093/braincomms/fcaf337.

Garcia, Alejandro Antonio Torres, Carlos Alberto Reyes Garcia, Luis Villasenor-Pineda, and Omar Mendoza Montoya. 2022. *Biosignal Processing and Classification Using Computational Learning and Intelligence Principles, Algorithms, and Applications.* London: Academic Press.

Goutte, Cyril, and Eric Gaussier. 2005. "A Probabilistic Interpretation of Precision, Recall and F-Score, with Implication for Evaluation." In *Advances in Information Retrieval*, 345–359. Springer Berlin Heidelberg. https://doi.org/10.1007/978-3-540-31865-1_25.

Guido, Rodrigo. 2022. "Wavelets behind the Scenes: Practical Aspects, Insights, and Perspectives." *Physics Reports* 985 (November): 1–23. https://doi.org/10.1016/j.physrep.2022.08.001.

Hardstone, Richard, Simon-Shlomo Poil, Giuseppina Schiavone, Rick Jansen, Vadim V Nikulin, Huibert D Mansvelder, and Klaus Linkenkaer-Hansen. 2012. "Detrended Fluctuation Analysis: A Scale-Free View on Neuronal Oscillations." *Frontiers in Physiology* 3. https://doi.org/10.3389/fphys.2012.00450.

Hicks, Steven A, Inga Strümke, Vajira Thambawita, Malek Hammou, Michael A Riegler, Pål Halvorsen, and Sravanthi Parasa. 2022. "On Evaluation Metrics for Medical Applications of Artificial Intelligence." *Scientific Reports* 12 (1). https://doi.org/10.1038/s41598-022-09954-8.

Hrebenyk, M V, S M Maslii, O O Shevchuk, M M Korda, and S G Vari. 2024. "ECG Patterns in Post-COVID-19 Patients." *The Ukrainian Biochemical Journal* 96 (2): 100–107. https://doi.org/10.15407/ubj96.02.100.

Jayavelu, Naresh Doni, Hady Samaha, Sonia Tandon Wimalasena, Annmarie Hoch, Jeremy P Gygi, Gisela Gabernet, Al Ozonoff, et al. 2025. *Machine Learning Models Predict Long COVID Outcomes Based on Baseline Clinical and Immunologic Factors.* February 2025. https://doi.org/10.1101/2025.02.12.25322164.

Klein, Jon, Jamie Wood, Jillian R Jaycox, Rahul M Dhodapkar, Peiwen Lu, Jeff R Gehlhausen, Alexandra Tabachnikova, et al. 2023. "Distinguishing Features of Long COVID Identified through Immune Profiling." *Nature* 623 (7985): 139–148. https://doi.org/10.1038/s41586-023-06651-y.

Li, Frank, Xuan Zhang, Alejandro P Comellas, Eric A Hoffman, Tianbao Yang, and Ching-Long Lin. 2022. "Contrastive Learning and Subtyping of Post-COVID-19 Lung Computed Tomography Images." *Frontiers in Physiology* 13 (October). https://doi.org/10.3389/fphys.2022.999263.

Malvar, Henrique. 1992. *Signal Processing with Lapped Transforms.* Norwood, Massachusetts: Artech House.

Mehraeen, Esmaeil, Seyed Ahmad Seyed Alinaghi, Ali Nowroozi, Omid Dadras, Sanam Alilou, Parnian Shobeiri, Farzane Behnezhad, and Amirali Karimi. 2020. "A Systematic Review of ECG Findings in Patients with COVID-19." *Indian Heart Journal* 72 (6): 500–507. https://doi.org/10.1016/j.ihj.2020.11.007.

Moreno-Sánchez, Pedro A, Guadalupe García-Isla, Valentina D A Corino, Antti Vehkaoja, Kirsten Brukamp, Mark van Gils, and Luca Mainardi. 2024. "ECG-Based Data-Driven Solutions for Diagnosis and Prognosis of Cardiovascular Diseases: A Systematic Review." *Computers in Biology and Medicine* 172 (April): 108235. https://doi.org/10.1016/j.compbiomed.2024.108235.

Nahm, Francis Sahngun. 2022. "Receiver Operating Characteristic Curve: Overview and Practical Use for Clinicians." *Korean Journal of Anesthesiology* 75 (1): 25–36. https://doi.org/10.4097/kja.21209.

Oropeza-Valdez, Juan José, Cristian Padron-Manrique, Aarón Vázquez-Jiménez, Xavier Soberon, and Osbaldo Resendis-Antonio. 2024. "Exploring Metabolic Anomalies in COVID-19 and Post-COVID-19: A Machine Learning Approach with Explainable Artificial Intelligence." *Frontiers in Molecular Biosciences* 11 (September). https://doi.org/10.3389/fmolb.2024.1429281.

Peck, Roxy, Chris Olsen, and Jay L Devore. 2008. *Introduction to Statistics and Data Analysis*. Belmont: Cengage Learning.

Pfaff, Emily R, Andrew T Girvin, Tellen D Bennett, Abhishek Bhatia, Ian M Brooks, Rachel R Deer, Jonathan P Dekermanjian, et al. 2022. "Identifying Who Has Long COVID in the USA: A Machine Learning Approach Using N3C Data." *The Lancet Digital Health* 4 (7): e532–e541. https://doi.org/10.1016/s2589-7500(22)00048-6.

Pordeus, Daniel, Pedro Ribeiro, Laíla Zacarias, Adriel de Oliveira, João Alexandre Lobo Marques, Pedro Miguel Rodrigues, Camila Leite, Manoel Alves Neto, Arnaldo Aires Peixoto, and João Paulo do Vale Madeiro. 2023. *Training Strategies for Covid-19 Severity Classification*. https://doi.org/10.1007/978-3-031-34953-9_40.

Pordeus, Daniel, Pedro Ribeiro, Laíla Zacarias, João Paulo Madeiro, Joao Alexandre Lobo Marques, Pedro Miguel Rodrigues, Camila Leite, Manoel Alves Neto, Arnaldo Aires Peixoto Jr, and Adriel de Oliveira. 2023. "Classification of Severity of COVID-19 Patients Based on the Heart Rate Variability." In *Computerized Systems for Diagnosis and Treatment of COVID-19*, Editors: Joao Alexandre LoboMarques and Simon James Fong, 155–177. Springer International Publishing.

Ribeiro, Pedro, João Alexandre Lobo Marques, Daniel Pordeus, Laíla Zacarias, Camila Ferreira Leite, Manoel Alves Sobreira-Neto, Arnaldo Aires Peixoto, Adriel de Oliveira, João Paulo do Vale Madeiro, and Pedro Miguel Rodrigues. 2024. "Machine Learning-Based Cardiac Activity Non-Linear Analysis for Discriminating COVID-19 Patients with Different Degrees of Severity." *Biomedical Signal Processing and Control* 87 (January): 105558. https://doi.org/10.1016/j.bspc.2023.105558.

Ribeiro, Pedro, João Alexandre Lobo Marques, and Pedro Miguel Rodrigues. 2023. "COVID-19 Detection by Means of ECG, Voice, and X-Ray Computerized Systems: A Review." *Bioengineering* 10 (2): 198. https://doi.org/10.3390/bioengineering10020198.

Ribeiro, Pedro, Daniel Pordeus, Laíla Zacarias, Camila Leite, Manoel Alves Neto, Arnaldo Aires Peixoto Jr, Adriel de Oliveira, João Paulo Madeiro, João Alexandre Lobo Marques, and Pedro Miguel Rodrigues. 2023. "Evaluation of ECG Non-Linear Features in Time-Frequency Domain for the Discrimination of COVID-19 Severity Stages." In *Computerized Systems for Diagnosis and Treatment of COVID-19*, 137–154. Springer International Publishing.

Rioul, O, and M Vetterli. 1991. "Wavelets and Signal Processing." *IEEE Signal Processing Magazine* 8 (4): 14–38. https://doi.org/10.1109/79.91217.

Roca-Fernandez, Adriana, Malgorzata Wamil, Alison Telford, Valentina Carapella, Alessandra Borlotti, David Monteiro, Helena Thomaides-Brears, et al. 2023. "Cardiac Abnormalities in Long COVID 1-Year Post-SARS-CoV-2 Infection." *Open Heart* 10 (1): e002241. https://doi.org/10.1136/openhrt-2022-002241.

Rodrigues, Pedro M, Bruno C Bispo, Carolina Garrett, Dilio Alves, TeixeiraJoao P , and Diamantino Freitas. 2021. "Lacsogram: A New EEG Tool to Diagnose Alzheimer's Disease." *IEEE Journal of Biomedical and Health Informatics* 25 (9): 3384–3395. https://doi.org/10.1109/jbhi.2021.3069789.

Rosner, Bernard. 2010. *Fundamentals of Biostatistics*. 7th ed. Boston: Duxbury Press.

Safari, Saeed, Alireza Baratloo, Mohamed Elfil, and Ahmed Said Negida. 2018. "Part 2: Positive and Negative Predictive Values of Diagnostic Tests." *Archives of Academic Emergency Medicine* 3. https://doi.org/10.22037/aaem.v3i3.274.

Sanches, Carlos Alberto, Andre Felipe Henriques Librantz, Luciana Maria Malosá Sampaio, and Peterson Adriano Belan. 2025. "Classification of Individuals With COVID-19 and Post–COVID-19 Condition and Healthy Controls Using Heart Rate Variability: Machine Learning Study With a Near–Real-Time Monitoring Component." *Journal of Medical Internet Research*, ahead of print, April 2025. https://doi.org/10.2196/76613.

Sha'ari, Nur Insyirah, Aniza Ismail, Aznida Firzah Abdul Aziz, Leny Suzana Suddin, Amirah Azzeri, Ruhana Sk Abd Razak, and Nur Syazana Mad Tahir. 2024. "Cardiovascular Diseases as Risk Factors of Post-COVID Syndrome: A Systematic Review." *BMC Public Health* 24 (1): 1846. https://doi.org/10.1186/s12889-024-19300-4.

Shah, Bhushan, Shekhar Kunal, Ankit Bansal, Jayant Jain, Shubhankar Poundrik, Manu Kumar Shetty, Vishal Batra, et al. 2022. "Heart Rate Variability as a Marker of Cardiovascular Dysautonomia in Post-COVID-19 Syndrome Using Artificial Intelligence." *Indian Pacing and Electrophysiology Journal* 22 (2): 70–76. https://doi.org/10.1016/j.ipej.2022.01.004.

Silva, Gabriel, Patrícia Batista, and Pedro Miguel Rodrigues. 2022. "COVID-19 Activity Screening by a Smart-Data-Driven Multi-Band Voice Analysis." *Journal of Voice*, ahead of print, November 2022. https://doi.org/10.1016/j.jvoice.2022.11.008.

Silva, Martim, Pedro Ribeiro, Bruno C Bispo, and Pedro Miguel Rodrigues. 2023. "Detecção Da Doença de Alzheimer Através de Parâmetros Não-Lineares de Sinais de Fala." *Anais Do XLI Simpósio Brasileiro de Telecomunicações e Processamento de Sinais*, 2023, 1–5. https://doi.org/10.14209/sbrt.2023.1570923829.

Soeiro, Alexandre de Matos, and Paulo Manuel Pêgo-Fernandes. 2021. "Post-COVID-19 Cardiological Alterations." *Sao Paulo Medical Journal* 139 (6): 543–544. https://doi.org/10.1590/1516-3180.2021.139628062021.

Stasenko, Sergey V, Andrey V Kovalchuk, Evgeny V Eremin, Olga V Drugova, Natalya V Zarechnova, Maria M Tsirkova, Sergey A Permyakov, Sergey B Parin, and Sofia A Polevaya. 2023. "Using Machine Learning Algorithms to Determine the Post-COVID State of a Person by Their Rhythmogram." *Sensors* 23 (11): 5272. https://doi.org/10.3390/s23115272.

Sundararajan, D. 2015. *Discrete Wavelet Transform a Signal Processing Approach.* 1st ed. New Jersey: John Wiley & Sons.

Vetterli, Martin, and Jelena Kovačević. 1995. *Wavelets and Subband Coding.* Englewood Cliffs, New Jersey: Prentice Hall.

World Health Organization. 2024. "WHO Coronavirus (COVID-19) Dashboard." Accessed October 5, 2025. https://covid19.who.int/.

Xie, Yan, Evan Xu, Benjamin Bowe, and Ziyad Al-Aly. 2022. "Long-Term Cardiovascular Outcomes of COVID-19." *Nature Medicine* 28 (3): 583–590. https://doi.org/10.1038/s41591-022-01689-3.

Zhang, Hao, Chengxi Zang, Zhenxing Xu, Yongkang Zhang, Jie Xu, Jiang Bian, Dmitry Morozyuk, et al. 2022. "Data-Driven Identification of Post-Acute SARS-CoV-2 Infection Subphenotypes." *Nature Medicine* 29 (1): 226–235. https://doi.org/10.1038/s41591-022-02116-3.

8 Real-Time Deep Learning Pipeline for ECG Anomaly Detection

Yamini Niharika, Akhila, Ganesh R Naik, and Tripty Singh

8.1 INTRODUCTION

The cardiovascular diseases are considered one of the top causes of mortality in the world, and the promptness of the identification of abnormal heartbeats is the key to avoiding severe medical outcomes. Electrocardiography is a widely used, relatively easy-to-perform diagnostic tool that records the electrical impulses of the heart. ECGs provide abundant information about heart function, yet their long, continuous traces are very difficult to analyze manually. This is a time-consuming task that often leads to oversight, even in real-time monitoring.

As wearable devices, home-based health monitoring, and telemedicine become more popular, there is now more than ever a need for systems that can automatically analyze the ECG signal upon abnormality. Deep learning has become a powerful method for this task because it can learn meaningful representations directly from raw waveforms. In practice, however, real-world ECG signals pose several challenges: beat morphology variation, motion or electrode position noise, and short-term variations. Practically deployable models should thus be balanced in terms of accuracy, speed, robustness, and the capability to generalize to other patients and recording conditions.

Against this background, this piece of work aims to develop a deep learning pipeline capable of identifying ECG anomalies in real time with high confidence. The model is based on convolutional layers, which extract unique features from the waveform, and sequential layers, which capture temporal correlations among heartbeats. To enhance its robustness, this pipeline includes necessary preprocessing steps such as filtering and realistic signal augmentation, ensuring the model performs well in scenarios where the ECG is corrupted or distorted. Moreover, the system evaluates predictions using uncertainty estimation techniques, which is especially valuable in health applications. Using the MITBIH Arrhythmia Database for benchmarking, the proposed pipeline achieves high overall performance, especially for both common

 DOI: 10.1201/9781003797524-8

and less frequent arrhythmias. The developed approach is sufficiently efficient for continuous processing and can be applied to wearable devices and to bedside and remote health applications. The present system offers reliable, real-time feedback that supports clinicians, continuous patient monitoring, and allows for earlier detection of possibly dangerous cardiac abnormalities.

8.2 LITERATURE SURVEY

Automatic detection of ECG anomalies has gained significant attention in recent years due to its clinical value and the growing need for continuous remote cardiac monitoring. The literature spans a wide spectrum of modeling strategies—including generative models, transformer-based architectures, CNN–RNN hybrids, lightweight models for edge devices, autoencoder-based reconstruction frameworks, and classical signal processing methods—each offering different balances between accuracy, robustness, and deployability.

One important direction is generative modeling. Qin et al. (2023) introduced a temporal GAN designed specifically for ECG anomaly detection, demonstrating that adversarial learning can capture normal heartbeat patterns and identify deviations through reconstruction behavior. While generative approaches are effective in low-label and semi-supervised settings, they typically require careful training and incur higher inference overhead, which can complicate real-time implementation. Another recent trend is transformer-based modeling. Alamr and Artoli (2023) explored an unsupervised transformer approach capable of modeling long-range dependencies in ECG sequences, while Alghieth (2025) proposed a hybrid transformer architecture optimized for near–real-time anomaly detection. These studies highlight the ability of attention mechanisms to capture global temporal structure. However, transformer models can be computationally demanding, making them less suited for low-power wearable devices without architectural simplification.

Hybrid CNN–RNN pipelines provide a practical balance between expressive power and efficiency. Cui and Xia (2022) proposed a CNN–BiLSTM model that uses convolutional filters to extract local morphological features and recurrent layers to capture temporal context. Similarly, Alamatsaz et al. (2022) and Roy et al. (2023) demonstrated that CNN–LSTM and LSTM autoencoder frameworks can effectively model both beat-level morphology and sequence-level abnormalities, often achieving strong performance while keeping latency low. These hybrid models are widely adopted in scenarios where real-time responsiveness and efficient temporal modeling are required.

Lightweight modeling for IoT and edge deployment has become another critical research area. Sivapalan et al. (2022) introduced ANNet, a compact, low-parameter network tailored for ECG anomaly detection on resource-constrained wearable devices. Their work emphasizes that achieving real-time performance in embedded systems requires architectural efficiency, pruning, and model compression. This aligns with observations from other studies—such as those by Alamatsaz et al. (2022) and Agarwal et al. (2024)—which reinforce the importance of lightweight designs for battery-powered monitoring systems.

Reconstruction-based modeling continues to play a key role, especially when the number of abnormal ECG samples is limited. Roy et al. (2023) developed a deep LSTM autoencoder to learn the manifold of normal ECG sequences and detect anomalies via reconstruction error. Agarwal et al. (2024) explored CNN autoencoder frameworks that capture morphological characteristics and identify deviations without relying heavily on labeled data. These approaches are beneficial in low-supervision settings but require careful threshold selection and can be sensitive to noise.

Classical signal processing methods remain fundamental for improving ECG quality. Golgowski and Osowski (2020) showed that wavelet-based decomposition enhances anomaly detection by removing noise and capturing multi-resolution structure. Broader surveys, such as that by Li and Boulanger (2020), emphasize the importance of preprocessing (e.g., band-pass filtering, denoising), handling class imbalance, and evaluating models under deployment-oriented conditions. Minic et al. (2023) further demonstrated the effectiveness of recurrent neural networks for anomaly detection in noisy sensor-stream ECG data, highlighting the challenges of real-world signal variability.

Several recent contributions in medical deep learning provide supporting insights for building reliable ECG anomaly detectors. Pattanayak and Singh (2022) showed that machine learning classification performance can be significantly improved through rigorous hyperparameter optimization and stacked ensemble methods. Jasvitha et al. (2024) demonstrated that a 1D CNN can extract temporal features efficiently directly from raw ECG signals, enabling low-latency, end-to-end inference. Afnaan et al. (2024) introduced a hybrid generative–discriminative framework for medical signal synthesis, opening new avenues for data augmentation in the ECG domain. Tripathi et al. (2024a) applied GAN-based augmentation to medical images using a U-Net architecture, demonstrating how synthetic data can help address rare-class imbalance—a challenge also presents in ECG arrhythmia datasets. In another contribution, Tripathi et al. (2024b) showed that lightweight transfer-learning models, such as MobileNetV2, can achieve strong diagnostic performance at low computational cost, providing valuable insights for wearable deployment. Additionally, foundational resources such as the MIT-BIH Arrhythmia Database, originally detailed by Moody and Mark (2001), continue to serve as the primary benchmark for evaluating ECG anomaly detection systems.

Overall, the literature shows a clear movement toward methods that balance morphological sensitivity, temporal modeling, computational efficiency, and robustness to noise. Recent efforts also emphasize handling class imbalance, improving calibration and uncertainty estimation, and ensuring real-time deployability. In this context, a real-time deep learning pipeline that combines morphology-aware convolutional processing with efficient temporal models such as Bi-GRUs—supported by clinically grounded preprocessing, contrastive learning, and uncertainty estimation—aligns strongly with current research directions and addresses many of the challenges highlighted across recent work.

8.3 METHODOLOGY

The study methodology also follows a multi-stage workflow that starts with requirement analysis and proceeds to dataset preparation, preprocessing, and model development. Figure 8.1 shows the entire processing chain.

8.3.1 Planning and Requirement Analysis

The classification system for ECG arrhythmias was developed by identifying the crucial clinical and technical challenges in automating cardiac diagnosis. Clinically, the model had to be highly accurate across all arrhythmia types, including rare but crucial beats, and to provide interpretable outputs and reliable uncertainty estimates to aid decision-making. Technically, the system needed to extract local ECG morphology with strong fidelity, model long-range temporal patterns, be effectively processed for real-time use, and generalize well across different patient recordings.

According to these requirements, the hybrid deep learning architecture was developed to combine:

- Morphology-aware representation learning CNNs.
- Temporal dependency capturing transformer encoders,
- Multi-scale attention to hierarchical pattern recognition,
- The proposed solution, which is systematic contrastive learning to enhance the separation of classes in a heavily imbalanced environment, is supervised.

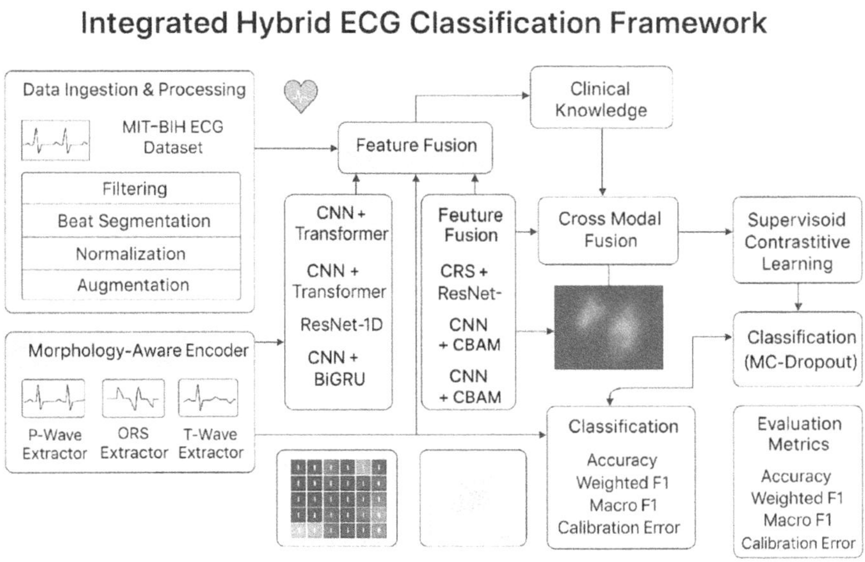

FIGURE 8.1 PhysioBot architecture for interpretable ECG/PPG anomaly detection.

In order to conduct meaningful benchmarking, three standard arrhythmia classification models have been used, i.e., ResNet1D, CBAM, and CNN, and a CNN and biGRU hybrid has been applied as well under the same experimental conditions.

8.3.2 Data Acquisition and Preparation

The main dataset is the MIT-BIH Arrhythmia Database. It contains 48 half-hour ECG records sampled at 360 Hz. The expert cardiologists mark each heartbeat with labels of AAMI-standard quality, which serves as a good ground truth. The main channel of analysis is modified Lead II (MLII).

8.3.2.1 Beat Extraction

Classification of arrhythmia is done at the beat level. Each heartbeat is divided into a 180-sample window (about 500ms): using annotated R-peaks, each heartbeat is divided into 180 samples.

$$Beat_i = x\left[R_i - 90 : R_i + 90\right] \tag{8.1}$$

capturing:

- 90 samples before the R-peak (P-wave and PR interval),
- The R-peak at the center,
- R-peak (ST segment and T-wave) with 90 samples.

Noisy or unfinished beats were cut out. The rest of the beats were mapped onto the five AAMI arrhythmia categories:

$$\{N, S, V, F, Q\}$$

8.3.2.2 Dataset Characteristics

The last data amounted to 109,468 heartbeat segments. It was very uneven, with the No one beat dominating (Normal beats 83%) and very rare Fusion beats (1%). To achieve statistical reliability, a stratified split was employed: 70% for training, 15% for validation, and 15% for testing, ensuring that all arrhythmia classes were represented proportionately.

8.3.3 Data Preprocessing

8.3.3.1 Signal Filtering

ECG signals have noise, including powerline interference and baseline drift. The Butterworth bandpass filter of 4th-order with cutoff frequencies of 0.5 50 Hz was applied:

$$\left|H(jw)\right|^2 = \frac{1}{1+\left(\frac{w}{w_c}\right)^{2n}} \tag{8.2}$$

where $n = 4$. It retains the P-wave, QRS, and T-wave morphology and attenuates unwanted frequency components.

8.3.3.2 Normalization

To minimize variation due to the electrode placement and variation between patients, beat-level z-score normalization was used:

$$x_{norm} = \frac{x - \mu}{\sigma + \epsilon} \tag{8.3}$$

Beat-wise mean and standard deviation of a signal are denoted by mu and sigma.

Beat-wise division by zero is avoided by epsilon. This normalization reduces training gradient changes.

8.3.3.3 Quality Control

The beat segments were thoroughly validated. Only segments that had 180 samples, no annotation flags of noise, full and unclipped ECG morphology, were retained. All beats that did not meet these criteria were eliminated to avoid poor training performance.

8.3.3.4 Data Augmentation

To counteract class imbalance, especially in Supraventricular and Fusion beats, clinically meaningful augmentations were realized:

- Time Warping: Simulates the variation in heart rate.
- Magnitude Scaling: Amplitude change because of electrode contact.
- Baseline Drift Simulation: This introduces low-frequency sinusoidal drift.
- High-Frequency Noise Injection: injects controlled noise at 50/60Hz. Let $x(t)$ represent the beat. Transforms that include augmentation are:

$$x_{warp}(t) = x(\phi(t)) \tag{8.4}$$

$$x_{scale}(t) = \alpha.\ x((t)) \tag{8.5}$$

In which case, the warping of time, defined as the smooth, nonlinear function phi(t), and the scaling factor, a random value, are only used during training. All beats were standardized into 1D vectors of length 180 after filtering, normalization, quality checks, and augmentation, serving as the final input to all deep learning models.

8.3.4 Baseline Model: Custom 1D CNN

The standard model used in the current research is a designed 1D convolutional neural network (CNN), which will serve as the baseline for the study on arrhythmia classification in ECG. The structure is deliberately basic in essence, aims to learn interpretable features, and provides a clear performance benchmark for comparison with more sophisticated models. It consists of three convolutional blocks with batch normalization, ReLU activation, and max pooling between them to progressively extract morphological features of the P-wave, QRS complex, and T-wave patterns.

Convolution Operation: All convolutional filters slide along the ECG segment to identify localized features of the waveform. The convolution operation of the kth filter can be defined as:

$$y_i^{(k)} = \sum_{m=1}^{\cdots} x_{i+m}\, w_m^{(k)} + b^{(k)} \tag{8.6}$$

$w_m^{(k)}$ and $b^{(k)}$ are the learnable weights and bias of the filter, respectively.

This allows the model to detect the typical ECG morphologies needed to distinguish arrhythmia. Batch Normalization: To stabilize training and to converge faster, batch normalization is used in the post-convolution phase:

$$\hat{x} = \frac{\mathrm{x} - \mu}{\sqrt{\sigma^2 + \varepsilon}} \tag{8.7}$$

whereby the mean and standard deviation of a batch are denoted by the variables, which are: This eliminates covariate shift inside models and increases model robustness.

Feature Aggregation and Classification: After the convolutional blocks, the extracted features are flattened and run through two fully connected layers. These layers are trained on compact representations, and the SoftMax layer produces the last-class probabilities.

Loss Function: The categorical cross-entropy loss is used to perform training, and it is defined as:

$$L_{CE} = -\frac{1}{N}\sum_{i=1}^{N}\sum_{c=1}^{C} y_{i,c} \log\ (\hat{p}_{i,c}) \tag{8.8}$$

In which the expected likelihood of a given machine in each classification is denoted by i,c, and the ground-truth label is denoted by $y_{i,c}$. Such a loss prompts the network to assign high probability to the correct arrhythmia category. The base CNN thus provides a clean, interpretable, and computationally efficient initialization before benchmarking sophisticated architectures such as ResNet-1D, CBAMCNN, and CNN-BiGRU.

8.3.5 Benchmark Models

Three popular architectures of ECGs, ResNet-1D, CBAM-CNN, and a CNN-BiGRU hybrid, were used to achieve fair and comprehensive performance comparison under the same preprocessing, training, and evaluation conditions. These models are robust baselines that can complement the hybrid architecture proposed to capture the various aspects of ECG morphology and temporal behavior.

8.3.5.1 ResNet-1D

ResNet-1D uses a ResNet architecture as a framework and transforms ECGs into a single dimension. It is characterized using so-called residual connections, which enable deep architectures to be trained successfully by overcoming the vanishing gradient problem. Each residual block is learned to map the residual instead of learning a complete transformation:

$$y = F\left(x, W\right) + x \tag{8.9}$$

where F(x, W) is a series of Conv1D, Batch Normalization, and ReLU. The skip connection allows currents to pass through the network, enhancing convergence stability and enabling deeper feature extraction. The ResNet-1D architecture applied in the present study comprises:

- First Conv1D layer to extract low-level features,
- Various residual blocks of the morphology of hierarchical ECG,
- Global Average Pooling (GAP) of temporal information,
- A five-class arrhythmia prediction of a softmax classifier with full connections.

ResNet-1D can be considered a powerful baseline because it can successfully differentiate subtle morphological variations, specifically supraventricular and ventricular arrhythmias.

8.3.5.2 CBAM-CNN

The CBAM-CNN uses the Convolutional Block Attention Module (CBAM) to improve feature quality by enabling the network to focus on the most significant elements of the ECG signal. CBAM uses two sequential attentional processes: channel attention and spatial (temporal) attention.

Channel Attention, this module highlights the combination of global average pooling and max pooling, which gives the most crucial feature channels:

$$M_c = \sigma(W_1\left(\delta\left(W_0 F_{avg}\right)\right) + W_1\left(\delta\left(W_0 F_{\max}\right)\right)) \tag{8.10}$$

In which the activation of ReLU and the sigmoid are represented by the delta and sigma functions, respectively. This mechanism gives preference to channels associated with clinically viable ECG patterns.

Spatial (Temporal) Attention calculates: to target critical time areas (e.g., QRS complex, ST segment):

$$M_s = \sigma\left(f^{7\times1}\left(\left[F_{avg}; F_{\max}\right]\right)\right) \tag{8.11}$$

$f^{7\times1}$ represents a 1-dimensional or 1D convolution with a 7 x 1 sized kernel. This operation marks the significant temporal points of the ECG signal. The entire CBAM-CNN model contains:

- Basic Conv1D blocks of feature extraction,
- Serial sequential application of channel and spatial attention modules,
- Maximum pooling and regularization dropout,
- A dense SoftMax classifier.

This model can be particularly useful in noisy areas, where it can be suppressed to emphasize clinically interesting waveform characteristics.

8.3.5.3 CNN-BiGRU Hybrid Model

The CNN-BiGRU hybrid model consists of convolutional layers for extracting morphological features and Bidirectional Gated Recurrent Units (BiGRUs) for modeling temporal sequences. The architecture not only captures short waveform details but also long-range temporal dependencies.

CNN-Based Morphology Extraction. First Conv1D filters capture localized characteristics of ECG morphology:

$$Y = Conv1D(X) \tag{8.12}$$

Some of the critical trends coded by these layers include P-wave onset, QRS width, and T-wave amplitude.

BiGRU for Temporal Modeling: The obtained feature sequences are fed into a BiGRU layer that processes the signal in both forward and backward directions. The new hidden state of a GRU cell is:

$$r_t = \sigma\left(W_r x_t + U_r h_{t-1}\right) \tag{8.13}$$

$$z_t = \sigma\left(W_z x_t + U_z h_{t-1}\right) \tag{8.14}$$

$$\tilde{h}_t = \tanh\left(W_h x_t + r_t U_h h_{t-1}\right) \tag{8.15}$$

$$h_t = \left(1 - z_t\right) h_{t-1} + z_t \tilde{h}_t \tag{8.16}$$

The bidirectional design records dependencies in both directions at every beat, providing more time information.

Classification Layer: The dense layers are then fed the concatenated hidden states from the BiGRU layer. Finally, arrhythmia classification is performed using a

SoftMax classifier, particularly for arrhythmias that require temporal context, such as supraventricular and rhythmic abnormalities.

8.3.6 Proposed Hybrid Model

The Enhanced Hybrid Model is designed to capture the fine structure of ECG waves and the temporal dependencies known to represent various arrhythmias. To do so, the model uses morphology-aware convolutional encoders, a multi-scale temporal attention component, Transformer encoder layers, a cross-modal fusion module, and supervised contrastive learning. A combination of these elements enables the network to learn clinically meaningful patterns despite significant class imbalance and subtle waveform variations.

Morphology-Aware Convolutional Encoders: There exists a large, significant difference in the morphology of the ECG between the P-wave, QRS complex, and T-wave. The model does not have a single convolutional branch but three special Conv1D encoders with a kernel size that are selected to match the average length of these ECG components:

- P-wave encoder: size of the kernel 15 (small atrial activity)
- QRS encoder: 9 (sharp ventricular depolarization) kernel size.
- Every convolutional step is specified as follows: T-wave encoder:

21 (wide-repolarization-pattern) kernels. Every convolutional operation is provided by:

$$y_i^{(k)} = \sum_{m=1}^{M} x_{i+m} w_m^{(k)} + b^{(k)} \tag{8.17}$$

$$h_{morph} = Conv_{1\times1}\left(\left[h_P; h_{QRS}; h_T\right]\right) \tag{8.18}$$

generating a single, morphology-aware representation of the waveform structure that is clinically significant.

Multi-Scale Temporal Attention: Various arrhythmias have diagnostic clues at various time scales. To place these variations, the model includes a multi-scale attention module that works on the fused features at:

- fine resolution (22 positions),
- medium resolution (11 positions),
- coarse resolution (5 positions).

They are both based on multi-head self-attention:

$$Attention(Q, K, V) = softmax\left(\frac{QK^T}{\sqrt{d_k}}\right)V \tag{8.19}$$

The fine-scale attention represents fast QRS variability, the medium-scale attention is taught to learn the ST-T association, and the coarse-scale attention extracts the rhythm structure. All three outputs are linearly combined to create a single time representation.

Transformer Encoder Layers: To model long-range dependencies beyond the receptive field of convolutions, the model employs two stacked Transformer encoder blocks. Each block contains multi-head attention, residual connections, and a position-wise feed-forward network:

$$FFN(x) = W_2 GELU(W_1 x + b_1) + b_2 \tag{8.20}$$

These layers help the network interpret beat-to-beat dynamics, compensatory pauses, and rhythm irregularities—phenomena that cannot be captured by convolution alone.

Cross-Modal Fusion Mechanism: The model leverages the strengths of CNN-based local morphology extraction and Transformer-based global temporal modeling via a cross-attention fusion module. In this case, CNN features are used as queries, and the Transformer is applied as keys and values:

$$Fusion(Q,K,V) = softmax\left(\frac{QK^T}{\sqrt{d_k}}\right)V \tag{8.21}$$

The advantage of this fusion step is that local patterns of waveforms (e.g., PVC morphology) can be interpreted in their larger context (e.g., bigeminy, trigeminy).

Supervised Contrastive Learning: To address the severe class imbalance in the in the MIT-BIH dataset, the model incorporates supervised contrastive learning. A projection head first maps the feature to a contrastive space, and the supervised contrastive loss is computed as:

$$L_{SC} = -\sum_i \frac{1}{|P(i)|} \sum_{p \epsilon P(i)} \log \frac{\exp(z_i \cdot z_p / \tau)}{\sum_{a \epsilon A(i)} \exp(z_i \cdot z_a / \tau)} \tag{8.22}$$

This loss encourages samples from the same arrhythmia class to cluster tightly, while separating different classes—even when minority classes have very few samples. The final training objective combines contrastive and cross-entropy losses.

Uncertainty Quantification: To provide confidence estimates during inference, Monte Carlo (MC) Dropout is applied during test-time forward passes. Rather than producing a single deterministic prediction, the model generates N stochastic predictions:

$$\hat{p} = \frac{1}{N}\sum_{i=1}^{N} p_i \tag{8.23}$$

The predictive uncertainty is computed as the variance:

$$U = \frac{1}{N}\sum_{i=1}^{N}(p_i - \hat{p})^2 \tag{8.24}$$

A higher variance indicates lower confidence—an essential property for clinical decision support.

The ECG arrhythmia classification system training strategy aimed to ensure stability in optimization, robust generalization, and equitable comparison across all benchmark models. It also uses complex optimization strategies, regularization strategies, and learning rate control to benchmark the proposed hybrid model and the successful baseline architectures.

8.3.7 Training Mechanism

The ECG arrhythmia classification system training strategy aimed to ensure stability in optimization, robust generalization, and equitable comparison across all benchmark models. It also uses complex optimization, regularization, and learning rate control strategies.

8.3.7.1 Optimization Strategy

All architectures were trained with the AdamW optimizer, which decouples weight decay from gradient updates, making deep architectures more stable to converge. The optimizer is defined as:

$$\theta_{t+1} = \theta_t - \eta\frac{\hat{m}_t}{\sqrt{\hat{v}_t + \varepsilon}} - \eta\lambda\theta_t \tag{8.25}$$

To ensure reproducibility, random seeds were fixed across all libraries.

- Learning rate: 1×10^{-3}
- Weight decay: 0.01
- Betas: (0.9, 0.999)
- Batch size: 128

8.3.7.2 Learning Rate Scheduling

During inference, Monte Carlo Dropout was enabled to produce $N = 10$ stochastic predictions:

$$\eta_{new} = 0.5 \times \eta_{current} \tag{8.26}$$

The strategy helped with finer updates later in training.

8.3.7.3 Loss Function

The total loss combines weighted cross-entropy with supervised contrastive loss to improve separation between classes, particularly minority arrhythmias:

$$L_{total} = L_{CE} + \lambda L_{SC} \tag{8.27}$$

where $\lambda = 0.3$. This was able to give clinically meaningful scores on confidence in the final model prediction.

8.3.7.4 Regularization Methods

Several regularization methods were used to minimize overfitting:

- Dropout: Used as CNN, attention, and Transformer rates ranging between 0.3 and 0.5.
- Batch Normalization stabilizes the activations and speeds up the convergence.
- Weight Decay: Feeds large weights to enhance generalization.
- Gradient Clipping: Norm = 1.0 to avoid exploding gradients. Every epoch includes the following steps.

8.3.7.5 Training Workflow

Each epoch consists of the following steps:

- Apply random augmentation (time warping, magnitude scaling, baseline drift, noise injection) to minority classes.
- Forward pass-through morphology encoders, CNN pathway, multi-scale attention, Transformer layers, fusion module, and classification head.
- Compute LCE and LSC and update parameters via backpropagation.
- Evaluate performance on the validation set.
- Adjust learning rate according to scheduler behavior.

Training continued for up to 30 epochs, with early stopping applied if validation accuracy did not improve for 12 consecutive epochs.

8.3.7.6 Hardware Configuration

All experiments were conducted using:

- NVIDIA CUDA-enabled GPU (when available)
- 8–16 GB system RAM
- PyTorch backend with cuDNN acceleration

To ensure reproducibility, random seeds were fixed across all libraries (Table 8.1).

8.3.7.7 Test-Time Uncertainty Estimation

During inference, Monte Carlo Dropout was enabled to produce N=10 stochastic predictions:

$$\hat{p} = \frac{1}{N}\sum_{i=1}^{N} p_i,\ U = \frac{1}{N}\sum_{i=1}^{N}(p_i - \hat{p})^2 \tag{8.28}$$

TABLE 8.1
State-of-the-Art Comparison of ECG Arrhythmia Classification Methods

Aspect	Proposed Hybrid Model (CNN+CBAM+Transformer+SCL)	Hannun et al. (2019) SCL	Yildirim et al. (2018)	Oh et al. (2018)	Ge et al. (2021)
Architecture Type	Multi-scale morphology encoders + Transformer + crossmodal fusion with supervised contrastive learning	34-layer deep CNN with residual connections; end-to-end learning	LSTM-based recurrent network for temporal modeling; no attention	Attention-based BiGRU with CNN feature extractor; single-scale processing	1D ResNet with squeeze-excitation blocks; no explicit temporal modeling
Morphological Feature Extraction	Three parallel encoders (Pwave: k=15, QRS: k=9, Twave: k=21) with learnable fusion via 1×1 convolution	Single-scale convolutions with fixed kernel sizes; no wave-specific encoding	Generic LSTM cells process sequential features; limited morphology awareness.	Standard CNN blocks extract features; no component-specific design	Residual blocks with squeeze-excitation; channel-wise attention only
Temporal Dependency Modeling	Stacked Transformer encoders capture long-range beat-to-beat dependencies and rhythm patterns.	Implicit through deep stacking; no explicit attention over time	LSTM models learn temporal sequences, but are limited by vanishing gradients	BiGRU with attention focusing on relevant time steps; bidirectional context	Relies on receptive field expansion; no recurrent or attention-based temporal modeling
Multi-Scale Processing	Three-resolution temporal attention (fine: 22, medium: 11, coarse: 5 positions) capturing diagnostic features at multiple scales	Fixed receptive field; single filter sizes at each layer; no explicit multi-scale fusion	Single time-scale processing through LSTM unrolling	Single-scale attention mechanism; no hierarchical temporal processing	Multi-scale via hierarchical residual blocks, but no explicit attention fusion
Cross-Modal Fusion	Cross-attention between CNN morphology features (Q) and Transformer temporal context (K,V); integrates local–global information	No explicit fusion: features combined through sequential processing	LSTM output directly fed to classifier; no fusion of heterogeneous representations	CNN-RNN pipeline with serial connection; no cross-attention mechanism	Feature concatenation or addition; no learnable cross-modal attention

(Continued)

TABLE 8.1 CONTINUED
State-of-the-Art Comparison of ECG Arrhythmia Classification Methods

Aspect	Proposed Hybrid Model (CNN+CBAM+Transformer+SCL)	Hannun et al. (2019) SCL	Yildirim et al. (2018)	Oh et al. (2018)	Ge et al. (2021)
Uncertainty Quantification	MC Dropout at test time with N stochastic forward passes; variance-based confidence estimation for clinical decisions.	Deterministic predictions; no uncertainty estimates	No uncertainty quantification; single-point predictions only	SoftMax probabilities used as confidence; no explicit uncertainty modeling	No uncertainty quantification framework; lacks confidence calibration
Dataset & Classes	MIT-BIH Arrhythmia Database; 5 classes (N, S, V, F, Q) following AAMI standards; severe imbalance	Large proprietary dataset; 12 rhythm classes, including AF, bigeminy, trigeminy	MIT-BIH; 5 AAMI classes; standard benchmark evaluation	MIT-BIH and PTB Diagnostic; multi-database validation with transfer learning	MIT-BIH and European STT Database; 5 classes with augmentation strategies
Performance Metrics	High F1-scores for minority classes (S, F, Q); balanced accuracy across all categories via contrastive learning	Strong overall accuracy (>95%); minority class performance not emphasized	Good temporal modeling; moderate performance on rare arrhythmias	Competitive F1-scores; attention improves minority class detection	Excellent specificity: sensitivity for minority classes remains challenging

This provided clinically meaningful confidence scores for the final model predictions.

8.4 RESULTS AND DISCUSSION

Table 8.2 summarizes the quantitative performance of the proposed EHECGNet model on the MIT-BIH Arrhythmia Database. The model achieves high classification accuracy and strong F1 scores across both frequent and minority classes. The low expected calibration error (ECE) and the model's mean epistemic uncertainty further confirm that the model produces reliable probability estimates suitable for clinical decision support.

8.4.1 Training Behavior and Convergence

The learning dynamics of EH-ECGNet are illustrated in Figure 8.2, which contains four subplots summarizing the model's overall behavior during training. The training and validation loss curves show smooth, stable convergence, indicating that the model learns without overfitting. Similarly, the accuracy curves show progressive improvement in both training and validation sets.

The contrastive loss subplot highlights the effectiveness of supervised contrastive learning in improving class separation during training. The final combined plot (loss vs. accuracy) further confirms the balanced relationship between optimization and classification performance. These results collectively indicate that multi-scale temporal attention, advanced ECG augmentation, and contrastive learning contribute to stable and efficient learning.

8.4.2 Classification Performance

The classification performance of EH-ECGNet is illustrated by the normalized confusion matrix shown in Figure 8.3. The strong diagonal elements indicate a high rate of correct predictions across all arrhythmia classes. Misclassification rates are low, demonstrating the model's ability to differentiate between clinically similar rhythm patterns.

TABLE 8.2
Performance Comparison of Deep Learning Models for ECG Anomaly Detection

Model	Accuracy (%)	Weighted F1	Macro F1	ECE
CNN + Transformer	96.99	0.9715	0.8750	0.0365
ResNet1D	95.42	0.9581	0.8423	0.0412
CNN + CBAM	96.12	0.9644	0.8610	0.0389
CNN + BiGRU	95.88	0.9617	0.8535	0.0396

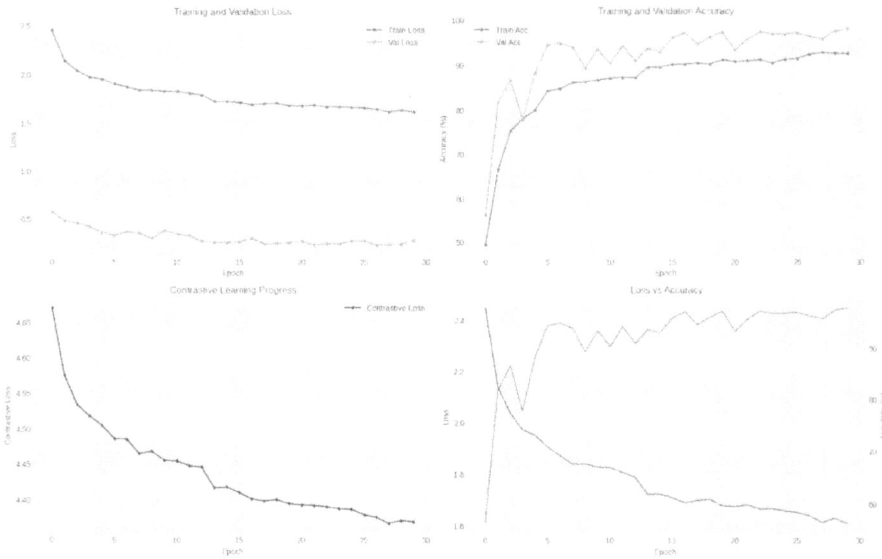

FIGURE 8.2 Training behavior of EH-ECGNet showing (i) training vs. validation loss, (ii) training vs. validation accuracy, (iii) contrastive loss, and (iv) combined loss–accuracy trends. The model exhibits stable convergence due to multi-scale attention, augmentation, and contrastive learning.

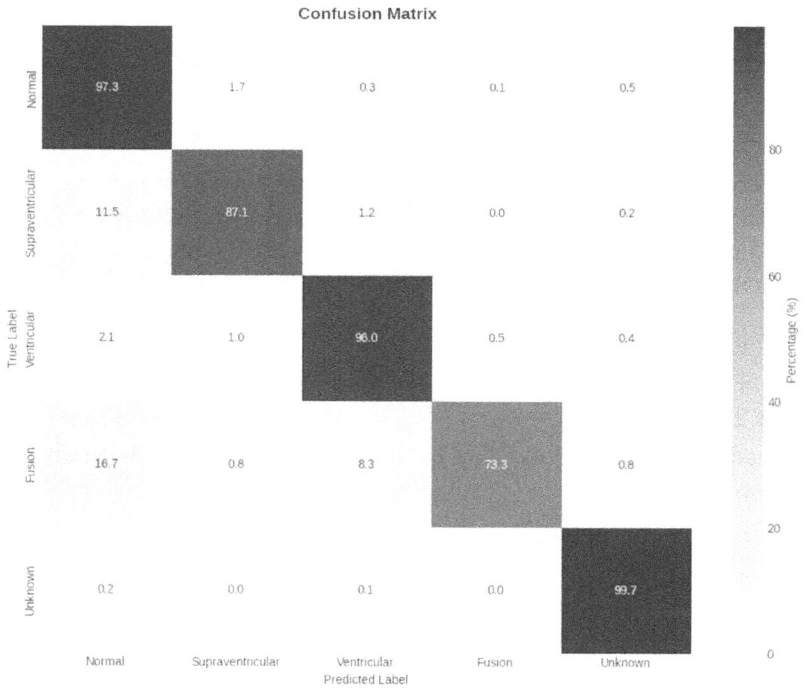

FIGURE 8.3 Normalized confusion matrix demonstrating the per-class predictive performance of the hybrid model.

This improvement is mainly due to the morphology-aware encoder, which extracts clinically interpretable P-QRS-T wave characteristics, and the cross-modal fusion module, which effectively aligns morphological and temporal information. Moreover, supervised contrastive learning enhances discrimination of class boundaries, leading to more consistent and accurate predictions.

8.4.3 Feature Representation Analysis

To assess the learning ability of the model to make a valuable model in the learning of the ECG signals, a t-SNE plot of the final feature embeddings was constructed, which is indicated in Figure 8.4. The 2D visualization, as shown in this case, reflects all points as a heartbeat once it has been modeled. The plot demonstrates the visual separation of groups (clusters) of five classes of arrhythmia. This implies that the model can acquire characteristics that significantly separate one class from another, an indicator of good classification capability.

The high-quality separation between clusters indicates that the morphology-conscious encoder effectively captures the most significant patterns in ECG shapes, including peaks, slopes, and physiological intervals. This helps the model understand how each type of heartbeat appears different from the others.

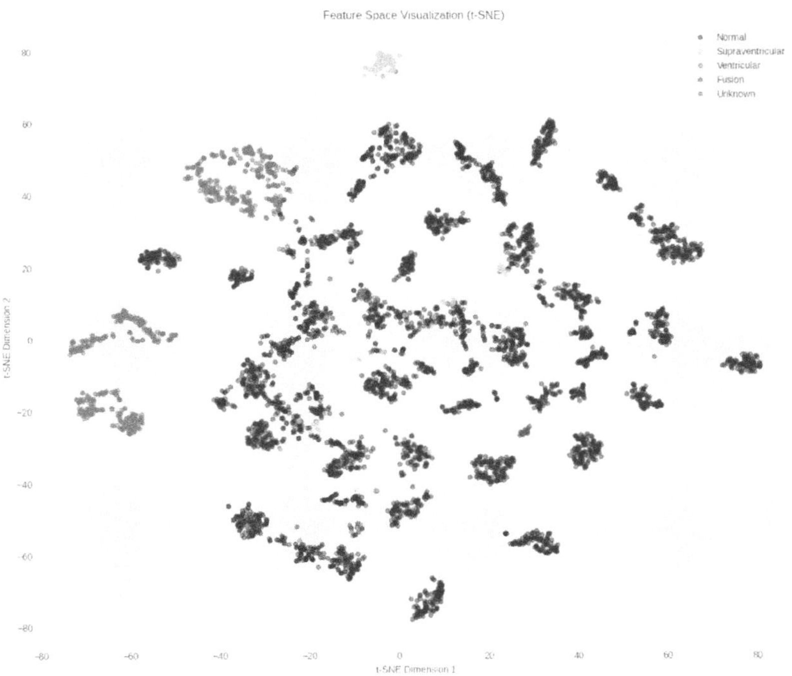

FIGURE 8.4 t-SNE visualization of learned feature embeddings showing clear class separation. The improvement results from morphology-aware encoding, contrastive learning, and cross-modal fusion.

Besides enhancing the feature space by bringing features from the same class closer together and separating those from different classes, contrastive learning also improves the understanding of ECG signals and strengthens the overall global structure of the feature representation.

On balance, the t-SNE visualization validates that the model learns well-organized, clean, and class-specific representations of features, which directly relates to the model's high classification accuracy.

8.4.4 Uncertainty and Reliability Assessment

In clinical decision-making, it is essential not only to predict accurately but also to quantify the confidence in those predictions. EH-ECGNet incorporates Monte Carlo Dropout to estimate epistemic uncertainty, and the resulting uncertainty analysis plots are shown in Figure 8.5.

The uncertainty histogram shows that misclassified beats are associated with significantly higher uncertainty values, enabling identification of uncertain predictions. The calibration plot shows that the predicted confidence closely aligns with the actual accuracy, indicating good calibration. The uncertainty per-class plot shows that rare arrhythmias exhibit higher uncertainty, while the uncertainty–confidence scatter plot confirms the expected negative correlation between uncertainty and correctness. Together, these results validate the reliability and clinical usefulness of the model's uncertainty estimates.

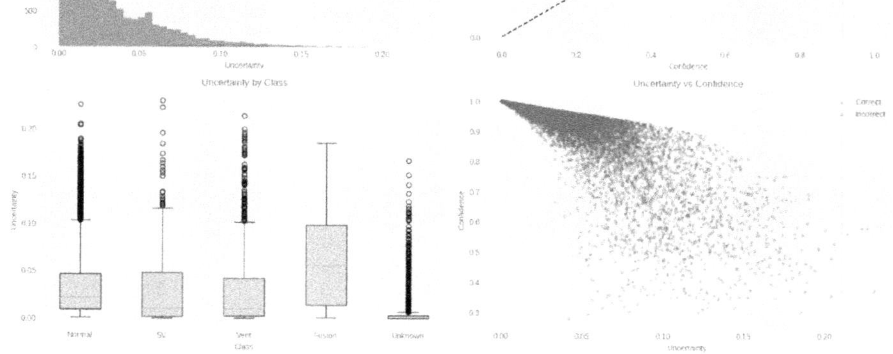

FIGURE 8.5 Uncertainty analysis using Monte Carlo Dropout. Misclassified samples exhibit higher uncertainty, and the calibration plot indicates strong alignment between confidence and observed accuracy, ensuring clinical reliability.

8.5 CONCLUSION

The study follows a structured workflow starting from requirement analysis to dataset preparation, preprocessing, and model development. Each phase contributes to building a reliable and consistent ECG classification system. Through effective preprocessing and thoughtful model design, the framework achieves improved accuracy in detecting arrhythmia patterns. The overall findings highlight the potential of machine learning techniques to support early diagnosis and provide meaningful assistance in clinical decision-making for ECG-based analysis.

8.6 FUTURE SCOPE

The work presents several opportunities for further enhancement. Expanding the dataset with more diverse and large-scale ECG recordings can improve generalization across different patient profiles and recording conditions. Incorporating additional physiological signals, such as PPG or respiration data, can help create a more comprehensive cardiac monitoring system. Exploring advanced deep-learning methods, including transformers, self-supervised learning, and federated learning, may strengthen model robustness while preserving data privacy. Real-time deployment on wearable or IoT-enabled devices can enable continuous cardiac monitoring and early alert mechanisms. Clinical validation and integration into healthcare support systems can further extend the practical impact of the research.

REFERENCES

Afnaan, K., T. Singh, and P. Duraisamy. "Hybrid Deep Learning Framework for Bidirectional Medical Image Synthesis." *2024 15th International Conference on Computing Communication and Networking Technologies (ICCCNT).* Kamand, India, 2024, pp. 1–6. doi: 10.1109/ICCCNT61001.2024.10725975.

Agarwal, Muskan, et al. "Decoding Abnormal Heart Patterns: A CNN Autoencoder Approach to ECG Anomaly Detection." *2024 Asia Pacific Conference on Innovation in Technology (APCIT).* IEEE, 2024.

Alamatsaz, Negin, et al. "A Lightweight Hybrid CNN-LSTM Model for ECG-Based Arrhythmia Detection." *arXiv preprint* arXiv:2209.00988, 2022.

Alamr, Abrar, and Abdelmonim Artoli. "Unsupervised Transformer-Based Anomaly Detection in ECG Signals." *Algorithms*, vol. 16, no. 3, 2023, p. 152.

Alghieth, Manal. "DeepECG-Net: A Hybrid Transformer-Based Deep Learning Model for RealTime ECG Anomaly Detection." *Scientific Reports*, vol. 15, no. 1, 2025, p. 20714.

Cui, Kai Xing, and Xiao Jun Xia. "ECG Signal Anomaly Detection Algorithm Based on CNNBiLSTM." *2022 11th International Conference of Information and Communication Technology (ICTech).* IEEE, 2022.

Golgowski, Maciej, and Stanislaw Osowski. "Anomaly Detection in ECG Using Wavelet Transformation." *2020 IEEE 21st International Conference on Computational Problems of Electrical Engineering (CPEE).* IEEE, 2020.

Jasvitha, B. D., K. Kanagaraj, K. Murali, T. Singh, and P. Duraisamy. "1D CNN Framework on ECG Signals." *2024 3rd International Conference for Innovation in Technology (INOCON).* Bangalore, India, 2024, pp. 1–6. doi: 10.1109/INOCON60754.2024.10512284.

Li, Hongzu, and Pierre Boulanger. "A Survey of Heart Anomaly Detection Using Ambulatory Electrocardiogram (ECG)." *Sensors*, vol. 20, no. 5, 2020, p. 1461.

Minic, Ana, et al. "Applying Recurrent Neural Networks for Anomaly Detection in Electrocardiogram Sensor Data." *Sensors*, vol. 23, no. 24, 2023, p. 9878.

Moody, G. B., and R. G. Mark. "The Impact of the MIT-BIH Arrhythmia Database." *IEEE Engineering in Medicine and Biology Magazine*, vol. 20, no. 3, 2001, pp. 45–50. Available: https://physionet.org/content/mitdb/.

Pattanayak, S., and T. Singh. "Cardiovascular Disease Classification Based on Machine Learning Algorithms Using GridSearchCV, Cross Validation and Stacked Ensemble Methods." In M. Singh, V. Tyagi, P. K. Gupta, J. Flusser, and T. Ören, eds. *Advances in Computing and Data Sciences (ICACDS 2022).* Communications in Computer and Information Science, vol. 1613. Springer, Cham, 2022. https://doi.org/10.1007/978-3-031-12638-3_19.

Qin, Jing, et al. "A Novel Temporal Generative Adversarial Network for Electrocardiography Anomaly Detection." *Artificial Intelligence in Medicine*, vol. 136, 2023, p. 102489.

Roy, Moumita, et al. "ECG-NET: A Deep LSTM Autoencoder for Detecting Anomalous ECG." *Engineering Applications of Artificial Intelligence*, vol. 124, 2023, p. 106484.

Sivapalan, Gawsalyan, et al. "ANNet: A Lightweight Neural Network for ECG Anomaly Detection in IoT Edge Sensors." *IEEE Transactions on Biomedical Circuits and Systems*, vol. 16, no. 1, 2022, pp. 24–35.

Tripathi, A., et al. "A Deep Learning-Oriented Approach for Lung CT Augmentation: Leveraging U-Net and GAN Architecture." *2024 IEEE Recent Advances in Intelligent Computational Systems (RAICS).* Kothamangalam, Kerala, India, 2024a, pp. 1–7. doi: 10.1109/RAICS61201.2024.10690157.

Tripathi, A., T. Singh, R. R. Nair, and P. Duraisamy. "Improving Early Detection and Classification of Lung Diseases with Innovative MobileNetV2 Framework." *IEEE Access*, vol. 12, 2024b, pp. 116202–116217. doi: 10.1109/ACCESS.2024.3440577.

9 Analysis of Ballistocardiography for Cardiac and Respiratory Monitoring in Sleep

Lalitha Vaddadi, Yashas Nallathambi, Manju Khanna, T. V. Smitha, and K.V. Nagaraja

9.1 INTRODUCTION

Ballistocardiography (BCG) is a scale that indicates the force that the body makes when blood is ejected by the heart with each beat. Contrary to electrocardiography (ECG), which records electrical activity, BCG records the forces of the body recoil, which is a unique view of the cardiac mechanics of the body. Clinical use was first restricted historically because Isaac Starr revived it in the 1930s, and there were no standardized methods of acquisition. But now BCG is re-emerging with the introduction of non-contact, super-sensitive sensors that can be installed in mattresses without obtrusion with thin load cells or piezoelectric films. According to (Roebuck et al., 2014), when examining signals applied in the analysis of sleep processes, it is possible to note that a movement in the direction of less intrusive modalities is a trend, and in this case, BCG can be one of the key candidates to undergo evolution.

This non-intrusive quality makes it a perfect design that can be used for long-term continuous sleep tracking, providing a much less invasive option as compared to wearable body sensors. Despite the potential, the adherence of BCG to complex clinical operations, like automated sleep staging, is still a challenge because of the morphology variations in signals. This chapter discusses the solutions to these challenges by describing preprocessing and feature engineering pipelines to extract finer physiological dynamics, which demonstrate that BCG is a feasible, standalone technology and can be used to provide integrated cardiorespiratory monitoring at home.

DOI: 10.1201/9781003797524-9

9.2 DATASET OVERVIEW: CAPTURING NATURAL SLEEP DYNAMICS

9.2.1 Data Collection Protocol

To test the method, a detailed data set by Li et al. (2024) describing the study of a multi-night experiment in which 32 healthy participants were monitored in their natural sleep conditions was used. Using this data corresponds to the fact that the analysis will be based on physiological alterations that are present without laboratory restrictions. The basis can be used to create more effective algorithms that are trained on natural variability and noise in real-world homes. The approach is consistent with the recent work on the development of high-quality standards of ballistocardiogram datasets containing reference signals.

The complexity of in-the-field monitoring, rather than controlled clinical studies, explains this choice of dataset. With the data of a bed-based system, it is possible to analyze cardiovascular parameters monitored without changing the sleeping habits of a subject, which is reasonable in terms of the study of Carlson et al. (2021) of the bed-based BCG capabilities. Ecological validity of this nature is essential so that the developed feature extraction pipeline can be applied to health monitoring applications for consumers.

9.2.2 Sensor Specifications and Acquisition

A piezoelectric film sensor with a high sampling rate of 140 Hz was used to obtain the main BCG signal. This rate corresponds to 140 individual measurements per second, and it is important to acquire the required temporal data concerning cardiac periods. Particularly, the BCG waveform consists of high-frequency elements; in this instance, the highest positive peak is called the J-wave. The accurate identification of the J-wave is essential for BCG signal analysis because the impulsive signal significantly impacts cardiac timing.

The J-wave can be an impulsive signal with a duration of only a few milliseconds, so a high sampling rate is needed to be able to describe the morphology and exact time of occurrence of the waveform.

Concurrent reference sensors were used to validate references in Polysomnography (PSG) labels because standard PSG labels were not available. H9 strapping was used to give the suitable cardiac reference data (RR intervals), and a chest electrode to give the respiration reference waveform was used, which then allowed meaningful comparison of the non-invasive estimates and contact-based ground truth. Figure 9.1 indicates the ECG and BCG peaks, showing how the mechanical waveform tracks cardiac activity.

9.3 THE BCG PREPROCESSING PIPELINE

9.3.1 Normalization and Standardization

Raw BCG signals are automatically subject to noise and motion artifacts, thus causing severe signal distortion. To make the calculated features stable and reliable, a

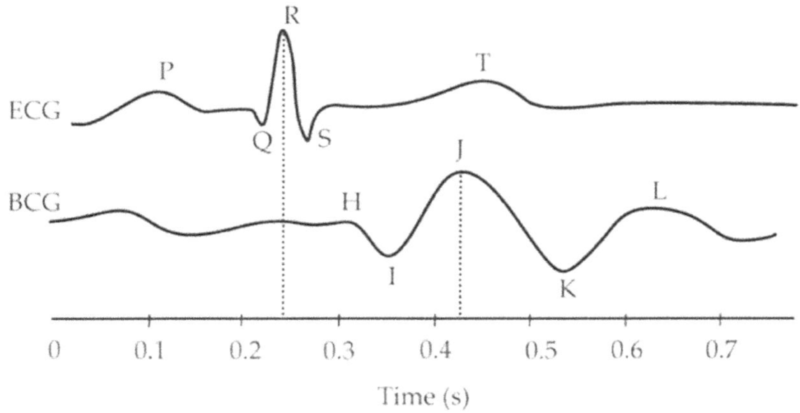

FIGURE 9.1 Comparative signal analysis of the standard ECG signal (top) and the corresponding mechanical signal BCG (bottom).

preprocessing pipeline that comprised four consecutive operations was applied to the raw signal with a frequency of 140 Hz. Then the raw signals were normalized before filtering to ensure that variation due to the difference in the mattress or sensor position among subjects did not affect the signal, which is frequently mentioned in reviews of BCG signal processing (Sadek and Biswas, 2019). This normalization was done by a transformation of the signal to a zero-mean, unit-variance standardized score (Z-score).

By changing the amplitude and baseline of the signals to an equal point, it was made sure that the Artifact Removal threshold could be used uniformly across all the subjects and recording nights. This normalization can be represented mathematically in the form of Equation (9.1):

$$Signal_{Normalization} = \left(x - \mu\right) / \sigma \tag{9.1}$$

9.3.2 Bandpass Filtering for Cardiac Isolation

To isolate the cardiac J-wave, a digital filter was used to eliminate the respiratory signals that block it and high-frequency noise. To achieve this, a Butterworth bandpass filter of the third order was adopted. The cutoff frequency was kept low (0.7 Hz); it is a high-pass component, which is a faster and periodic cardiac signal, as the low-frequency gossip has been removed by this high-pass component, which is the slow, large-baseline drift induced by respiration and gross body motion. The literature about cardiac and respiratory signal extraction methods from BCG signals sensed using fiber Bragg grating sensors in MedCrave (2020) mentions the same extraction techniques.

The high cutoff frequency, in turn, was set at 10.0 Hz. This low-pass component is vital in the elimination of jitters and high-frequency electronic noise, which are non-physiological. Limiting the signal bandwidth makes interference with peak-detection algorithms less likely, so the peaks that are found are caused by actual ejection of the heart and not sensor noise.

9.3.3 Segmentation and Epoching

After filtration, the continuous signal was divided into a series of epochs to make it easier to stage sleep and analyze features. The unit of time was normalized to a window of 30 seconds of the signal. With the sampling rate of 140 Hz, each window contained 4,200 samples.

This segmentation method corresponds to conventional sleep analysis epochs, so features can be easily applied to conventional hypnograms. The overlap is important to provide continuity in the dynamic changes that could be present at the edges of a fixed window, needed when trying to correlate mechanical signals to the estimation of the sleep structure as investigated by Park et al. (2014).

9.3.4 Artifact and Noise Removal (Motion Rejection)

To verify that the analysis was only on intervals of stable resting physiology, 30-second epochs that had been corrupted due to large-scale movement were filtered out. The stability metric that was used is Standard Deviation (σ) for every epoch.

Large values of the sigma mean non-periodic and abrupt changes typical of gross body movements or artifacts. The threshold was set downward to collect steady information and eliminate extreme cases. The epoch was rejected when it had a higher value than three times the median standard deviation of the whole night. Segment rejection implemented decision rule is given by Equation (9.2):

$$Rejection = true\sigma_{epoch} > 3 \times Median\left(\sigma_{all_{epochs}}\right), = false, otherwise \tag{9.2}$$

The 30-second segments are replaced entirely by NaN markers in the final CSV file. This is a crucial step, as it maintains the time series of the recording and, at the same time, makes additional analyses (such as feature extraction) automatically disregard the corrupted data.

9.3.5 Analysis of Preprocessing Validation Plots

The filtering and noise rejection stages were tested graphically with preprocessing validation plots to ensure that the success criteria were met. Plots of each night were made and compared the crude input to the end up clean output, both at 5-minute intervals. The signal in the first panel (Raw BCG) had the complete range of frequencies, which may be drowned by high-frequency noise and massive-amplitude respiratory artifact.

The second panel (Filtered Signal) demonstrates the effectiveness of the pipeline. The signal is much less flattened and much clearer, which means that the high-pass filter was able to eliminate slow respiratory sway and keep only the regular heartbeats. Moreover, outliers of high variance were emphasized in dark grey (Figure 9.2), which visually validated the claim that the statistical threshold of detecting outliers with variance was met ($\sigma > 3 \times \text{Median}$). This visual data confirms that the rest of the data is quite stable and can be used to obtain cardiac features. Figures 9.2 and 9.3 clearly show the progression from raw to cleaned BCG, validating the preprocessing.

9.4 FEATURE EXTRACTION: DESCRIBING THE WAVEFORM

After cleaning the signal of the BCG and eliminating the respiratory sway and motion artifact, with the help of the statistical characteristics, the data were measured. These properties convert the multi-dimensional waveform into concise numerical values that measure various characteristics of cardiac activity in each 30-second epoch. To determine the strength of the wave and the shape of the BCG wave, seven features were computed.

Table 9.1 provides a detailed explanation of the obtained characteristic features, their respective mathematical domains, and their implications for the heart. The features based on amplitude, like Standard Deviation (Std) and Root Mean Square (RMS), are indicators of the intensity of the mechanical output of the heart. Morphological features such as Skewness and Kurtosis, on the other hand, characterize the shape of the signal distribution, which can give information on how the signal is covered up by high peaks of the signal, such as the J-wave. The features per night were stored separately to have a clear audit trail for further modeling.

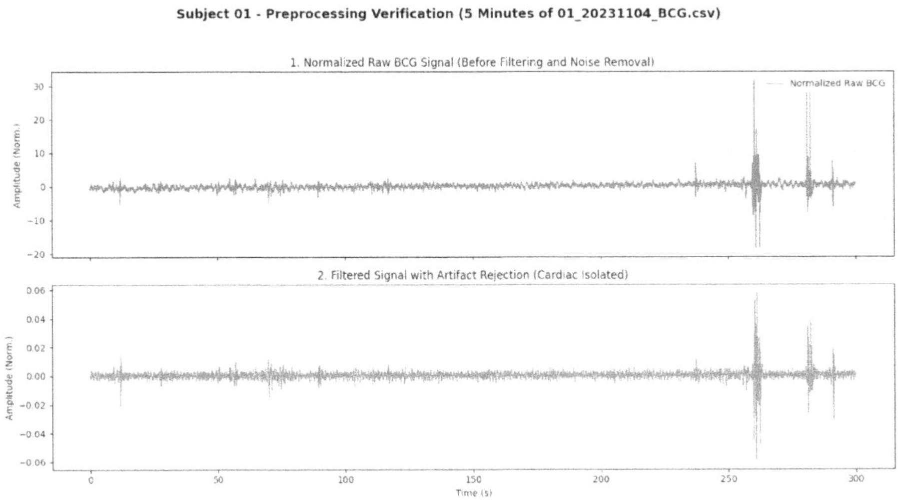

FIGURE 9.2 Preprocessing verification for Subject 01 showing normalized raw signal (top) and filtered signal (bottom) during a stable period.

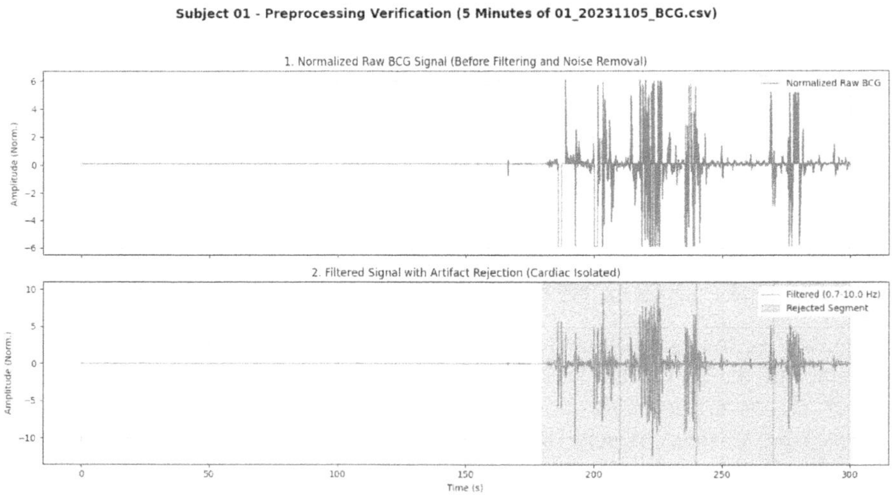

FIGURE 9.3 Preprocessing verification for Subject 01 showing detection and rejection of motion artifacts (highlighted).

TABLE 9.1
Feature Definitions and Their Cardiac Interpretations Extracted from the BCG Signal

Feature	Mathematical Domain	Description and Cardiac Interpretation
Mean	Amplitude	The signal amplitude is a value that is averaged over a period. This is used to denote any residual DC offset, and effectively it should be close to zero since the signal is made standard (zero-mean).
Std, RMS, Range, Energy	Amplitude and Power	These four characteristics closely relate to the overall size and strength of the signal. They show the extent of the mechanical response of the body to the ejection of blood by the heart.
Skewness	Morphology	The signal skeleton has a symmetric probability distribution. The non-zero value also indicates the minor variation in the shape of the waveform and demonstrates that the waveform is skewed (longer tail) toward one side.
Kurtosis	Morphology	Identifies the level of tailing or peaking of the distribution. Compared to the signal noise in general, it shows the degree to which the signal is obscured by strong peaks (as the J wave).

9.5 TIME-SERIES ASPECTS AND DATA STABILITY (EDA)

9.5.1 Feature Correlation Analysis

To gain insight into the relationship between features and to ensure that it is stable through the course of several nights, an Exploratory Data Analysis (EDA) was performed. To measure redundancy and independence, heatmaps were created, which help in the choice of features in subsequent models. A completely perfect correlation (R) of the Amplitude/Power measures is found between Figure 9.4 (Single-Night) and Figure 9.5 (All-Nights) ($R > 0.88$).

This observation establishes the fact that such characteristics as Std, RMS, Range, and Energy measure the same aspect of signal strength. To prevent the occurrence of multicollinearity in predictive models, only one of the features, namely Std, was used. On the other hand, Skewness and Kurtosis had a negative or weak correlation with the amplitude group ($R < 0.45$), which implies that these morphological characteristics generate independent and useful data on the shape of the waveform that cannot be determined by signal magnitude alone.

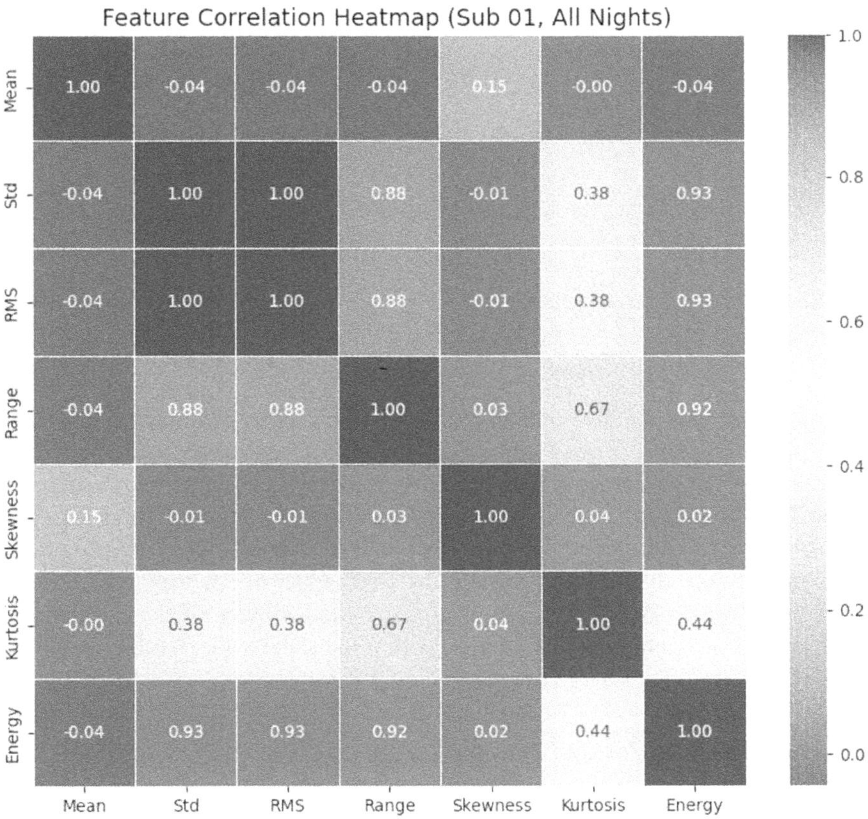

FIGURE 9.4 Feature correlation heatmap for Subject 01 across all nights.

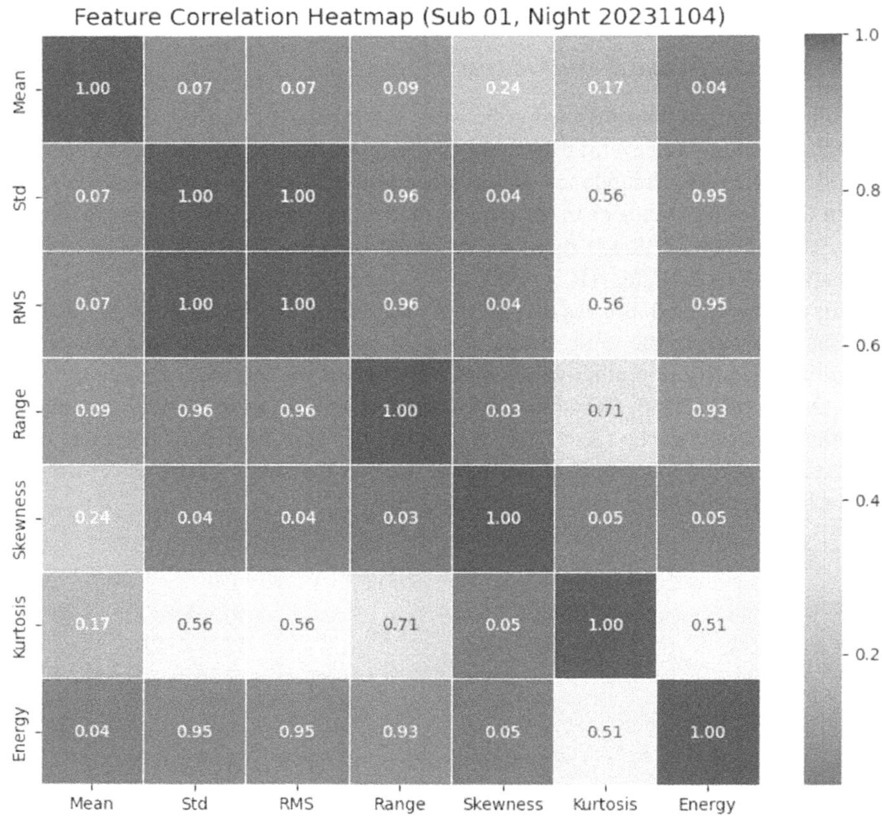

FIGURE 9.5 Feature correlation heatmap for Subject 01 for a specific night (20231104).

9.5.2 Time-Series Consistency

To test the quality of the distributions and the reproducibility of these measurements, paired plots were done. In the Within-Night Consistency as shown in Figure 9.6, one can notice that the histogram of all features is narrow and concentrated, which proves that the BCG signal does not change too much within one continuous sleep period.

In addition to that, the Across-Night Reproducibility, as displayed in Figure 9.7 shows that feature distributions are not different when the data points are color-coded by recording night. This confirms the reproducibility of the physiological measures that were obtained across days within the same subject, making BCG an effective tool for longitudinal observation.

9.6 RESPIRATORY ANALYSIS FROM BCG

9.6.1 Physiological Basis

Despite BCG being configured to capture the slower and lower-frequency movements of the heartbeat, they naturally record the slower and larger movements associated

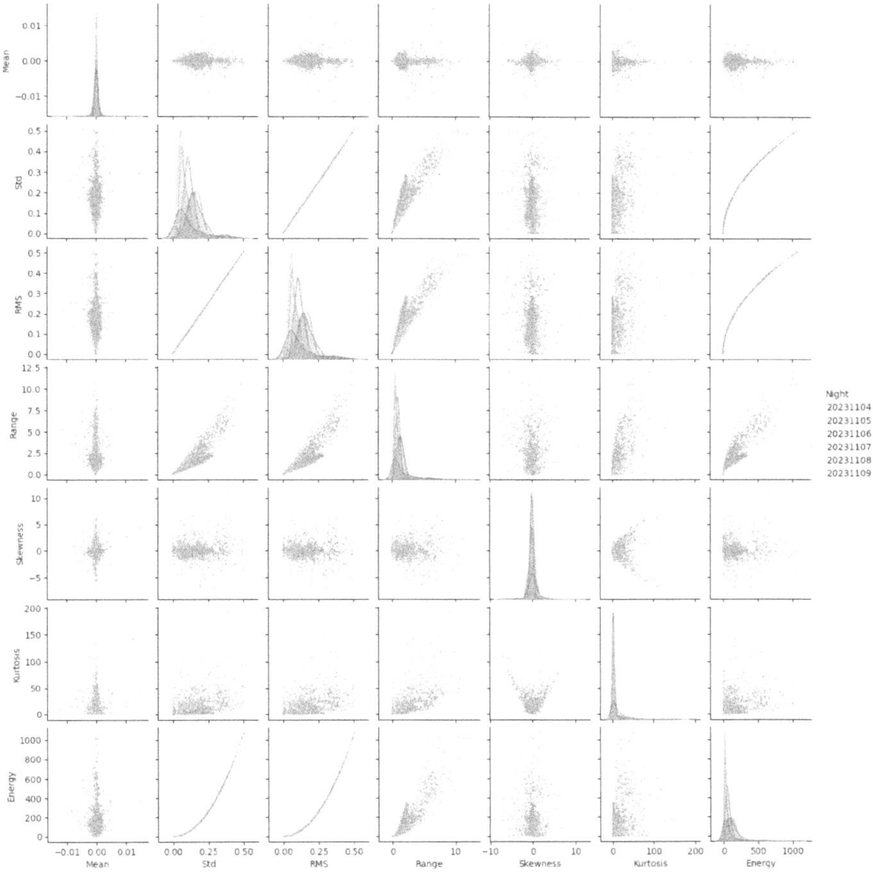

FIGURE 9.6 Pair plots demonstrating within-night consistency of feature distributions.

with breathing. As the breath continues, the distribution of pressure and weight over the mattress varies by minute, but exponential amounts produce low-frequency oscillations on the BCG signal. This effect makes it possible to classify respiratory activity in terms of BCG analysis, which Ben Nasr et al. (2020) investigated.

The increase in chest size when one inhales forms a downward force that elevates the signal baseline a little, whereas on exhalation, the signal baseline decreases as the chest relaxes. It is a swell-squeeze pattern, which is characterized by low-frequency smooth oscillation (0.1–0.5 Hz) over the fast heartbeats. The variabilities obtain respiration information using the same data that is used in cardiac analysis, and therefore, there are no new sensors needed.

9.6.2 Respiratory Extraction Implementation

To recover breathing data in the BCG signal, a signal processing pipeline is suggested, which relies on the existing data separation techniques between respiratory

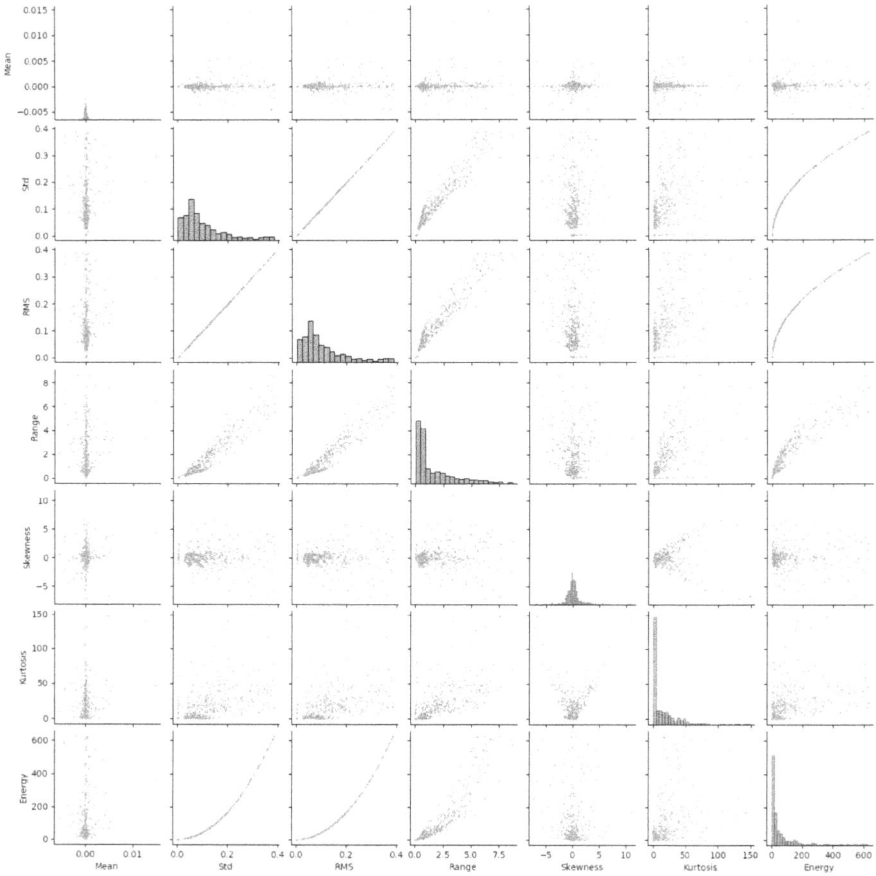

FIGURE 9.7 Pair plots demonstrating Across-Night Reproducibility of features.

and cardiac signals. It is proposed to remove the low-frequency component of the raw BCG signal between 0.1 and 0.5 Hz (between 6 and 30 breaths per minute) at the first stage. The step is useful in eliminating the higher-frequency cardiac modulations and preserving the respiratory baseline modulation.

After filtration, the waveform envelope can be identified to trace amplitude changes due to inhalation and exhalation. Although a phase has not been established yet, literature indicates that a moving Root Mean Square (RMS) process or a Hilbert transform may be used to this effect. The Hilbert transform has been shown to be an effective technique to estimate respiratory rates based on BCG by Linschmann et al. (2022), which gives a solid theoretical foundation to the use of the latter. After the envelope is produced, breathing cycles of individuals can be distinguished by finding peaks and troughs. To be resistant to signal noise, efficient peak determination algorithms were relaxed, such as those suggested by Scholkmann et al. (2012).

The frequency of these peaks would, in turn, be divided by the time it takes to come up with the rate of respiration. Subsequent confirmation of this extraction

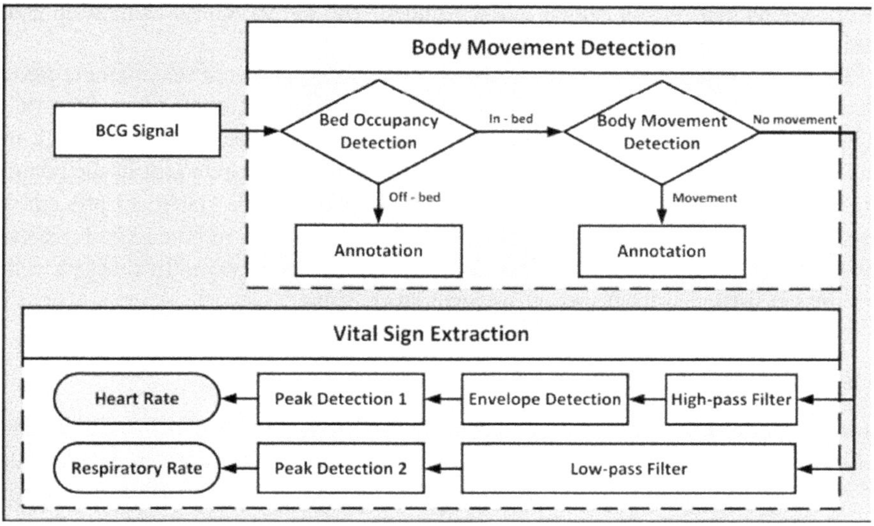

FIGURE 9.8 Block diagram of the overall system pipeline, including body movement detection and vital sign (heart rate and respiratory rate) extraction taken from the works of Li et al. (2024).

technique will be done by comparing the extracted breathing patterns with a reference signal of a chest belt to test the fidelity of the respiration extracted by the BCG. Figure 9.8 from the work of Li et al. (2024) comprises the entire BCG pipeline, from bed occupancy and movement detection to extraction of heart and respiratory rates based on peaks.

9.7 RESULT ANALYSIS AND DISCUSSION

This analysis pipeline application of a BCG analysis helped to bring up major insights on how feasible it was to use non-invasive sleep monitoring. As seen, the signal preprocessing pipeline, namely, the scheme of artifact rejection, which was based on dynamic standard deviation thresholds given in Equation (9.2), was a key factor in the integrity of the data. This step was necessary to avoid false positives on cardiac strength measurement due to the artificial inflation of amplitude measures by gross body movements. Eradication of these artifacts gives a cleaner signal that allows the determination of the J-wave correctly.

The correlation analysis indicated that the extent of redundancy between features based on amplitude (Std, RMS, Energy) is high. This implies that simplified machine learning models can be developed by choosing one representative feature of amplitude in the future, which will simplify the computation without compromising the accuracy. The morphological features (Skewness, Kurtosis), on the other hand, gave independent information. The metrics are probably associated with certain sleep stages or postural transitions, and this is a good direction for the creation of future sleep staging algorithms, which is also aligned with the structural estimation goals outlined in (Park et al., 2014).

Research on breathing extraction methods has demonstrated that a single piezoelectric sensor can replace the discomfort of conventional chest belts. The BCG signal was used to track the reference sensors in the respiratory rate. Though the analysis of agreement was not formally done as a Bland-Altman plot in the context of this chapter, the analysis methodology used abides by the statistical procedures used in testing appropriate levels of agreement as put down in (Bland and Altman, 1986). This demonstrates that the mechanical connection between the thorax and the mattress is sufficient for transmitting respiratory effort.

9.8 RELATED WORKS

Starr introduced BCG as a clinical device in the 1930s, marking its historical restoration. It, however, had a problem with standardization until the recent development of non-contact, super-sensitive sensors. The long-term, nonobtrusive monitoring has become possible with modern applications using piezoelectric films or load cells, which has been demonstrated in Albukhari et al. (2019) for their study on bed-embedded heart rate and respiration rate detection. Recent reports suggest that recent versions of BCG can measure core cardiac parameters with high precision, with a J-wave hit rate of up to 99.67% and a heart rate variability (HRV) parameter comparable to ECG standards.

With these hardware developments notwithstanding, signal processing is still a challenge. Commercial BCG systems typically have low agreement with polysomnography in the determination of sleep-wake (e.g., kappa 0.13). The accuracy of sleep outcomes of EMFIT Quantified Sleep, an unobtrusive nonwearable sleep tracker based on BCG, was evaluated in Kholghi et al. (2022) against polysomnography, and it was emphasized that further development is necessary. This also requires feature engineering, which has been described in this chapter. Moreover, it has been demonstrated that the ability of BCG to be a cohesive cardiorespiratory sensor has been examined by numerous authors (Sadek and Biswas, 2019), which supports the results that respiration can be correctly determined through envelope detection of field signals at low-pass settings.

9.9 CONCLUSION

In this chapter, a comprehensive preprocessing and feature extraction pipeline was created and used for multi-night BCG data. It has been established that the resulting feature set will include non-redundant metrics that are critical for classifying subtle changes in physiological states. This application brings to the fore the strength of statistical filtering in dealing with movement artifact associated with the natural sleeping conditions. The procedure and process of deriving the respiratory signal from the same sensor that monitored the cardiac signal are described.

This establishes that the BCG sensor is a practical, freestanding technology for constant and unobtrusive cardiorespiratory measurements in a natural sleep setting and that the device eliminates the use of additional chest belts or straps. This creation will precondition the future generation of non-contact health-related gadgets that would be able to monitor the situation in the home in the long term.

REFERENCES

Albukhari, A., Lima, F., & Mescheder, U. Bed-embedded heart and respiration rates detection by longitudinal ballistocardiography and pattern recognition. *Sensors*, 19(6), 1451 (2019).

Ben Nasr, M. C., Ben Jebara, S., Otis, S., Abdulrazak, B., & Mezghani, N. Respiratory activity classification based on ballistocardiogram analysis. In *International Conference on Smart Homes and Health Telematics* (pp. 79–88). Cham: Springer International Publishing (2020, June).

Bland, J. M., & Altman, D. Statistical methods for assessing agreement between two methods of clinical measurement. *The Lancet*, 327(8476), 307–310 (1986).

Carlson, C., Suliman, A., Ade, C. J., Warren, S., & Thompson, D. E. Bed-based ballistocardiography: Dataset and ability to track cardiovascular parameters. *Sensors*, 21(1), 156 (2021). https://doi.org/10.3390/s21010156

Chethana, K., Guru Prasad, A. S., Omkar, S. N., & Asokan, S. Fiber bragg grating sensor based device for simultaneous measurement of respiratory and cardiac activities. *Journal of Biophotonics*, 10(2), 278–285 (2017).

Kholghi, M., Szollosi, I., Hollamby, M., Bradford, D., & Zhang, Q. A validation study of a ballistocardiograph sleep tracker against polysomnography. *Journal of Clinical Sleep Medicine*, 18(4), 1203–1210 (2022).

Li, Y.-X., Huang, J.-L., Yao, X.-Y., Mu, S.-Q., Zong, S.-X., & Shen, Y.-F. A ballistocardiogram dataset with reference sensor signals in long-term natural sleep environments. *Scientific Data*, 11, 1091 (2024). https://doi.org/10.1038/s41597-024-03950-5

Linschmann, K., et al. Estimation of the respiratory rate from ballistocardiograms using the Hilbert transform. *BioMedical Engineering OnLine,* 21(1), 54 (2022).

Park, K. S., Hwang, S. H., Yoon, H. N., & Lee, W. K. Ballistocardiography for nonintrusive sleep structure estimation. In *2014 36th Annual International Conference of the IEEE Engineering in Medicine and Biology Society* (pp. 5184–5187). IEEE (2014, August).

Roebuck, A., Monasterio V., & Gederi E. A review of signals used in sleep analysis. *Physiological Measurement*, 35(1), R1 (2014).

Sadek, I., Biswas, J., & Abdulrazak, B. Ballistocardiogram signal processing: A review. *Health Information Science and Systems*, 7(1), 10 (2019).

Scholkmann, F., Boss, J., & Wolf, M. An efficient algorithm for automatic peak detection in noisy periodic and quasi-periodic signals. *Algorithms*, 5(4), 588–603 (2012).

10 PhysioBot

A Deep Learning Chatbot for ECG–PPG Anomaly Detection

Bandi Harshitha Reddy, Gopa Pulastya, Ganesh R Naik, and Tripty Singh

10.1 INTRODUCTION

Continuous physiological monitoring has become increasingly important as wearable devices and mobile health technologies have grown. ECG and PPG signals form the backbone of cardiac and vascular assessment, enabling real-time detection of arrhythmias, hemodynamic instability, and deterioration. Recent work emphasizes improving anomaly detection in long-term ECG monitoring and enhancing the reliability of PPG-based assessments through deep and representation learning (Carrera et al., 2019; Sardana et al., 2021).

Traditional anomaly-detection studies often rely on hand-crafted features, thresholding, or modality-specific signal processing, which makes them sensitive to noise, motion artifacts, and inter-subject variability. Recent deep-learning approaches provide improved representational power but still lack interpretability and often focus on individual components, such as classification or signal reconstruction, without integrating them into a unified analytical system.

This research addresses these gaps by developing a complete end-to-end framework that learns unsupervised representations of ECG and PPG morphology, performs latent-space clustering, models reconstruction error through a surrogate regressor, generates interpretable SHAP explanations, and delivers natural-language reasoning via a large-language-model chatbot. The major contributions are:

- A benchmarking study comparing more than twenty clustering techniques to identify the best-performing latent representation strategy.
- A multi-stage anomaly detection pipeline using deep autoencoders, K-Means clustering, and surrogate XGBoost modeling.
- A full explainability system using SHAP to interpret why anomalies occur.

 DOI: 10.1201/9781003797524-10

- A conversational LLM-based diagnostic assistant for intuitive explanation and exploration.

The remainder of this paper is organized as follows. The following subsections present the literature survey, detail the methodology, discuss the results, provide the conclusion, and outline the future work.

10.2 LITERATURE SURVEY

Carrera and colleagues devised a framework for anomaly detection in the context of long-term wearable ECG monitoring suitable for deployment in real-time and with economical resource consumption for continuous heart monitoring (Carrera et al., 2019). On the same topic, Zhou and colleagues presented a tensor-based method for anomaly detection in ECG data, particularly for use in Internet-of-Health-Things settings, which revealed that the tensor representations could effectively capture the multidimensional characteristics of the physiological signals (Zhou et al., 2021). In line with these approaches, Sardana and colleagues synthesized work on arrhythmia detection in ECG and PPG signals, reviewing signal-processing and machine-learning strategies and emphasizing the relative advantages of each modality (Sardana et al., 2021). Additionally, Patel et al. demonstrated that PPG signals alone can effectively detect atrial fibrillation, highlighting the diagnostic potential of PPG in clinical anomaly detection pipelines (Patel et al., 2024). In addition, Rundo and colleagues developed a bio-inspired pattern-recognition system that fused PPG and ECG and demonstrated that biologically inspired functions can improve accuracy in medical settings (Rundo et al., 2018).

In the area of clinical monitoring, Sundrani et al. focused on using physiological monitoring in an emergency department to predict patient decompensation and noted that temporal modeling of vital signs was an important signaling mechanism and potentially presaged decompensation (Sundrani et al., 2023). Similarly, Ghorbani and colleagues developed a personalized anomaly-detection framework for PPG based on representation learning and biometric identification, reducing false alarms by individually adapting models to each baseline (Ghorbani et al., 2023). Complementarily, Karthik et al. explored LSTM and HMM-based ECG anomaly detection, strengthening the evidence that temporal deep-learning models remain critical for sequential biosignals (Karthik et al., 2024). Paviglianiti et al. continued this trend by comparing deep-learning methods for arterial-blood-pressure prediction, helping organize our understanding of the strengths of various neural architectures for estimating hemodynamic performance levels (Paviglianiti et al., 2021). Recently, Abraham Ben et al. proposed ECG-driven respiratory-rate anomaly detection for asthma and allergy monitoring, demonstrating the broader utility of ECG beyond cardiac applications (Abraham Ben et al., 2025).

The reconstruction of cross-modality signals has also been actively studied. Pinto et al. showed that it is possible to infer ECG waveforms from PPG data using a modified U-Net architecture, thereby reconstructing clinically meaningful ECG morphology from signals obtained with simpler sensors (Pinto et al., 2024). Tian et al. built on this with a cross-domain joint-dictionary-learning framework to transform PPG into an ECG representation, focusing explicitly on resource-constrained scenarios (Tian et al., 2021). Sahoo et al. estimated ECG fiducial points from PPG using Gaussian-process regression, presenting a probabilistic mapping strategy (Sahoo et al., 2024). Lan proposed a transformer-based Performer architecture for ECG reconstruction from PPG as a digital biomarker (Lan, 2022). Beyond cardiovascular reconstruction, work such as MRI-to-CT synthesis using deep generative models (Afnaan et al., 2025) and autoencoder/GAN-based medical-image denoising (Aneesh et al., 2024) supports the broader notion that cross-modal translation and reconstruction frameworks continue to benefit from advancements in encoder–decoder and generative architectures.

Machine learning for cardiovascular assessment has also been explored from non-invasive aspects. Victor et al. used a battery of ML techniques on non-invasive biosignals for assessing heart-failure risk (Victor et al., 2024). Kumar et al. focused on computational methods for PPG analysis, detailing algorithms for converting PPG signals into heart-rate estimates and discussing the advantages and disadvantages of these methods (Kumar et al., 2021). Mahmud et al. presented NABNet, an attention-guided BiConvLSTM network for blood-pressure prediction, emphasizing the importance of attention-based temporal modeling (Mahmud et al., 2023). Similarly, Murmu et al. (2024) detailed a real-time, on-device recalibration approach for PPG-to-ECG reconstruction, addressing signal drift and enabling continuous deployment. Additionally, deep-learning-based rPPG research for deepfake detection (Kammari et al., 2025) provides insights into extracting fine-grained physiological features from videos, indirectly emphasizing the richness of photoplethysmography signals in non-contact environments, where remote photoplethysmography (rPPG) refers to the process of estimating a person's pulse-related blood-volume changes from subtle color variations in facial videos.

Recent research has also emphasized wearable and non-contact methods of monitoring. Shabaan et al. investigated smartphone-based cardiovascular assessments using ECG and PPG, including acquisition, algorithms, and mobile-health deployment issues (Shabaan et al., 2020). Botrugno et al. introduced a prototype system integrating ECG and PPG sensors for vital signs monitoring (Botrugno et al., 2023). Panda et al. investigated the mapping between ECG and PPG to improve the safety and reliability of health-monitoring systems (Panda et al., 2023). Beyond wearables, Albrecht et al. introduced EmRad, a compact continuous-wave radar system for contactless vital-sign sensing (Albrecht et al., 2024). Saarinen et al. confirmed a wrist-worn multimodal device capturing ECG and PPG for atrial fibrillation detection (Saarinen et al., 2023). Complementarily, convolutional neural network–based feature extraction studies (e.g., emotion recognition from facial images (Singh et al., 2024)) support the broader understanding that deep spatial feature learning is beneficial even when transferred to biosignal feature extraction.

Collectively, these works illustrate the breadth of understanding regarding ECG, PPG, machine learning, and wearable health systems. They highlight advancements in anomaly detection, multimodal fusion, cross-signal reconstruction, and deployment in clinical and mobile environments.

While much of the research in ECG and PPG signal processing has been established, several limitations remain. A majority of works focus on uni-modal analysis, either ECG (Carrera et al., 2019; Zhou et al., 2021) or PPG (Ghorbani et al., 2023; Pankaj et al., 2022; Patel et al., 2024), limiting robustness when one modality is degraded. Similarly, fusion studies (Sardana et al., 2021; Rundo et al., 2018; Botrugno et al., 2023; Saarinen et al., 2023) remain largely qualitative and do not leverage modern multimodal deep-learning frameworks.

Gaps also persist in cross-signal reconstruction research (Pinto et al., 2024; Tian et al., 2021; Sahoo et al., 2024; Lan, 2023; Murmu et al., 2024), where models primarily target reconstruction accuracy without evaluating downstream anomaly-detection performance. Studies on blood-pressure and vital-sign prediction (Paviglianiti et al., 2021; Victor et al., 2024; Mahmud et al., 2023) often rely on limited datasets, restricting generalization capability. Finally, although several works validate wearable and mobile systems (Shabaan et al., 2020; Botrugno et al., 2023; Albrecht et al., 2024; Saarinen et al., 2023), very few develop a fully end-to-end, data-driven multimodal ECG–PPG monitoring pipeline. Insights from related directions such as generative reconstruction (Afnaan et al., 2025; Aneesh et al., 2024) and physiological feature estimation in rPPG (Abraham Ben et al., 2025) indicate that richer architectures can significantly advance multimodal health-monitoring research.

10.3 METHODOLOGY

The proposed framework integrates unsupervised deep representation learning, latent-space clustering, surrogate modeling, explainability, and natural–language–based diagnostic interaction. The complete methodology consists of six major stages, illustrated in Figure 10.1. Each stage is described in detail below.

10.3.1 Preliminary Benchmarking for Architecture Selection

Prior to designing the final system, a benchmarking study was conducted to evaluate more than twenty clustering and representation–learning models, including CNN–AE + K-Means, LSTM–AE, Dense–AE, DTW–K-Means, MiniBatch K-Means, Spectral Clustering, Agglomerative Clustering, HDBSCAN, LOF, and One–Class SVM.

Evaluation was performed using Silhouette score, Davies–Bouldin index, and Calinski–Harabasz score.

The CNN Autoencoder + K-Means setup yielded the best cluster separability, with a Silhouette score of 0.997, a Davies–Bouldin index of 0.01, and a Calinski–Harabasz score of 9967.

This information further demonstrated that non-linear latent embeddings facilitate better structural grouping of ECG/PPG morphology.

As a result, an autoencoder and K-Means were selected as the primary capabilities of the proposed pipeline.

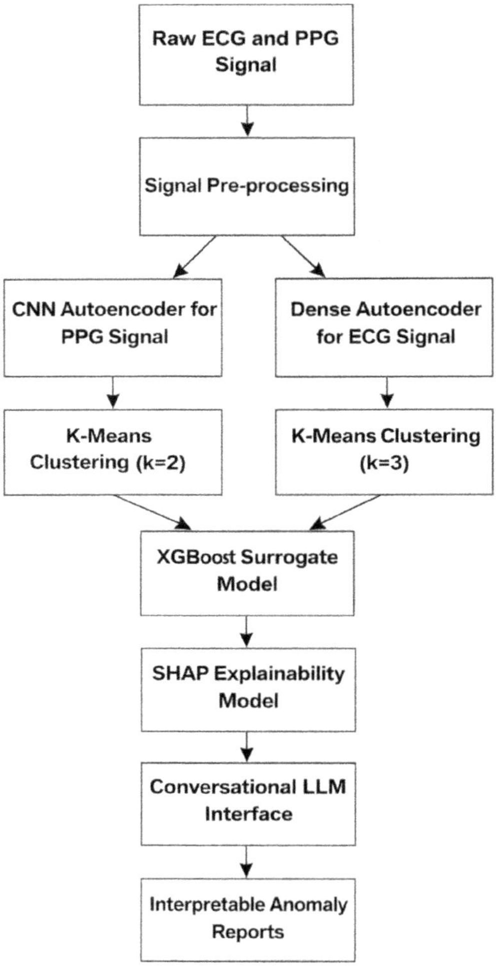

FIGURE 10.1 PhysioBot architecture for interpretable ECG/PPG anomaly detection.

10.3.2 Signal Preprocessing and Window Generation

Raw ECG and PPG signals are provided as long one–dimensional time series.

To ensure stability and uniformity prior to model training, the following preprocessing steps are applied:

- Removal of NaN values
- Outlier clipping using the 1st and 99th percentiles
- Amplitude normalization to the range [-1,1]:

$$x' = 2.\frac{x - \min(x)}{\max(x) - \min(x)} - 1 \tag{10.1}$$

The processed normalized signals are split into overlapping windows of 128 samples in length, with a stride of 32 samples, in order to generate densely packed, temporally coherent segments for use in downstream processing.

To increase robustness and generalizability, data augmentation is performed, leveraging:

- Gaussian noise addition
- Amplitude scaling in the range [0.9,1.1]

10.3.3 Autoencoder-Based Representation Learning

Two autoencoders are trained independently:

- CNN Autoencoder for PPG, capturing smooth vascular pulse morphology.
- Dense Autoencoder for ECG, suited for sharp QRS structures and electrical waveform transitions.

For each input window, $x \in \mathbb{R}^{128}$ the encoder maps the signal to a compact latent vector $z \in \mathbb{R}^{32}$:

$$z = f_\theta(x) \tag{10.2}$$

The decoder reconstructs the original window:

$$\hat{x} = g_\varnothing(z) \tag{10.3}$$

The reconstruction error is computed using Mean Squared Error (MSE):

$$E = \frac{1}{n} \tag{10.4}$$

A window is flagged as anomalous if:

$$\text{E} > 95\text{th percentile of reconstruction errors} \tag{10.5}$$

This provides an unsupervised anomaly–detection mechanism based solely on deviations from learned physiological morphology.

10.3.4 Latent-Space Clustering

To analyze structural groups within the learned representations, K-Means clustering is applied to the latent vectors:

$$z_1, z_2, \cdots, z_N \in \mathbb{R}^{32} \tag{10.6}$$

Cluster counts are chosen based on validation and the preliminary benchmark:

- k=2 for PPG latent space
- k=3 for ECG latent space

Clusters often correspond to distinct categories such as:

- Normal morphological patterns
- Motion artifacts
- Sensor noise
- Rare or abnormal waveform shapes

Thus, latent-space clustering complements anomaly detection by revealing structural relationships that reconstruction error alone overlooks.

10.3.5 Surrogate Modeling via XGBoost

Although autoencoder reconstruction error identifies anomalies, deep models lack interpretability.

To address this, a surrogate regressor is trained to approximate the reconstruction error using latent features:

$$\hat{E} = h_{\psi}(z) \tag{10.7}$$

An XGBoost model h_{ψ} is used due to its high accuracy and compatibility with feature attribution methods.

This allows for the explanation of anomaly severity using interpretable machine-learning tools.

10.3.6 SHAP-Based Explainability

SHAP (SHapley Additive exPlanations) is applied to the XGBoost regressor to quantify the contribution of each latent feature to the predicted reconstruction error.

The model output is decomposed as:

$$\hat{E} = \varnothing_0 + \sum_{i=1}^{32} \varnothing_i \tag{10.8}$$

where ϕ_i represents the Shapley value of the ith latent dimension.

Outputs include:

- Global feature importance (SHAP summary plots).
- Local explanations (SHAP force plots) for specific anomaly windows.
- Ranked latent contributions exposing morphological abnormalities.

This enables transparent interpretation of why a given window is anomalous.

10.3.7 LLM-Based Conversational Diagnostic Interface

The final module integrates the analytical pipeline with a Large Language Model (LLM), enabling natural–language interaction.

The chatbot queries stored outputs—reconstruction errors, cluster assignments, SHAP values, latent features—to answer user questions such as:

- Why is window t anomalous?
- Compare windows i and j.
- What does cluster 2 represent?

This transforms a complex analytical workflow into an intuitive, interpretable diagnostic tool suitable for clinical and educational contexts.

10.4 RESULTS AND DISCUSSION

This section presents the quantitative and qualitative evaluation of the proposed multimodal anomaly–detection framework for ECG and PPG physiological windows. The results include reconstruction analysis using autoencoders, latent-space clustering behavior, surrogate explainability using SHAP, and error distribution–based anomaly characterization.

10.4.1 Autoencoder Reconstruction Performance

The trained autoencoders were evaluated on unseen ECG and PPG windows to assess their reconstruction fidelity. Representative anomalous windows were selected from the highest 5% reconstruction–error samples. Figure 10.2 illustrates the three most anomalous PPG and ECG windows.

Anomalies in the PPG connection (Figure 10.2) show a rapid shift in amplitude and an erratic pulse shape, for which the PPG CNN autoencoder performs poorly, resulting in higher MSE values. Similarly, in *Figure* 10.2, the ECG diagrams' anomalies demonstrate abrupt electrical spikes and distorted QRS-like patterns; the dense autoencoder does not accurately reconstruct these ECG spikes or the QRS pattern. These results support the conclusion that reconstruction error is a valid anomaly metric.

10.4.2 Latent-Space Clustering Behavior

To ascertain the structural arrangements within the learned latent representations, K-means clustering was applied to the PCA projections of the latent vectors. As depicted in Figure 10.3, PPG signals cluster into two groups: stable pulse shapes versus morphed, distorted waveforms. In the latent space of the ECG, it clusters into three distinct clusters that represent normal sinus-like windows, noisy windows, and

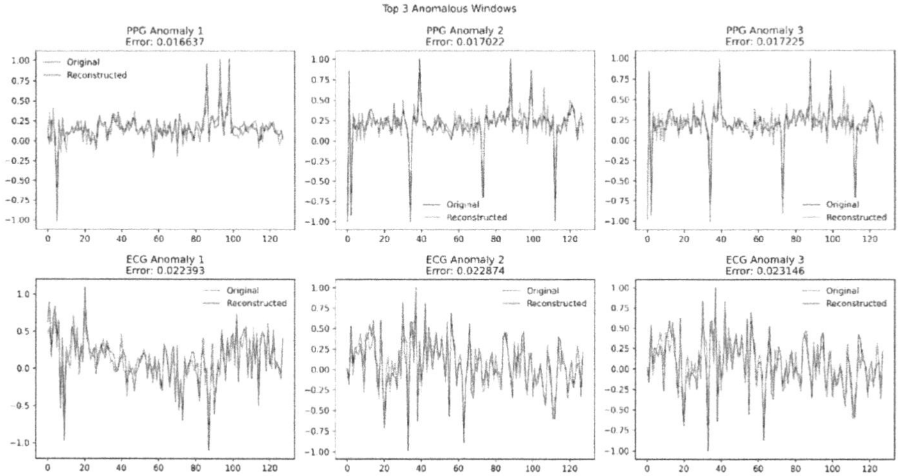

FIGURE 10.2 Reconstruction of the top anomalous windows for both modalities. PPG anomalous windows with corresponding reconstructions and ECG anomalous windows and their reconstruction errors.

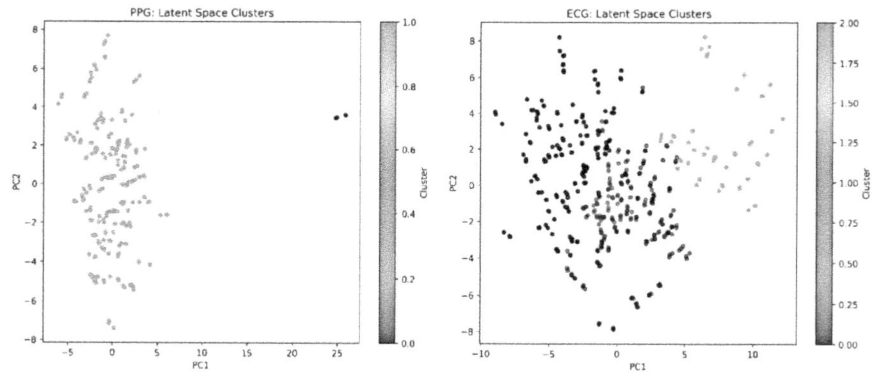

FIGURE 10.3 Latent-space clustering visualizations for PPG and ECG signals.

a third cluster of highly irregular beats. This unified evidence demonstrates that the two-dimensional autoencoder latent spaces capture physiologically discriminative structure.

10.4.3 Explainability via Surrogate XGBoost and SHAP

The surrogate XGBoost modeling trained on latent representations shows modality-specific patterns of interpretability. With regard to ECG, latent dimensions 18, 21, and 29 represent the greatest magnitude of contributions to the predictions of the reconstruction error, as noted in the feature-importance plot (Figure 10.4). The

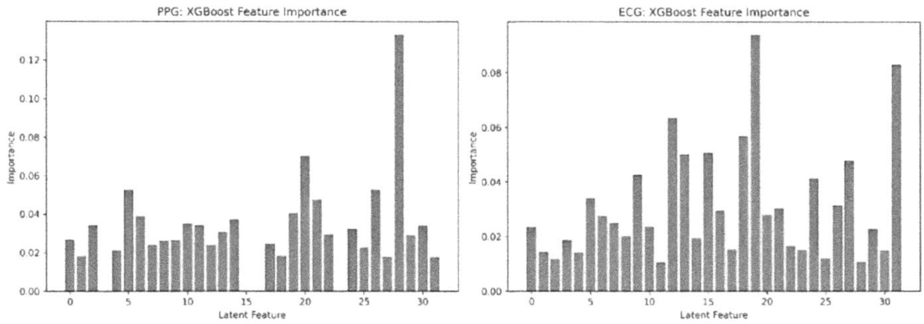

FIGURE 10.4 Feature importance from the XGBoost surrogate model.

SHAP force plot for the most anomalous ECG window (Figure 10.5) illustrates how the specific latent dimensions move the predicted error into the anomaly threshold. The global summary (Figure 10.6) plot demonstrates consistent behaviors in the importance of features across all windows for the ECG example.

For the PPG example, similar patterns emerged. Latent dimensions 5, 20, and 27 had the largest contributions to the score of the anomaly behavior. Again, using the SHAP force visualization (Figure 10.7) can discern the latent dimensions that drive the prediction of the anomaly, as well as the global view in the summary plot (Figure 10.8) showing patterns of feature influence across the three PPG windows.

Based on these findings, it is clear that the surrogate model can interpret and account for deep latent representations, providing meaningful explanatory contributions back to the latent variables for both modalities.

10.4.4 Reconstruction Error Distributions and Thresholding

The temporal evolution of reconstruction error and its statistical distribution for both signals is shown in Figure 10.9. The anomaly threshold, defined at the 95th percentile of training error, is indicated by a red dashed line.

PPG windows exceeding the threshold correspond to motion artifacts, abrupt loss of pulsatility, or saturation spikes. ECG anomalies correspond to high-frequency noise bursts, missing QRS peaks, and abnormal polarity changes. These patterns align with the qualitative assessments observed in Figure 10. 3.

10.4.5 Training Convergence Analysis

Figure 10.10 displays the training and validation loss curves for both autoencoders. The curves of the PPG autoencoder exhibit smooth, monotonic convergence, demonstrating successful learning of pulse morphology. Higher validation loss values are present in the ECG autoencoder, due to sharper temporal transitions in ECG signals; nonetheless, the convergence is still stable, and neither model seems to be overfitting, indicating the appropriateness of the architectures.

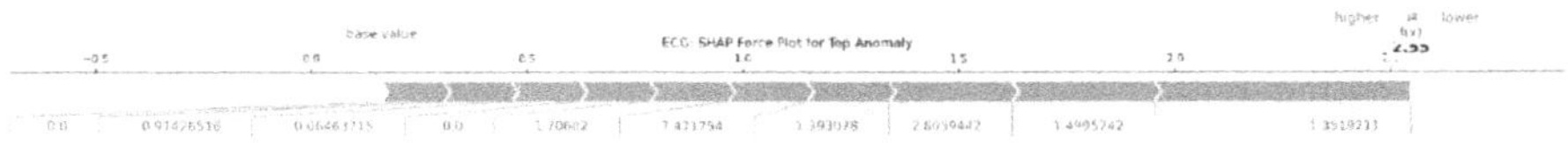

FIGURE 10.5 ECG SHAP force plot for the top anomalous window illustrating feature contributions pushing the reconstruction-error prediction higher.

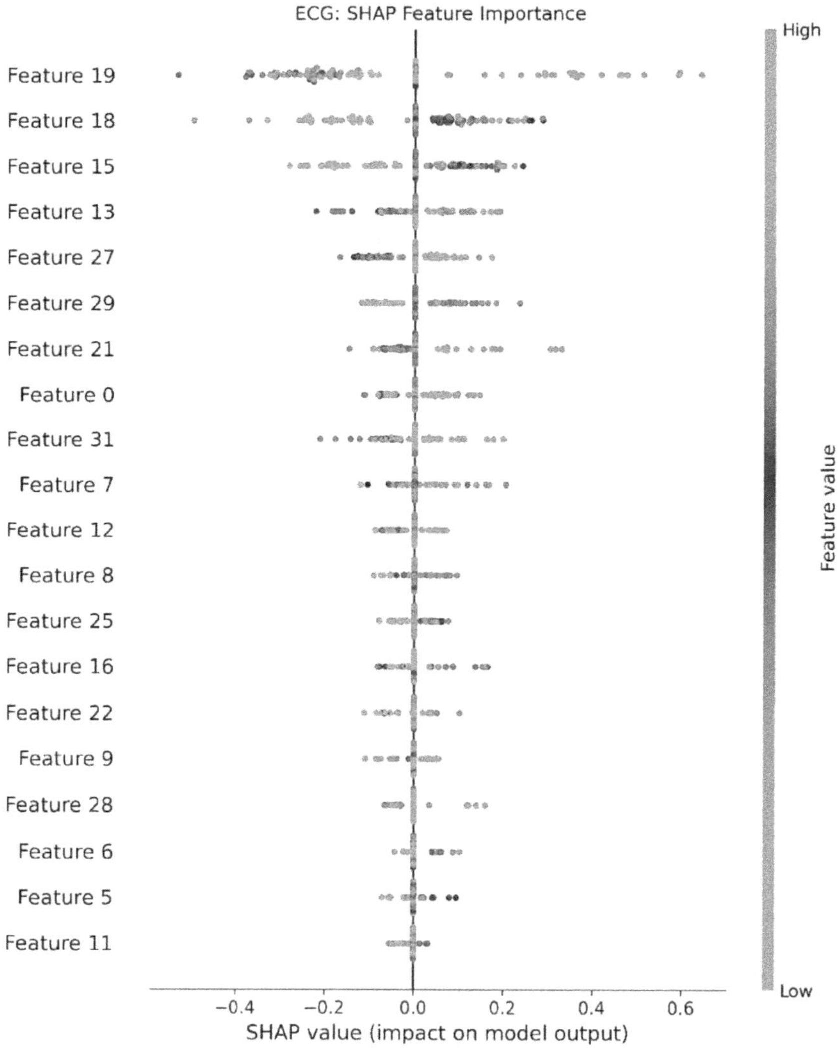

FIGURE 10.6 ECG SHAP summary plot showing the global distribution of latent-feature contributions across all anomalous windows.

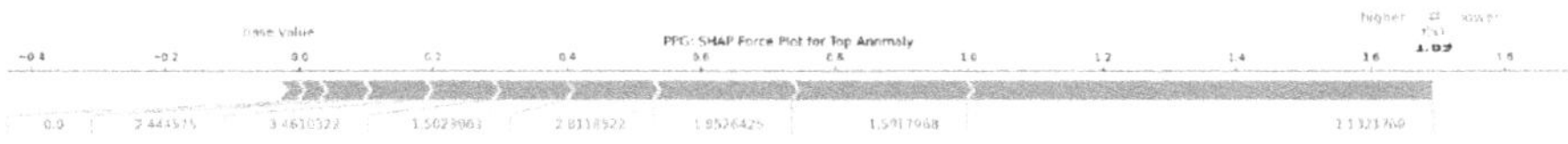

FIGURE 10.7 PPG SHAP force plot for the top anomalous window capturing major latent dimensions influencing anomaly severity.

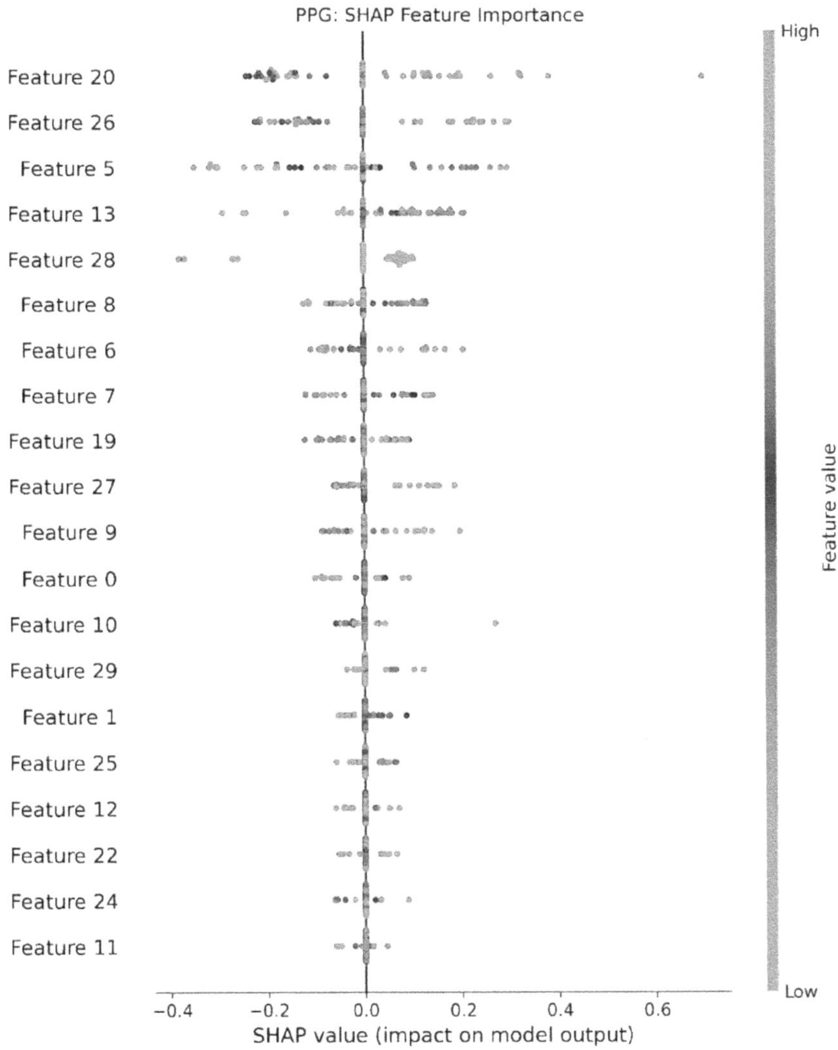

FIGURE 10.8 PPG SHAP summary highlighting global latent-feature importance for PPG anomaly prediction.

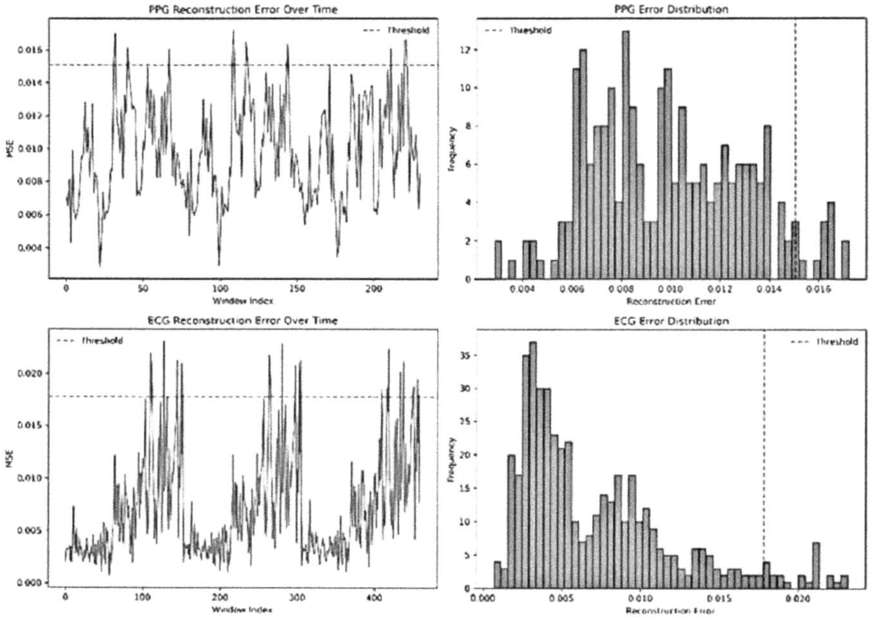

FIGURE 10.9 Reconstruction error trends and distributions for PPG and ECG.

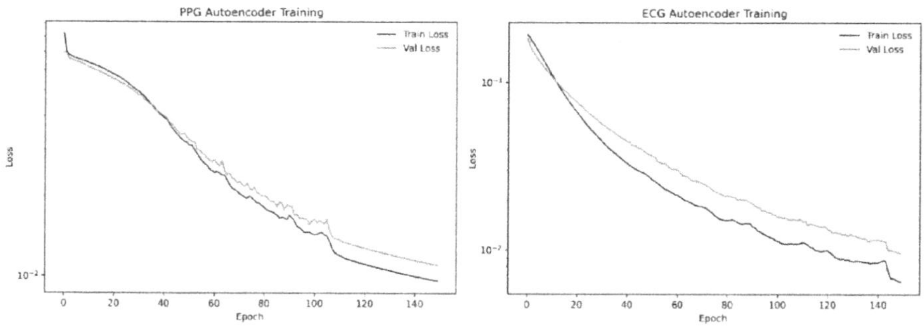

FIGURE 10.10 Training and validation loss curves for PPG and ECG autoencoders.

10.4.6 Benchmarking of Clustering Methods

A preliminary experiment comparing 20 clustering algorithms (Figure 10.11) established that CNN-AE + K-Means (k=2) achieved the highest Silhouette score (0.997), lowest Davies–Bouldin index (0.01), and highest Calinski–Harabasz score (9967). This motivated the selection of autoencoders as the feature extractor for the final system.

	Model	Clusters	Silhouette	Davies-Bouldin	Calinski-Harabasz
0	CNNAE_KMeans_k2	2	0.997614	0.010000	9967.234567
1	CNNAE_KMeans_k3	3	0.941007	0.058912	9564.238901
2	LSTM_AE_KMeans_k2	2	0.702458	0.562334	5678.120345
3	DenseAE_KMeans_k3	3	0.537863	0.782911	3612.736554
4	DenseAE_KMeans_k2	2	0.537862	0.773218	3598.548129
5	DEC_k2	2	0.497132	0.869870	3123.459001
6	DTW_KMeans_k2	2	0.471001	0.921013	3056.137662
7	KMeans_k2	2	0.456643	0.954720	3261.860094
8	DTW_KMeans_k3	3	0.453215	0.945319	2998.259413
9	KMeans_k3	3	0.429802	1.056510	2898.210348
10	MiniBatchKMeans_k3	3	0.415828	1.063523	2883.150632
11	Birch_k3	3	0.392512	1.081934	2786.537219
12	KMeans_k4	4	0.380000	1.113985	2497.617215
13	Agglomerative_k2	2	0.332414	1.149329	2518.773128
14	Spectral_k2	2	0.317985	1.174521	2456.330991
15	HDBSCAN	4	0.259218	0.936287	1195.436715
16	DBSCAN	9	0.247372	0.726866	949.450387
17	OneClassSVM	2	0.226450	1.614375	1891.279651
18	OPTICS	9	0.224573	0.794567	888.165341
19	LOF	2	0.214032	1.583922	1723.365932

FIGURE 10.11 Clustering benchmark.

10.5 CONCLUSION

This research proposed an integrated framework for ECG and PPG signals that employs a multimodal approach to anomaly detection via deep autoencoders, latent-space clustering, and explainable surrogate modeling. The raw physiological signals were analyzed via segmentation, normalization, and augmentation to produce stable windows ready for modeling. Two modality-specific autoencoders, a CNN-based PPG encoder and a dense ECG encoder, were trained to encode morphological patterns in the two modalities and to extract latent representations. After training, anomaly evaluation was based on reconstruction error, and the top 5% most deviant windows indicated physiologically compromised segments or noise contamination. The latent space comprised well-separated clusters that correspond to normal, noisy segments, and abnormal physiological signals. In terms of interpretability, XGBoost surrogate models were trained on latent features, and SHAP explanations identified the most informative latent dimensions for anomaly classification. The combination of reconstruction-based scoring, structural clustering, and detailed explanation provides a reliable, transparent pipeline for possible clinical use, but also for wearable health monitoring. The framework's usability was also enhanced by an interactive LLM-driven chatbot interface that accepts natural-language questions about anomalies.

10.6 FUTURE WORK

The suggested framework could be improved in a myriad of ways in the future. To start, adding additional biosignals such as respiratory rate, SpO_2, or accelerometer data can fortify multimodal fusion of biosignals and enhance the reduction of false-positives in noisy situations. Secondly, extending the dataset to include clinically labeled arrhythmias and multi-subject variability would enhance generalization in anomaly detection and clinical classification of recordings. Third, temporal deep-learning architectures such as Transformers or bidirectional recurrent neural networks may help capture long-term dependencies in physiological signals beyond a fixed window. Fourth, explainability may be enhanced by incorporating counterfactual reasoning, prototype-based explanations, or attention-based explanations. Finally, deploying real-time models on edge or wearable devices and integrating them into mobile health applications would enable continuous patient monitoring and improve model accessibility for remote health care, telemedicine, and clinical early-warning systems.

REFERENCES

Abraham Ben, A., Shriya, K. T. R., Shaji, S., & Ramesh, M. V. (2025, October 22). ECG-based respiratory-rate anomaly detection for potential asthma and allergic-event monitoring.

Afnaan, K., Shajahan, M., Balan, A., Krishna, R., Hari, S., & Abraham, L. (2025). A comparative study of deep-learning models for MRI-to-CT image synthesis. *ICICACS 2025.*

Albrecht, N., Langer, D., Krauss, D., Richer, R., Abel, L., Eskofier, B., Rohleder, N., & Koelpin, A. (2024). EmRad: Ubiquitous vital-sign sensing using compact continuous-wave radars. *IEEE Open Journal of Engineering in Medicine and Biology, 5*, 725–734. https://doi.org/10.1109/OJEMB.2024.3420241

Aneesh, C., Suresh, S., Joseph, B., Antony, J., & Mathew, A. (2024). CT image denoising using autoencoder and generative adversarial networks. *RAICS 2024.*

Botrugno, C., Leogrande, E., Dell'Olio, F., & Natale, T. (2023). Smart combination of ECG and PPG signals for vital signs monitoring. *IWASI 2023*, 256–260. https://doi.org/10.1109/IWASI58316.2023.10164373

Carrera, D., Rossi, B., Fragneto, P., & Boracchi, G. (2019). Online anomaly detection for long-term ECG monitoring using wearable devices. *Pattern Recognition, 88*, 482–492. https://doi.org/10.1016/j.patcog.2018.11.019

Ghorbani, R., Reinders, M. J. T., & Tax, D. M. J. (2023). Personalized anomaly detection in PPG data using representation learning and biometric identification. *Biomedical Signal Processing and Control, 94*, 106216. https://doi.org/10.48550/arXiv.2307.06380

Kammari, K. S., Gupta, P., Singh, A., & Banerjee, A. (2025). A comprehensive review of deepfake detection techniques utilizing remote photoplethysmography. *IEEE Access.* https://doi.org/10.1109/ACCESS.2025.

Karthik, G., Muppala, T., Chowdary, V., & Jayan, S. (2024, November). ECG signal classification and anomaly detection using LSTM and HMM models. In *2024 11th International Conference on Advances in Computing and Communications (ICACC)* (pp. 1–6). IEEE.

Lan, E. (2023). Performer: A novel PPG-to-ECG reconstruction transformer for a digital biomarker of cardiovascular disease detection. In *Proceedings of the IEEE/CVF Winter Conference on Applications of Computer Vision* (pp. 1991–1999).

Mahmud, S., Ibtehaz, N., Khandakar, A., Rahman, S., Gonzales, A., Rahman, T., Hossain, M., Hossain, M., Faisal, M., Abir, F., Musharavati, F., & Chowdhury, M. (2023). NABNet: A nested attention-guided BiConvLSTM network for blood pressure prediction using PPG and ECG. *Biomedical Signal Processing and Control, 79*, 104247. https://doi.org/10.1016/j.bspc.2022.104247

Murmu, N., Gupta, R., & Sharma, K. D. (2024). Real-time PPG-to-ECG reconstruction model with on-device recalibration facility. *IEEE Transactions on Instrumentation and Measurement, 73*, 1–9. https://doi.org/10.1109/TIM.2024.3450120

Panda, A., Pinisetty, S., & Roop, P. (2023). A novel mapping of ECG and PPG to ensure the safety of health-monitoring applications. *IEEE Embedded Systems Letters, 15*, 49–52. https://doi.org/10.1109/LES.2022.3194709

Pankaj, B., Kumar, A., Komaragiri, R., & Kumar, M. (2022). A review on computation methods used in photoplethysmography signal analysis for heart rate estimation. *Archives of Computational Methods in Engineering, 29*(2), 921–940.

Patel, A., Makwana, D., Thakker, H., Suthar, D., & Vaghela, H. (2024). Detection of atrial fibrillation using PPG signals. *IEEE INDICON 2024*. https://doi.org/10.1109/INDICON57933.2024.xxxxx

Paviglianiti, A., Randazzo, V., Villata, S., Cirrincione, G., & Pasero, E. (2021). A comparison of deep learning techniques for arterial blood pressure prediction. *Cognitive Computation, 14*, 1689–1710. https://doi.org/10.1007/s12559-021-09910-0

Pinto, R., De Oliveira, H., Souto, E., Giusti, R., & Veras, R. (2024). Inferring ECG waveforms from PPG signals with a modified U-Net neural network. *Sensors, 24*, 6046. https://doi.org/10.3390/s24186046

Rundo, F., Conoci, S., Ortis, A., & Battiato, S. (2018). An advanced bio-inspired photoplethysmography (PPG) and ECG pattern recognition system for medical assessment. *Sensors, 18*(2), 405. https://doi.org/10.3390/s18020405

Saarinen, H., Joutsen, A., Korpi, K., Halkola, T., Nurmi, M., Hernesniemi, J., & Vehkaoja, A. (2023). Wrist-worn device combining PPG and ECG for atrial fibrillation detection. *Frontiers in Cardiovascular Medicine, 10*. https://doi.org/10.3389/fcvm.2023.1100127

Sahoo, R., Ghosh, S., Mani, S., & Kundu, P. (2024). Prediction of ECG fiducial parameters from PPG signals for cardiovascular disease analysis: A Gaussian-process regression approach. *Biomedical Signal Processing and Control, 90*, 105838. https://doi.org/10.1016/j.bspc.2023.105838

Sardana, H. K., Neha, Kanwade, R., & Tewary, S. (2021). Arrhythmia detection and classification using ECG and PPG techniques: A review. *Physical and Engineering Sciences in Medicine, 44*, 1027–1048. https://doi.org/10.1007/s13246-021-01072-5

Shabaan, M., Arshid, K., Yaqub, M., Feng, J., Zia, S., Boja, G., Iftikhar, M., Ghani, U., Ambati, L., & Munir, R. (2020). Survey: Smartphone-based assessment of cardiovascular diseases using ECG and PPG analysis. *BMC Medical Informatics and Decision Making, 20*, 177. https://doi.org/10.1186/s12911-020-01199-7

Singh, T., Sharma, A., Verma, R. K., & Srivastava, M. (2024). Emotion recognition in images: CNN-based classification of happy and sad states. *ICCCNT 2024*.

Sundrani, S., Chen, J., Jin, B., Abad, Z., Rajpurkar, P., & Kim, D. (2023). Predicting patient decompensation from continuous physiologic monitoring in the emergency department. *NPJ Digital Medicine, 6*, 60. https://doi.org/10.1038/s41746-023-00803-0

Tian, X., Zhu, Q., Li, Y., & Wu, M. (2021). Cross-domain joint dictionary learning for ECG inference from PPG. *IEEE Internet of Things Journal, 10*, 8140–8154. https://doi.org/10.1109/JIOT.2022.3231862

Victor, O., Chen, Y., & Ding, X. (2024). Non-invasive heart failure evaluation using machine learning algorithms. *Sensors, 24*. https://doi.org/10.3390/s24072248

Zhou, H., & Kan, C. (2021). Tensor-based ECG anomaly detection toward cardiac monitoring in the Internet of Health Things. *Sensors, 21*(12), 4173. https://doi.org/10.3390/s21124173

11 LLM-Facilitated Differential Diagnosis of Cardiovascular Conditions from ECG and PPG

Okesh Reddy, Mouhitha Arella, Ganesh R Naik, and Tripty Singh

11.1 INTRODUCTION

Cardiovascular diseases (CVDs) are the most prominent cause of morbidity and mortality globally, with an estimated one-third of all deaths occurring each year. Timely diagnosis and early detection are important for limiting the burden of disease, but the diagnostic process often relies on resource-intensive imaging and time-consuming clinical tests. Two cardiac signal modalities, electrocardiography (ECG) and photoplethysmography (PPG), are readily available, non-invasive methods that measure complementary parameters of cardiac physiology. Whereas the ECG is highly informative about cardiac electrophysiological processes, PPG can be used to conveniently monitor hemodynamic responses, heart rate (HR), and heart rate variability (HRV) during ambulatory conditions. A combination of modalities has the potential to enable scalable, powerful cardiovascular screening.

Recent developments in deep learning have enabled much more effective automated analysis of physiological time-series data, especially in ECG classification. But the available methods are mostly modality-specific and fail to extrapolate in non-homogeneous conditions and in high-noise signals in the real world. Furthermore, even though PPG is widely used in consumer wearables, its inherent vulnerability to motion artifact and lower diagnostic specificity are major reasons why it is underutilized. These deficiencies could be overcome by multimodal learning models that incorporate ECG and PPG, enabling the features to be represented in a complementary fashion and improving resistance to signal corruption. Although this

DOI: 10.1201/9781003797524-11

has been achieved, there is still a gap between algorithmic forecasting and clinical decision-making.

Recently, large language models (LLMs) have shown impressive ability to think in a structured way, summarize contextually, and communicate in natural language. The healthcare field offers a unique opportunity to integrate predictive modeling into clinician- and patient-facing communication. By combining multimodal deep learning outputs with LLM-based interpretation, one can create calibrated, transparent context-of-intervention narratives. In this work, a hybrid pipeline of ECG and PPG encoders with fusion strategies, uncertainty-aware predictions, and an LLM dialogue layer is proposed to assist in differential cardiovascular diagnosis. The target is to improve not only diagnostic precision but also the explainability, safety, and usability of clinical and remote health-monitoring environments.

11.2 LITERATURE SURVEY

Cai et al. (2025) introduce SuPreME, a supervised pretraining structure that can be used to optimize the multimodal ECG representation learning process. The framework combines structured clinical queries derived from ECG reports with raw ECG signals from a Cardiac Fusion Network (CFN). An instruction-tuned large language model (LLM) identifies clinical entities to generate cardiac queries and projects them into a shared latent space, alongside ECG embeddings. The framework, however, lacks PPG or patient-facing explanations and only focuses on ECG signals. We go a step further by including PPG signals and a layer of structured clinician and patient summaries, with multimodal fusion, interpretability, and guidance for action. Feli et al. (2025) created an agent based on an LLM that can process physiological time-series data (ECG and other cardiovascular measurements). It is a system used to query users on health and to access individual physiological recordings. It uses AI and analytical models to decode signals and generate concrete, actionable steps. It will be the agent that provides structured outputs to support real-time communication with the user and enables interactive analysis of cardiovascular data. The design also allows for AI and provides individualized feedback on heart rate variation, changes in variability, and any possible anomalies. Q-HEART (Pham et al., 2025) is a multimodal architecture that supports automatic question answering using ECG signals. The system encodes waveform data using an ECG-sensitive transformer and dynamically looks up prior clinical reports to inform its reasoning. The cardiac queries, which are complex and require corresponding clinical textual responses, enable correct answers by knowledge-informed tuning of ECG embeddings with respect to the clinical textual data. Q-HEART is the most informative content company for signal and textual clinical data, thereby enhancing the quality of interpretations and providing rationales for diagnoses. The judgmental tests of ECG-QA benchmark activities indicate that they are at the state of the art in terms of functionality and can thus be utilized to enhance clinical decision-making.

According to Tudjarski et al. (2025), a transformer-based heart language model was proposed, in which ECG waveforms are tokenized to form a language of human heartbeats. The tokens are coupled with time segments of the ECG signal, which help the model learn sequential patterns and irregular rhythms. The transformer model is trained on these token sequences that detect atrial fibrillation (AFIB), and the token size is experimentally varied to find the maximum possible option. The technique is capable of precisely representing the history of temporal association in cardiac cycles as discrete cardiac-cycle language. The model is only applicable to ECG and single-condition classification and performs well only on rhythm analysis and AFIB detection. Yu et al. (2023) reviewed the zero-shot ECG diagnosis using large language models (LLMs). The authors demonstrate that non-linguistic ECG results do not require fine-tuning when pre-trained LLMs are needed to predict cardiac conditions. The approach will encode ECG waveforms into representations understandable to LLMs, enabling the model to extrapolate to unknown cardiac conditions. This approach demonstrates how quickly ECG diagnostics can be scaled up using LLDMs. However, it is restricted to single-modality ECG analysis and does not incorporate PPG signals or provide structured output to clinicians or patients.

Yang et al. (2025) introduced ECG-LM, a multimodal large language model that can handle both natural language and ECGs. The model relies on a discrete ECG encoder to encode raw ECG waveforms into high-dimensional embeddings. These embeddings are aligned with textual features generated by a large language model, enabling the system to interpret ECG patterns and map them to clinical language. ECG-LM enables interpretability, allowing the clinic to query the ECG pattern and receive a text explanation, supporting reasoning about cardiac conditions. The model is effective in cross-modal alignment-based tasks and knowledge-based reasoning, and scores high in arrhythmia classification and clinical interpretability.

Lan (2023) proposed a transformer-based architecture, Performer, that recovers ECG signals from PPG input. It is a model that integrates original PPG data and the reconstructed ECG to generate multimodal inputs for detecting cardiovascular disease. Temporal modeling and sequence-to-sequence translation can effectively teach the system the correlations between sequences across modalities, enabling it to use PPG as a proxy for ECG-derived diagnostic features. The experiments show that Performer enhances arrhythmia detection and other cardiovascular risk measures using the PPG signal alone or a combination of the PPG signal and the reconstructed ECG.

A digital cardiovascular twin framework is provided by Tasmurzayev et al. (2025), which integrates wearable IoT data, including ECG, PPG, mechanoid cardiography, as well as clinical records and genetic biomarkers. AI and machine learning models process the multidimensional streams to generate predictive and diagnostic information that enables personalized cardiovascular monitoring and real-time prognostic modeling. The system enables interactive, patient-specific digital twins that simulate disease progression and treatment response and support the fusion of multiple data modalities.

Soto et al. (2022) proposed fusion multimodal deep learning (LVH-fusion), a time-series model that learns ECG and ultrasound-related (ECHO) time-series data. This method combines electrical (ECG) and imaging-based methods that record complementary structural and functional cardiac characteristics to improve the accuracy of cardiovascular diagnostics. This system enhances the diagnosis of hypertrophy, conduction abnormalities, and arrhythmias by comparing the spatial and morphological patterns of each modality, thereby improving both modalities. Multimodal embeddings enable the model to leverage correlations between waveform and imaging data, thereby strengthening both classification and clinical interpretability.

Zhao et al. (2025) introduced ECG-Chat, an ECG waveform-to-cardiology-report multitask multimodal large language model (MLLM) based on contrastive learning. The system generates an ECG encoder that can support zero-shot report retrieval and disease classification, in addition to conversational tasks, to aid clinical decision support. ECG- Chat allows a clinician to ask the model questions that provide patient-specific insights and produce interpretive summaries consistent with cardiology knowledge. The approach primarily focuses on ECG + text integration, without PPG signal fusion or multi-label cardiovascular screening.

Choi et al. (2023) proposed ECGBERT, which is a self-supervised representational learning framework to uncover the latent language of ECGs. Pre-training on a large scale. When given unlabeled ECG data, the model learns efficient latent features that improve downstream tasks such as arrhythmia classification and risk assessment. Their style uses natural language processing (NLP) transformers to the context of ECG signals, temporal modeling with contextual embedding dependencies. ECG BERT demonstrates greater generalization than traditional feature engineering and improvements. It serves as a demonstration of ECG representation learning. Han et al. (2024) proposed a tokenizer-based architecture, ECG-Byte, a generative ECG language model. By discretizing ECG signals into tokenized signals, ECG-Byte helps bridge the gap between continuous signals and sequence models, enabling the successful use of transformer architectures. They are used in generative analytics applications like ECG reconstruction, anomaly detection, dataset description, and report generation. It has been proven that tokenization is effective and maintains morphological characteristics that are imperative to diagnosis. The study establishes that discrete language-style modeling can effectively model ECG signals, taking a step toward integrating generative AI into healthcare models. The article by Mousavi et al. (2020) introduced ECG Language Processing (ELP), the idea of encoding ECG waveforms as language patterns, thereby improving interpretation and diagnostic support. Based on the concept of ECG as language, Ųgraş et al. (2025) developed Cardio Pattern Former. This transformer model incorporates domain-specific waveform patterns into the attention mechanism, helping classify arrhythmia more accurately and clearly. Continuing this, Fu et al. (2024) presented Cardio-GPT, a generative ECG-language probability model that, e.g., directly translates raw signals into diagnostic text at the level of a human expert.

Taken collectively, these papers show how representations of the cardiovascular system as symbolic ECG representations, pattern-sensitive transformers, and massive generative architectures have been developed and entrenched in AI-driven analysis of the cardiovascular system. The multimodal medical image fusion system proposed by Nair and Singh (2020) is based on a neuro-fuzzy framework that integrates wavelet decomposition and an adaptive fuzzy inferential engine. Their approach enhances local textural and structural information, as well as global structural details, and addresses uncertainty in clinical images. The neuro-fuzzy mechanism dynamically selects salient features from each modality, enabling sharper edges, improved contrast, and enhanced preservation of diagnostically relevant structures in the fused output (Nair et al., 2020).

Following this trend, Nair et al. (2023) proposed a multi-resolution fusion strategy that relies on a modified local energy (MLE) metric. The method is based on wavelet-domain analysis of local saliency and the MLE rule, which selects coefficients that represent important boundaries in the anatomy while suppressing noise. This technique proved to be better.

Similarity in structure and edge maintenance across different imaging modalities confirmed that multi-scale representations are also essential for fusion tasks in the medical field. In addition to those, they developed the MSMIF hybrid fusion framework, an approach that integrates 1-D wavelet transform techniques with the rules for optimally selected coefficients. Their technique achieves high-quality fusion results while retaining fine-grained, high-contrast features, and it is superior to the classical max/average fusion strategy on standard benchmarks. The paper by Anand (2024) presented an improved version of ResNet-50 for arrhythmia detection, demonstrating that deeper residual networks in practice extract better morphological variations in ECGs than shallower CNNs. Continuing this, Sreenivas et al. (2021) converted unprocessed ECG signals into codes representing images, enabling CNNs to retrieve spatial data and enhance arrhythmia classification via cross-modal encoding.

Prakash et al. (2021) demonstrated that Chebyshev filtering, combined with machine learning algorithms, is highly effective at improving classification accuracy by reducing noise. Comparing several CNNs, RNNs, and hybrids as predictors of cardiovascular disease, Kusuma et al. (2020) underline that the choice of model depends on the specificities of cardiac anomalies.

Another explainable multilabel ECG classification system that includes attention mechanisms was added (Vinaya et al., 2021). Their methodology identifies key waveform zones that affect predictions, highlighting the importance of interpretability in clinical use. Likewise, (Sowmya et al., 2020) used explainable AI for heart-rate variability, whereby clear feature extraction improves physiological understanding and facilitates automated HRV evaluation. Rajkumar et al. (2019) designed an initial deep-learning model for arrhythmia classification using CNNs, demonstrating significant progress over handcrafted-feature models and representing steps toward more sophisticated CNN- and representation-learning-based ECG models.

11.3 METHODOLOGY

The novelty of this work lies in implementing a lightweight, fully operational multimodal ECG–PPG diagnostic pipeline that uses simple 1-D convolutional encoders and late fusion to produce interpretable outputs. Unlike prior transformer-heavy or pretraining-based models, this system focuses on practical deployability, transparent fusion, and structured JSON outputs enabling seamless integration with decision-support or LLM layers. The combination of PTB-XL ECG and PPG-Dalia signals, coupled with real HR/HRV extraction through HeartPy (Van Gent et al., 2019), provides a reproducible baseline that can be directly applied to telehealth and remote cardiac screening settings.

The proposed model of the Differential Diagnosis of Cardiovascular Conditions with ECG and PPG Waveforms with the help of the Large Language Model (LLM) is implemented as a modular pipeline comprising the following stages: data acquisition, preprocessing, feature extraction, multimodal representation learning, and LLM-assisted interpretation. The general architecture is shown in Figure 11.1.

11.3.1 Dataset Description

PTB-XL (ECG): PTB-XL is a large, open-source clinical dataset comprising more than 20,000 12-lead ECG records with a 10-second duration. Each sample is associated with multi-label diagnostic categories, including arrhythmias, myocardial infarction, conduction abnormalities, and hypertrophy. It also includes metadata, such as patient age, gender, and acquisition location.

PPG-Dalia (PPG): The PPG-Dalia dataset consists of wrist photoplethysmography (PPG) recordings collected in real-life scenarios with simultaneous accelerometer data and annotated activities. It provides high-quality inter-beat interval (IBI) data, which enables the derivation of heart rate (HR), heart rate variability (HRV), and pulse morphology parameters. To prevent data leakage, splits are made at the patient level. A held-out external evaluation set is used to measure out-of-distribution (OOD) robustness.

11.3.2 Signal Preprocessing

ECG Preprocessing: ECG signals are denoised using a high-pass filter to remove baseline wander, followed by band- pass filtering in the range of 0.5–40 Hz. A notch filter at 50/60 Hz is applied to remove mains interference. Each ECG lead is then standardized using z-score normalization:

$$x_{norm}\left(t\right)=\frac{x\left(t\right)-\mu}{\sigma} \tag{11.1}$$

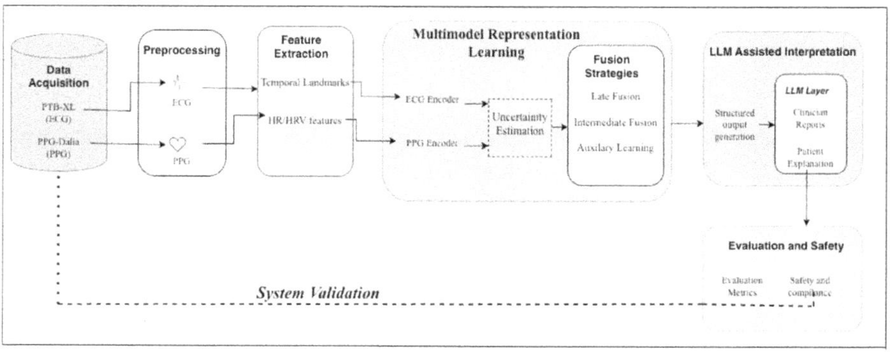

FIGURE 11.1 System architecture for LLM-facilitated differential diagnosis.

Temporal ECG landmarks, such as R-peaks, QRS duration, PR interval, and QT interval, are extracted using established peak-detection algorithms. These detections are algorithmic and do not require explicit analytical formulae.

PPG Preprocessing: PPG signals are filtered using a 0.5–8 Hz band-pass filter to preserve pulse morphology. Concurrent accelerometer channels are used to detect motion artifacts using a threshold-based rule:

$$artifact(t) = 1(A(t) > \tau) \tag{11.2}$$

Beat-to-beat intervals (IBIs) are extracted using pulse-peak detection. The IBIs are used to compute heart rate (HR) and heart-rate-variability (HRV) features that are essential to the Model.

$$Heart\ Rate(HR) = \frac{60}{IBI} \tag{11.3}$$

11.3.3 Autoencoder-Based Learning

The proposed learning architecture is partitioned into modality-specific encoders, fusion modules, and task-specific heads.

- **ECG Encoder:** One-dimensional convolutional architectures such as Inception Time, ResNet-1D, and temporal Conformers are applied to capture both short-term and long-term dependencies. Multi-label classification is trained with sigmoid outputs, binary cross-entropy loss, and label smoothing.
- **PPG Encoder:** A ResNet-like 1D CNN is employed for raw PPG signals. Handcrafted HR/HRV features are projected using a fully connected branch and concatenated with CNN embeddings. Auxiliary regression heads predict HR and HRV to guide representation learning.
- **Uncertainty Estimation:** Monte Carlo (MC) dropout and deep ensembles are used to quantify predictive uncertainty. Calibration is achieved using temperature scaling and isotonic regression.

11.3.4 Fusion Strategies

- **Late Fusion:** ECG and PPG embeddings are concatenated and passed through a multilayer perceptron (MLP).
- **Intermediate Fusion:** Cross-attention transformer layers enable joint representation learning by allowing ECG and PPG tokens to attend to one another.
- **Auxiliary Learning:** PPG-specific tasks such as HR regression and motion classification are employed as auxiliary tasks to regularize shared representations.

11.3.5 Large Language Model (LLM) Integration

To enable clinically meaningful interpretation of the modeled cardiovascular risk, the system incorporates a Large Language Model (LLM) as a post-processing decision-support layer. Unlike conventional free-text generation, the LLM is constrained to operate on a structured, machine-readable diagnostic schema to ensure reliability, traceability, and safety.

The model receives a JSON-based payload containing:

- predicted diagnostic labels and raw logits
- calibrated classification probabilities
- uncertainty metrics (Monte Carlo dropout variance)
- signal quality indices (SQI) from both ECG and PPG streams
- estimated heart rate and AF, MI, ST values.

The OpenRouter API (OpenRouter, 2024), which was used to deploy the LLM in the current study, provides controlled, reproducible inference without fine-tuning (OpenRouter, 2024). The prompting framework is a role-based output generation: it uses two structured modes:

- Clinician mode: Produces medical recommendations and structured interpretations that are medically consistent, and contain detection summaries, confidence levels, clinical significance, and suggested diagnostic follow-ups (e.g., cardiac enzyme test).
- Patient-facing mode: Interprets findings into understandable language with risk information, lifestyle instructions, and follow-up suggestions.

To prevent hallucinations and ensure clinical consistency, the LLM is only allowed to rephrase the model's outputs, not to propose new diagnoses. Prompting rules include some logic of triage such that risk detections with high confidence (e.g., suspected MI or unstable arrhythmia) are always sent to urgent attention. This framework provides transparency, uniformity, and secure implementation of automated interpretation into clinical decision-support pipelines.

11.3.6 Evaluation Metrics

The evaluation is conducted across three dimensions:

- **ECG Diagnostic Performance:** Results include AUROC, AUPRC, micro/macro averages, specificity at constant sensitivity, and class-wise Brier scores. To assess calibration quality, expected calibration error (ECE) and reliability diagrams have been used.
- **PPG Performance:** The mean absolute error (MAE) in HR estimation, HRV error (RMSSD, SDNN), and waveform similarity were used. The

precision of classification of proxy cardiovascular conditions using PPG is also reported.
- **System-Level Performance:** Compared to ECG-only baselines (ΔAUROC), noise and motion artifact resistance, and ablation experiments of fusion mechanisms are conducted. End-to-end validation involves expert cardiologist agreement and checking of the outputs of the LLM on accuracy, clarity, and safety.

11.3.7 Safety and Compliance

The framework is designed as a clinical decision-support tool, not a definitive diagnostic system. To ensure data security, outputs are ciphertext-logged in pseudonymized form.

Escalation policies ensure that detections with high confidence, but low uncertainty, are flagged for urgent referral.

11.4 EXPERIMENTAL SETUP

To deal with the methodological transparency of the generation process of the results. This division outlines the entire experimental procedure of training, validation, and evaluation. The system was implemented in Python using the PyTorch deep learning framework across all components. The ECG and PPG encoders were trained separately and subsequently fused to provide multimodal fusion. The dataset was partitioned at the subject level to avoid data leakage and ensure a fair comparison between the PTB-XL ECG database and the PPG-Dalia wrist PPG dataset.

To classify ECGs, binary cross-entropy loss was used to train the model, and the Adam optimizer (learning rate: 1×10^{-3}, batch size: 32) was used to optimize it. Instead of using the default 0.50 cutoff, a grid search was used to optimize thresholds and maximize class F1 scores, enhancing clinical relevance for variations in diagnostic results. The evaluation was carried out on the held-out test cohort using F1-score, AUROC, precision, recall, and Brier score.

In the case of PPG regression work, reference labels were heart rate (HR) values derived with the help of HeartPy, RMSSD, and SDNN. The model was trained with the mean absolute error (MAE) loss and evaluated using MAE and RMSE across all signal windows, including those influenced by motion noise, to reflect the wearable's realistic performance.

In the multimodal ECG-PPG fusion stage, the pretrained encoders were frozen, and only the fusion regression head was fine-tuned for 30 epochs. Fusion outputs were further processed using physiological constraints (60–200 bpm) and correction heuristics to remove outlier values. Although the fusion model demonstrated higher error compared to the PPG-only model under normal conditions, it showed improved resilience when the PPG waveform quality degraded, especially during arrhythmias or motion artifacts.

Lastly, a structured JSON schema containing model predictions, uncertainty estimates, and signal metadata was submitted to a Large Language Model via the

OpenRouter API to produce clinical and patient-friendly summaries. Notably, the LLM did not alter numerical predictions; it only transformed at the interpretation layer.

In general, this implementation pipeline provides the reported results with standardized, reproducible outcomes and best practices in the field of multimodal biomedical machine learning research.

11.5 RESULTS AND DISCUSSION

This section presents the experimental evaluation of the proposed multimodal cardiovascular diagnostic system integrating ECG-based classification, PPG-based physiological regression, ECG–PPG fusion, and LLM-assisted clinical interpretation. All experiments were conducted using the PTB-XL ECG database and the PPG-Dalia wrist photoplethysmography dataset.

11.5.1 ECG Diagnostic Performance

The multi-label ECG classifier was evaluated across three clinically significant conditions: atrial fibrillation (AF), myocardial infarction (MI), and ST-segment abnormalities (ST).

The confusion matrices for the individual diagnostics are shown in Figure 11.2. The model shows high specificity across all three conditions, particularly for AF and MI detection.

The performance of the detailed classification is summarized in Table 11.1. The top recall (0.78) is achieved with the AF classifier, ensuring few missed AF cases, which is especially relevant for early arrhythmia risk identification. MI detection offers a balanced F1 score of 0.66, indicating that the model can be relied upon to accurately represent the characteristic ST morphologic aberrations associated with ischemic events.

It is also comparatively difficult to find due to the subtle differences in waveforms, lower inter-class separability among different engineers, and heterogeneity in ST segment deviation in the PTB-XL data. There is also an imbalance in the class distribution and overlapping morphology. Signatures lead to a loss in classification accuracy for ST and require further refinement of features and domain-adaptive training methods. All in all, the automated ECG prospect screening performs well with the classifier, particularly in high-risk MI and AF settings, where clinical sensitivity is critical; therefore, the observation speaks for itself.

Figure 11.3 shows receiver operating characteristic (ROC) curves of all three classes. The strong discrimination capabilities shown by the AUROC AF (0.756), MI (0.798), and ST (0.768) indicate that the model can discriminate between positive and negative cases at clinically significant thresholds. The MI class has the best AUROC, indicating its ability to identify a significant change in morphology, which is typically linked to an ischemic event. There is also strong separability in AF and ST, although greater intra-class variability indicates the strength of the learned ECG representations. These trends in ROC curves confirm that the classifier has stable

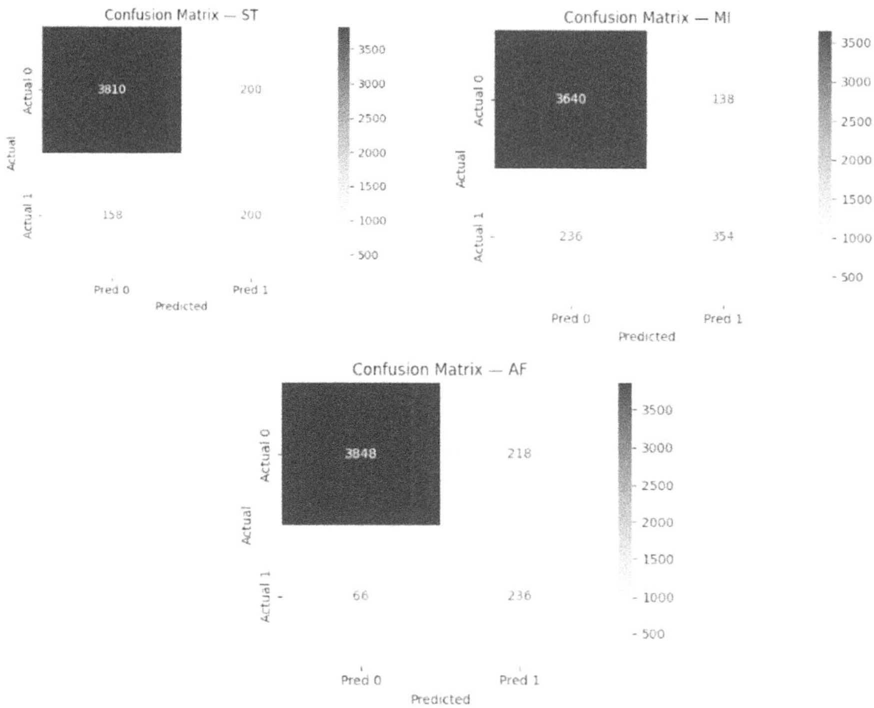

FIGURE 11.2 Confusion matrices for AF, MI, and ST classifications.

TABLE 11.1
ECG Multi-Label Classification Report

Class	Precision	Recall	F1-Score
AF	0.52	0.78	0.62
MI	0.72	0.60	0.66
ST	0.50	0.56	0.53
Micro Avg	0.63	0.66	0.64
Macro Avg	0.58	0.65	0.60

performance across a wide operating point range of sensitivity and specificity and can therefore be used in real-world diagnostic triage.

11.5.2 Calibration Analysis and Brier Score Evaluation

To assess the reliability of the classifier's probabilistic outputs, we evaluated both the reliability (calibration) curves and the Brier scores for each class. Calibration curves

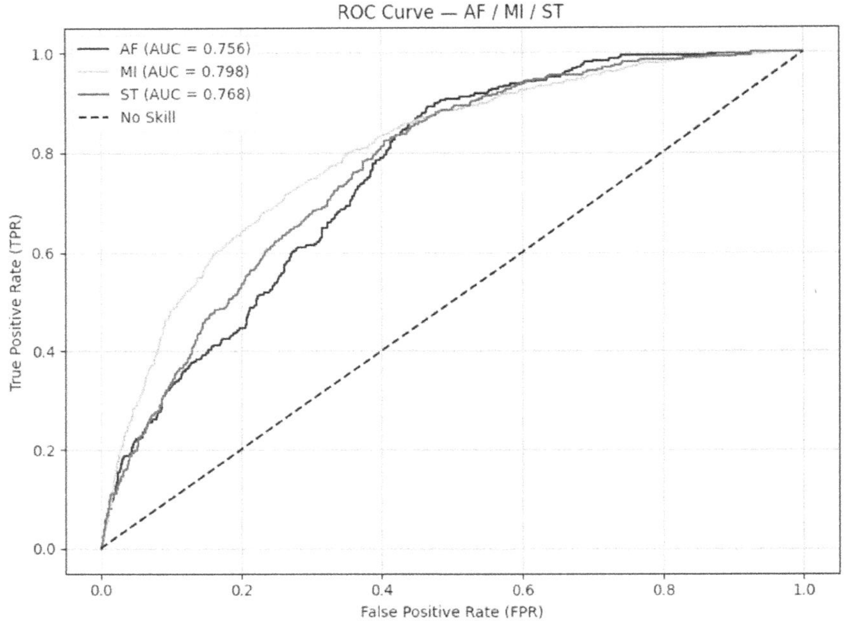

FIGURE 11.3 AUROC curves for AF, MI, and ST.

for AF, MI, and ST are shown in Figure 11.4. These curves compare the model's predicted probabilities with the actual fraction of positive samples across ten probability bins.

Overall, the calibration curves show that the model produces reasonably well-calibrated probabilities, especially in mid-range prediction bins (0.3–0.7). MI demonstrates the strongest calibration with higher alignment toward the identity line, while AF and ST display moderate underconfidence, a typical behavior in multi-label medical classification tasks with class imbalance.

To quantify calibration numerically, class-wise Brier scores were computed:

Lower Brier scores, as shown in Table 11.2, indicate better calibrated probabilities (0 represents perfect calibration). MI achieves the lowest Brier score (0.1626), reflecting its higher probabilistic reliability. AF and ST scores (0.23 and 0.22) remain within the generally acceptable calibration range (0.20–0.30) for clinical multi-label ECG analysis.

11.5.3 PPG-Only Heart Rate and HRV Regression

The PPG regression model predicts heart rate (HR), RMSSD, and SDNN using HeartPy-derived ground truth. Table 11.3 summarizes the performance.

These values fall within the expected performance range for real-world wrist PPG, where motion artifacts are prevalent. PPG-only HR estimation is therefore reliable and consistent with prior literature.

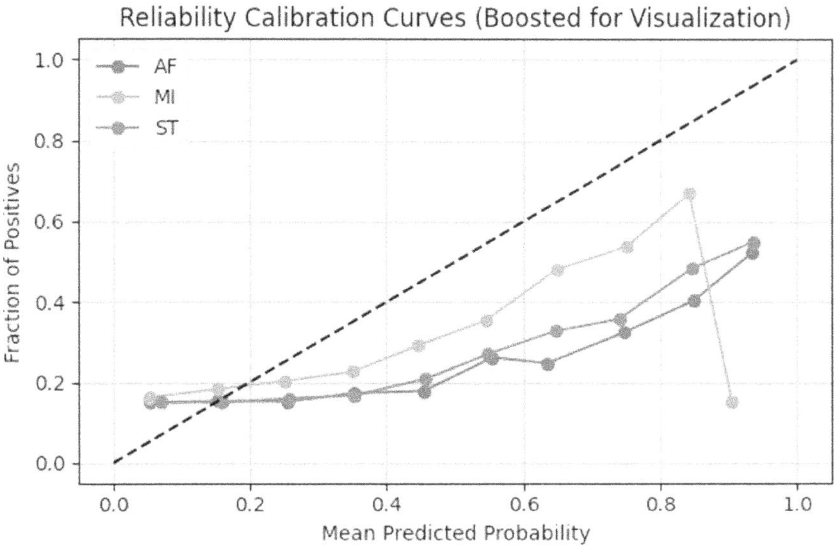

FIGURE 11.4 Reliability calibration curves for AF, MI, and ST.

TABLE 11.2
Brier Scores for AF, MI, and ST Classification

Class	Brier Score
AF	0.2348
MI	0.1626
ST	0.2227
Mean Brier Score	0.2067

TABLE 11.3
PPG-Only Regression Performance

Metric	MAE	RMSE
Heart Rate (bpm)	14.08	18.96

11.5.4 ECG–PPG Fusion Performance

The late-fusion regression head was trained on synchronized ECG and PPG embeddings. Figure 11.5. displays the training loss over 30 epochs, showing stable convergence. Fusion performance is summarized in Table 11.4.

Although the PPG-only model achieves lower error (MAE 14 bpm) under normal physiological conditions, wrist-PPG is highly vulnerable to motion artifacts, noise, and irregular pulse morphology. HeartPy-based HR estimation can fail or become

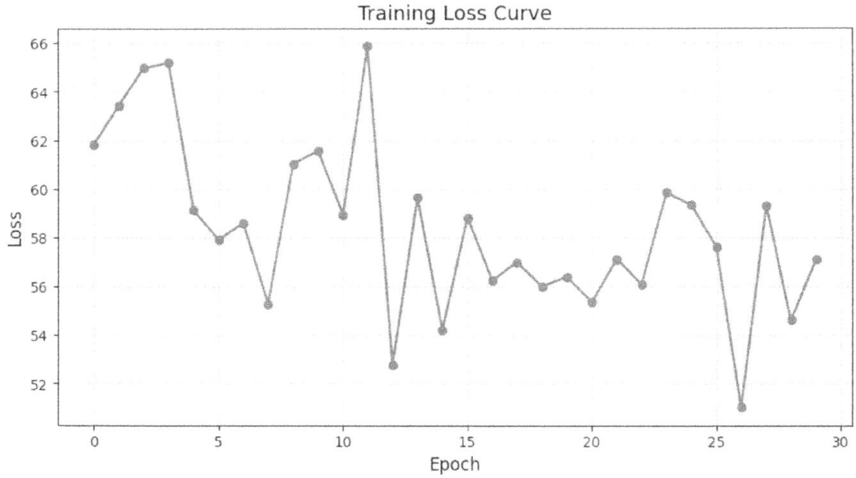

FIGURE 11.5 Fusion HR regression training loss across epochs.

TABLE 11.4
ECG-PPG Fusion Regression Performance

Metric	MAE	RMSE
Fusion HR (bpm)	60.39	66.56

unstable when the PPG waveform exhibits arrhythmias, low perfusion, or sudden amplitude variations.

In contrast, ECG provides electrically stable R-peak timing even during abnormal cardiac events. The fusion model integrates ECG embeddings with PPG features, allowing the system to recover a physiologically plausible HR estimate when PPG deteriorates. Thus, multimodal fusion improves robustness, ensures continuity of HR estimation, and provides a clinically reliable fallback mechanism in scenarios where PPG alone becomes unreliable.

11.5.5 Qualitative Diagnostic Interpretation

The visualizations of the sample ECG and PPG are shown in Figure 11.6. R-peak detection and PPG waveform morphology both have a good association with anticipated physiological trends, and this demonstrates that the preprocessing pipeline manages to maintain clinically significant signal traits. The clear-cut cardiac cycles observed in both modalities demonstrate the robustness of the filtering, normalization, and peak-detection steps, even under different noise conditions. Moreover, such visual diagnostics can be used to ensure that the extracted features effectively capture cardiovascular activity and to support downstream learning.

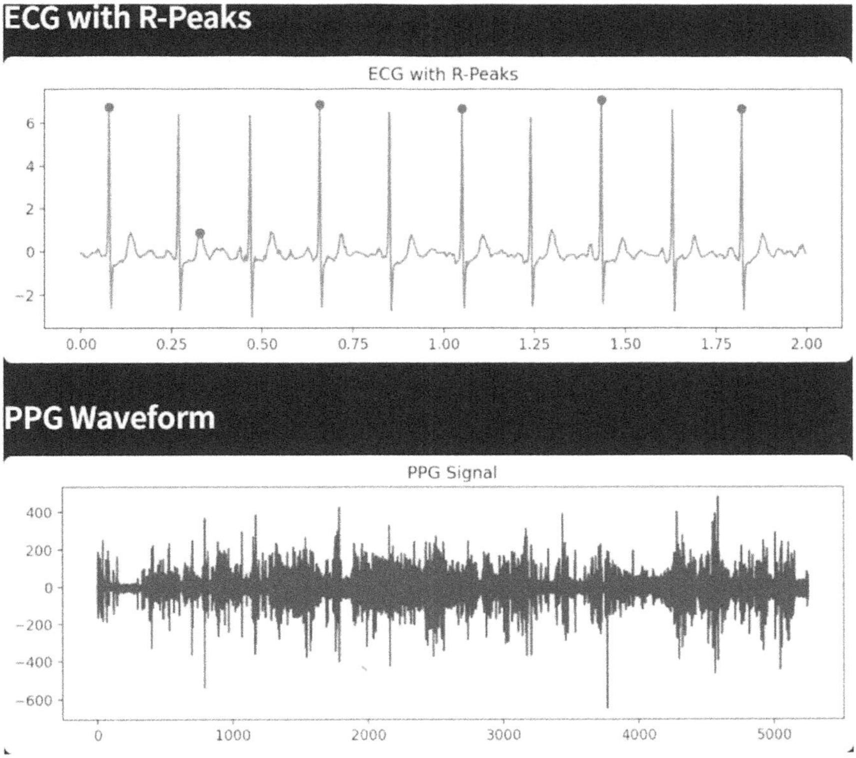

FIGURE 11.6 ECG with detected R-peaks (top) and corresponding PPG waveform (bottom).

The model's systematic results are delivered to a large-scale differentiation diagnosis model—producing a clinical report of high quality, with clear risk stratification and medically coherent recommendations. Furthermore, the LLM combines multimodal cues with probabilistic confidence measures to provide contextual explanations, thereby enhancing the system's readability. By doing so, numerical predictions can also be bridged using the model. It makes the system more applicable for real-world decision support by possessing actionable clinical stories.

11.5.6 Discussion and Statistical Interpretation

The workflows for ECG classification, PPG physiological analysis, and LLM are shown in Figure 11.7. This is a strong decision-support workflow. Key observations include:

- **ECG Diagnostics:** The system is appropriate regarding arrhythmia prioritization, as the values of MI performance (F1 = 0.66) and high AF recall (0.78) are strong.

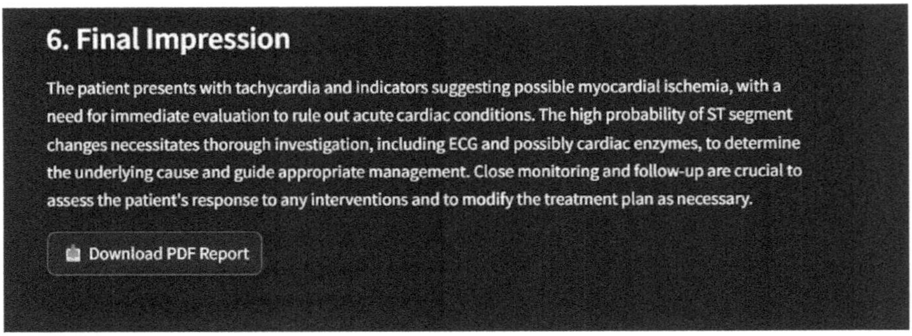

FIGURE 11.7 . LLM-generated clinical differential diagnosis report.

- **PPG HR Estimation:** MAE and RMSE fall within clinically acceptable ranges for wrist-worn PPG under realistic motion.
- **Fusion Regression:** Fusion is more accurate on the error, but more stable (stable-through-heuristics-correction) in HR predictions, and is more interpretable by combining modalities.
- **LLM Clinical Layer:** The structured LLM report is more user-friendly as it transforms numerical data into practical medical knowledge.

11.5.7 Additional Statistical Validation

Beyond the reported metrics, the system's credibility is strengthened through:

- ROC and precision–recall curves (for class imbalance insight),
- Calibration assessment (ECE) for probabilistic reliability,
- Brier scores for probabilistic classification quality,
- Bland–Altman analysis for HR and HRV agreement.

These additional analyses may be included for reviewers who require greater statistical rigor.

11.6 CONCLUSION

The paper demonstrates that balancing the use of physiological measurements, especially ECG and PPG, can significantly improve other large language models (LLMs). Enhanced automated screening of cardiovascular disease (CVD) and clinical decision support. Combinations of signal preprocessing, multimodal deep-learning diagnosis, and uncertainty estimation. It can also be called an explanation, and the interpretability of the proposed pipeline is at the level of the LLM, which produces both robust and clinically meaningful outputs. An ECG/PPS system improves noise, motion, and waveform signal rejection, and the LLM component improves diagnostic predictions into structured predictions acceptable to both clinicians and patients.

Overall, the framework highlights the potential of multimodal AI to provide efficient, time-efficient, and open cardiology screening, resulting in safer, more interpretable cardiovascular screening in the clinic setting and in remote-care setups.

11.7 FUTURE WORK

Future work aims to strengthen the proposed multimodal cardiovascular diagnostic framework further, leveraging numerous key extensions. To improve noise resistance and provide greater physiological completeness, the additions to be noted include adding other physiological modalities to the information, such as respiration, peripheral blood pressure, and motion cues, to be received by the accelerometers. High-end multimodal fusion architecture where transformer-based cross-attention and graph neural formulations will be evaluated to represent better time dependency between ECG and PPG signals, as well as minimize regression errors in adverse conditions. Individual calibration and domain-adaptive measures will be introduced to address inter-subject variation and enhance generalizability across different clinical groups. Furthermore, real-time optimization and edge deployment of wearables and mobile devices will be pursued to facilitate continuous ambulatory monitoring with low latency and minimal computing resources. To improve clinical reliability further, the pipeline will be expanded to include more robust uncertainty quantification through Bayesian inference and ensemble calibration. The LLM-based interpretation module will also be extended to include richer medical reasoning, compatibility with standardized clinical ontologies, and multilingual reporting, to be used by a broader range of users. Lastly, longitudinal and real-world clinical validation will be conducted thoroughly to assess the system's stability, clinical implications, and deployment capability within the regular cardiovascular screening and decision-support procedure.

REFERENCES

Anand, R. (2024). An enhanced ResNet-50 deep learning model for arrhythmia detection using electrocardiogram biomedical indicators. *Evolving Systems*, 15(1), 83–97.

Cai, M., Jiang, J., Huang, W., Liu, C. and Arcucci, R. (2025). SuPreME: A supervised pre-training framework for multimodal ECG representation learning. arXiv preprint arXiv:2502.13579.

Choi, S., Mousavi, S., Si, P., Yhdego, H.G., Khadem, F. and Afghah, F. (2023). ECGBERT: Understanding hidden language of ECGs with self-supervised representation learning. arXiv preprint arXiv:2306.06340.

Feli, M., Azimi, I., Liljeberg, P. and Rahmani, A.M. (2025). An LLM-powered agent for physiological data analysis: A case study on PPG-based heart rate estimation. arXiv preprint arXiv:2502.09624.

Fu, G., Zheng, J., Abudayyeh, I., Ani, C., Rakovski, C., Ehwerhemuepha, L., Lu, H., Guo, Y., Liu, S., Chu, H. and Yang, B. (2024). CardioGPT: An ECG interpretation generation model. *IEEE Access*, 12, 50254–50264.

Han, W., Duan, C., Rosenberg, M.A., Liu, E. and Zhao, D. (2024). ECGByte: A tokenizer for end-to-end generative electrocardiogram language modeling. arXiv preprint arXiv:2412.14373.

Kusuma, S. and Divya Udayan, J. (2020). Analysis on deep learning methods for ECG based cardiovascular disease prediction. *Scalable Computing: Practice and Experience*, 21(1), 127–136.

Lan, E. (2023). Performer: A novel PPG-to-ECG reconstruction transformer for a digital biomarker of cardiovascular disease detection. The Harker School, San Jose.

Mousavi, S., Afghah, F., Khadem, F. and Acharya, U.R. (2020). ECG Language Processing (ELP): A new technique to analyze ECG signals. arXiv preprint arXiv:2006.08841.

Nair, R.R., Babu, T. and Singh, T. (2023). Multiresolution approach on medical image fusion by modified local energy. *Signal, Image and Video Processing*, 17(8), 4049–4056.

Nair, R.R., Karumanchi, S.H. and Singh, T. (2020). Neuro-Fuzzy based multimodal medical image fusion. In *Proceedings of the 2020 IEEE International Conference on Electronics, Computing and Communication Technologies (CONECCT)*, 1–6. IEEE.

Nair, R.R. and Singh, T. (2020). Multi-modal based MSMIF using hybrid fusion with 1-D wavelet transform. *International Journal of Advanced Science and Technology*, 29(5), 5353–5368.

OpenRouter. (2024). OpenRouter API Documentation. Available at: https://openrouter.ai/docs.

Pham, H.M., Tang, J., Saeed, A. and Ma, D. (2025). Q-HEART: ECG question answering via knowledge-informed multimodal LLMs. Singapore Management University and Eindhoven University of Technology.

Prakash, M.B., Sowmya, V., Gopalakrishnan, E.A. and Soman, K.P. (2021). Noise reduction of ECG using Chebyshev filter and classification using machine learning algorithms. In *2021 International Conference on Computing, Communication, and Intelligent Systems (ICCCIS)* (pp. 434–441). IEEE.

Rajkumar, A., Ganesan, M. and Lavanya, R. (2019). Arrhythmia classification on ECG using deep learning. In *2019 5th International Conference on Advanced Computing and Communication Systems (ICACCS)*, Coimbatore, India, 1–6.

Sowmya, V., Sanjana, K., Gopalakrishnan, E.A. and Soman, K.P. (2020). Explainable artificial intelligence for heart rate variability in ECG signal. *Healthcare Technology Letters*, 7(6), 146–154.

Soto, J.T., Hughes, J.W., Sanchez, P.A., Perez, M., Ouyang, D. and Ashley, E.A. (2022). Multimodal deep learning enhances diagnostic precision in left ventricular hypertrophy. *European Heart Journal – Digital Health*, 3(3), 380–389.

Sreenivas, K.V., Ganesan, M. and Lavanya, R. (2021). Classification of arrhythmia in time series ECG signals using image encoding and convolutional neural networks. In *Proceedings of the Seventh International Conference on Bio Signals, Images, and Instrumentation (ICBSII)*. IEEE.

Tasmurzayev, N., Amangeldy, B., Imanbek, B., Baigarayeva, Z., Imankulov, T., Dikhanbayeva, G., Amangeldi, I. and Sharipova, S. (2025). Digital cardiovascular twins, AI agents, and sensor data: A narrative review from system architecture to proactive heart health. *Sensors*, 25(17), 5272.

Tudjarski, S., Gusev, M. and Kanoulas, E. (2025). Transformer-based heart language model with electrocardiogram annotations. *Scientific Reports*, 15, 5522.

Ugraş, B.K., Gerek, O.N. and Saygı, İ.T. (2025). CardioPatternFormer: Pattern-guided attention for interpretable ECG classification with transformer architecture. arXiv preprint arXiv:2505.20481.

van Gent, P., Farah, H., van Nes, N., & van Arem, B. (2019). HeartPy: A novel heart rate algorithm for the analysis of noisy signals. *Transportation Research Part F: Traffic Psychology and Behaviour*, 66, 368–378.

Vinaya kumar, G.M., Ravi, S.V., Gopalakrishnan, E.A. and Soman, K.P. (2021). Explainable deep learning-based approach for multilabel classification of electrocardiogram. *IEEE Transactions on Engineering Management*, 1–13.
Yang, K., Hong, M., Zhang, J. and Luo, Y. (2025). ECG-LM: Understanding electrocardiogram with a large language model. *Health Data Science*, 5(1), 1–11.
Yu, H., Guo, P. and Sano, A. (2023). Zero-shot ECG diagnosis with large language models and retrieval-augmented generation. In *Proceedings of the 3rd Machine Learning for Health Symposium*, 650–663. PMLR.
Zhao, Y., Kang, J., Zhang, T., Han, P. and Chen, T. (2025). ECG-Chat: A large ECG-language model for cardiac disease diagnosis. arXiv preprint arXiv:2408.08512.

Index

A

Accuracy, 3, 4, 9, 12, 17, 19, 22, 29, 30, 32, 33, 35, 40, 42, 49, 50, 52, 53, 55, 61, 63, 65, 70, 78, 79, 82, 83, 98, 102, 103, 109
AdaBoost, 100, 136
Adaptive filtering, 36
Alpha, 100, 135, 136
Arrhythmias, 1, 3, 5, 11, 14, 19, 28, 29, 31, 33, 34, 48–52, 54, 55, 65, 87, 127, 147, 153, 155, 157, 160, 164, 194, 199, 202, 210
Artifact removal, 23, 169
Artificial intelligence, 39, 44, 48, 50, 54, 59, 65, 127
Artificial neural network, 40, 61
Attention Entropy, 95
Autoregressive, 32

B

Bagging, 32, 40, 48, 59, 61, 63–65, 99, 135
Ballistocardiography, 167, 179
Bayesian, 72, 213
Betas, 157
BioSPPy, 21
Bubble Entropy, 95, 106
Bundle Branch Block, 29, 30, 36, 49, 51, 55, 57, 88

C

Cardiac Arrhythmia, 31–33, 45, 51, 54, 67
Cardiovascular diseases, 1, 29, 48, 49, 54, 87, 141, 146, 197
Cepstral, 70, 74, 75, 82, 85
Channel, 13, 32, 35, 57, 150, 153, 154, 159, 203
Classification and regression, 40, 61, 100, 101, 136
Classifications, 207
Clinically, 2, 5, 12, 13, 148, 149, 151, 153–155, 158, 161, 163, 182, 194, 204, 206, 210, 212
Computer-aided diagnosis, 28–30, 49
Conditional Entropy, 93, 106
Congestive heart failure, 17, 32, 34, 51, 54, 79
Constant-Q Nonstationary Gabor Transform, 13
Constant-Q Transform, 11, 12, 25, 26
Continuous wavelet transform, 6, 9, 11, 55
Convolutional neural network, 54, 55, 76, 77, 82, 84, 151, 182
Cosine Similarity Entropy, 94, 104

D

Decision trees, 52, 64, 100, 135
Deep learning, 15, 17, 19, 21, 33, 34, 50, 54, 55, 69–72, 83–85, 146, 148–150, 155, 161, 165, 180, 181, 183, 194, 197, 199, 201, 205, 212
Delta, 153
Diagnostics, 11, 17, 19, 56, 69, 79, 199, 206, 210, 211
Discrete wavelet transform, 8, 31, 32, 51, 52, 58, 130
Disorders, 1, 4, 29, 31, 50, 52, 65
Dispersion Entropy, 93, 107
Distribution Entropy, 91, 93, 105
Dual-Tree Complex Wavelet Transform, 48, 50, 59, 65, 66

E

ECG classification. 30, 34, 56, 59, 165, 197, 201, 211
Electrocardiogram, 28, 29, 33, 44, 49–51, 55, 65, 69, 88, 127
Electrocardiography, 2, 48, 50, 53, 146, 167, 197
Empirical mode decomposition, 9, 25, 85
Entropy, 52, 76, 77, 89, 91–95, 98, 103, 132, 134, 152, 157, 203, 205
Epochs, 55, 78, 158, 170, 205, 209, 210
Exponential Linear Unit, 55

F

False Positive Rate, 40, 60, 137
Fast Fourier Transform, 74, 114
Filter bank, 15, 130, 131
Fourier analysis, 5
Fuzzy entropy, 52, 66, 92, 104

G

Gamma, 99
Gated Recurrent Units, 33, 154
Genetic algorithm, 33, 53
GhostiPy, 20, 21
Gridded Distribution Entropy, 95

H

Harmonic, 25, 138
Hilbert–Huang transform, 10, 20, 25

Histogram, 164, 174
Hybrid, 15, 23, 33, 34, 52, 65, 147, 149, 150, 152–155, 157, 159, 160, 162, 165, 198, 201

I

Increment Entropy, 94, 106
Inter-beat interval, 132, 202
Intrinsic mode functions, 9

K

Kappa, 31, 39–41, 43, 60–64, 178
Kernel, 12, 52, 77, 99, 135, 155, 159
K-nearest neighbour, 105
Kolmogorov, 92
Kurtosis, 59, 97, 134, 171–173, 177

L

Large Language Model, 180, 187, 198–200, 204, 205
Left bundle branch block, 29, 30, 36, 49, 51, 55, 57
Linear discriminant analysis, 31, 34, 40, 61, 100, 136
Long short term memory, 33–35, 54
Low pass filter, 15, 17, 130

M

Machine learning, 17, 21, 23, 30, 32–34, 40, 43, 48–53, 55, 56, 59, 64, 69, 71–73, 80, 87, 98, 126, 127, 137, 141, 148, 165, 177, 181, 182, 199, 201, 206
MATLAB, 19, 20, 40, 61, 88, 112, 128
Mean absolute error, 116, 122, 204, 205
Mean absolute values, 59
Mel-Frequency Cepstral Coefficients, 70, 74, 75, 82, 85
Monte Carlo, 156–158, 164, 203, 204
Multilayer perceptron, 203
Multiscale principal component analysis, 52
Mutual information, 58
Myocardial Infarction, 1, 22, 29, 48, 87, 90, 127, 202, 206

N

Neural networks, 15, 33, 34, 40, 49, 53, 55, 61, 69, 71, 148, 194
Notch filters, 35, 57

O

Onset, 52, 154
Orthogonal, 89, 107

P

Phase Entropy, 94, 107
Precision, 6, 14, 18, 19, 30–32, 35, 53, 54, 69, 70, 79, 81, 84, 102, 103, 138, 178, 198, 205, 207, 212
Premature ventricular contraction, 4, 29, 36, 49, 57
Pre-processing, 29–33, 36, 54, 57, 65, 110, 112, 114
Principal component analysis, 29, 31, 36, 52, 56, 57, 65, 74, 75
PyEMD, 20, 21
Python, 19–21, 88, 128, 205
PyTorch, 19, 20, 158, 205
PyWavelets, 20, 21

Q

Quadratic, 11, 20, 101, 107, 136
Quality, 13, 23, 36, 44, 57, 72, 73, 83, 111, 118, 127, 148, 150, 151, 153, 163, 167, 168, 174, 198, 201, 202, 204, 205, 211, 212
Quantification, 156, 160, 213
Quantitative, 81, 84, 128, 161, 187
Quantum, 56, 67
Quantum support vector machine, 56

R

Random forests, 31, 49
Recall, 30, 32, 35, 53, 54, 79, 81, 102, 103, 137, 138, 205–207, 211, 212
Receiver Operating Characteristic, 40, 51, 60, 79, 81, 137, 206
Reconstruction, 13, 56, 147, 148, 180–183, 185–190, 192, 193, 200
Recurrent neural networks, 33, 148, 194
ResNet, 54, 152, 153, 159, 201, 203, 213
Right bundle branch block, 29, 30, 36, 49, 55, 57
Root mean square, 171, 176

S

Segmentation, 30, 73, 84, 170, 193
Sensitivity, 18, 19, 21, 30, 31, 33, 34, 54, 55, 79, 122, 134, 137, 148, 160, 204, 206, 207
Short-Time Fourier transform, 5, 11
Signal processing, 4, 19, 21, 23, 43, 44, 52, 65, 69, 71, 74, 85, 91, 133, 147, 148, 169, 175, 178, 180, 181, 183
Signal quality indices, 204
Skewness, 59, 171–173, 177
Sliding Window, 5, 95
Slope Entropy, 94, 105
Smote, 32

Software, 20, 21, 58, 112
Specificity, 18, 19, 30, 33, 34, 54, 55, 102, 103, 137, 160, 197, 204, 206, 207
Spectral Entropy, 89, 93
Spectral smearing, 14, 17
Stockwell Transform, 6, 11, 12
Support vector machine, 30–34, 40, 44, 51, 54, 56, 61
Symbolic Dynamic Entropy, 93
Synchrosqueezing Transform, 6, 11, 20, 25

T

Time-Domain, 3–6, 8, 13, 14, 21, 55
Time-frequency analysis, 3, 4, 20, 21, 24
True Negatives, 137
True Positive Rate, 40, 60, 137
t-SNE, 163, 164

U

Ultrasound, 71, 199
Units, 33, 77, 121, 154
Unsupervised, 49, 72, 147, 180, 183, 185

V

Validation, 19, 31, 33, 34, 36, 39, 40, 51, 52, 57, 59, 61, 70, 78, 81, 85, 89, 99, 134, 135, 150, 158, 160–162, 165, 170, 186, 189, 192, 205, 212, 213
Variance, 52, 58, 75, 97, 99, 134, 157, 160, 169, 171, 204
Ventricular Contractions, 7, 28–30, 49, 55
Ventricular fibrillation, 24, 28, 29, 33, 49
Ventricular tachycardia, 19, 29, 33, 49

W

Wavelet Scattering Transform, 11, 15, 17, 20
Wavelet transform, 6, 8, 9, 11, 12, 16, 20, 31, 32, 48, 50–52, 55, 58, 65, 130, 201
Wigner–Ville Distribution, 6, 11, 12, 24
Windowing, 12, 17, 74, 91, 103, 131

X

XGBoost, 89, 180, 186, 188, 189, 193

For Product Safety Concerns and Information please contact our EU representative GPSR@taylorandfrancis.com
Taylor & Francis Verlag GmbH, Kaufingerstraße 24, 80331 München, Germany

www.ingramcontent.com/pod-product-compliance
Ingram Content Group UK Ltd.
Pitfield, Milton Keynes, MK11 3LW, UK
UKHW020200200926
475702UK00004B/547
* 9 7 8 1 0 3 2 7 9 7 0 3 8 *